Co-morbidities in Heart Failure

Editors

FAIEZ ZANNAD
HECTOR O. VENTURA

HEART FAILURE CLINICS

www.heartfailure.theclinics.com

Consulting Editors
MANDEEP R. MEHRA
JAVED BUTLER

Founding Editor
JAGAT NARULA

April 2014 • Volume 10 • Number 2

ELSEVIER

1600 John F. Kennedy Boulevard • Suite 1800 • Philadelphia, Pennsylvania, 19103-2899

http://www.theclinics.com

HEART FAILURE CLINICS Volume 10, Number 2
April 2014 ISSN 1551-7136, ISBN-13: 978-0-323-29694-6

Editor: Adrianne Brigido
Developmental Editor: Susan Showalter

Heart Failure Clinics (ISSN 1551-7136) is published quarterly by Elsevier Inc., 360 Park Avenue South, New York, NY 10010-1710. Months of publication are January, April, July, and October. Business and editorial offices: 1600 John F. Kennedy Boulevard, Suite 1800, Philadelphia, PA 19103-2899. Periodicals postage paid at New York, NY, and additional mailing offices. Subscription prices are USD 235.00 per year for US individuals, USD 382.00 per year for US institutions, USD 80.00 per year for US students and residents, USD 280.00 per year for Canadian individuals, USD 442.00 per year for Canadian institutions, USD 300.00 per year for international individuals, USD 442.00 per year for international institutions, and USD 100.00 per year for Canadian and foreign students/residents. To receive student and resident rate, orders must be accompanied by name of affiliated institution, date of term, and the *signature* of program/residency coordinator on institution letterhead. Orders will be billed at individual rate until proof of status is received. Foreign air speed delivery is included in all *Clinics* subscription prices. All prices are subject to change without notice. **POSTMASTER:** Send address changes to *Heart Failure Clinics*, Elsevier Health Sciences Division, Subscription Customer Service, 3251 Riverport Lane, Maryland Heights, MO 63043. **Customer Service: 1-800-654-2452 (US and Canada). From outside of the US and Canada, call 314-447-8871. Fax: 314-447-8029. For print support, E-mail: JournalsCustomerService-usa@elsevier.com. For online support, E-mail: JournalsOnlineSupport-usa@elsevier.com.**

Reprints. For copies of 100 or more of articles in this publication, please contact the Commercial Reprints Department, Elsevier Inc., 360 Park Avenue South, New York, NY 10010-1710. Tel.: 212-633-3874; Fax: 212-633-3820; E-mail: reprints@elsevier.com.

Heart Failure Clinics is covered in *MEDLINE/PubMed (Index Medicus).*

Printed and bound by CPI Group (UK) Ltd, Croydon, CR0 4YY

Contributors

CONSULTING EDITORS

MANDEEP R. MEHRA, MD
Co-Director, BWH Cardiovascular, Executive Director, Center for Advanced Heart Disease, Brigham and Women's Hospital, Professor of Medicine, Harvard Medical School, Boston, Massachusetts

JAVED BUTLER, MD, MPH
Professor of Medicine, Director, Heart Failure Research, Emory University, Atlanta, Georgia

EDITORS

FAIEZ ZANNAD, MD, PhD, FESC
Professor of Medicine; Head, Division of Hypertension and Heart Failure, Institut Lorrain du Coeur et des Vaisseaux, Center Hospitalier Universitaire of Nancy; Coordinator, Clinical Investigation Centre, Inserm, University of Lorraine, Nancy, France

HECTOR O. VENTURA, MD, FACC, FAHA, FRCPE, FACCP
Professor of Medicine, Department of Cardiovascular Diseases, Head of Heart Failure and Heart Transplant, John Ochsner Heart and Vascular Institute, Ochsner Clinical School, University of Queensland School of Medicine, New Orleans, Louisiana

AUTHORS

MARTIN A. ALPERT, MD
Division of Cardiovascular Medicine, University of Missouri School of Medicine, Columbia, Missouri

NATASHA P. ARORA, MD
Division of Cardiovascular Services, Saint John Hospital and Medical Center, Detroit, Michigan

DAN ATAR, MD, PhD
Department of Cardiology, Oslo University Hospital Ullevål; Institute of Clinical Sciences, University of Oslo, Oslo, Norway

CYNTHIA S. CROWSON, MS
Associate Professor of Medicine, Division of Rheumatology, Departments of Medicine and Health Sciences Research, Mayo Clinic, Rochester, Minnesota

ALBAN DE SCHUTTER, MD
Department of Cardiovascular Diseases, John Ochsner Heart and Vascular Institute, Ochsner Clinical School, University of Queensland School of Medicine, New Orleans, Louisiana

AKSHAY S. DESAI, MD, MPH
Division of Cardiology, Department of Medicine, Brigham and Women's Hospital, Harvard Medical School, Boston, Massachusetts

LUCA DI LULLO, MD, PhD
Department of Nephrology and Dialysis, L. Parodi-Delfino Hospital, Colleferro, Roma, Italy

JAVIER DÍEZ, MD, PhD
Full Professor of Medicine, School of Medicine; Director, Department of Cardiovascular Sciences, Centre of Applied Medical Research; Consultant and Head of Research, Department of Cardiology and Cardiac Surgery, University Clinic; University of Navarra, Pamplona, Spain

MONA FIUZAT, PharmD
Duke University Medical Center, Duke Clinical Research Institute, Durham, North Carolina

SHERINE E. GABRIEL, MD, MSc
Professor of Medicine and Epidemiology, Division of Rheumatology, Departments of Medicine and Health Sciences Research, Mayo Clinic, Rochester, Minnesota

JALAL K. GHALI, MD
Division of Cardiology, School of Medicine, Mercer University, Macon, Georgia

WEI JIANG, MD
Associate Professor of Medicine, Associate Professor of Psychiatry and Behavioral Sciences, Duke University Medical Center, Durham, North Carolina

AMIT N. KESWANI, MD
Department of Cardiology, Ochsner Clinic Foundation, Ochsner Clinical School, University of Queensland, New Orleans, Louisiana

ANURADHA LALA, MD
Division of Cardiology, Department of Medicine, Brigham and Women's Hospital; Assistant Professor of Medicine, Harvard Medical School, Boston, Massachusetts; Division of Cardiology, Department of Medicine, New York University School of Medicine, New York, New York

CARL J. LAVIE, MD, FACC, FACP, FCCP
Department of Cardiovascular Diseases; Medical Director, Cardiac Rehabilitation, Director, Exercise Laboratories, John Ochsner Heart and Vascular Institute, Ochsner Clinical School, University of Queensland School of Medicine, New Orleans; Department of Preventive Medicine, Pennington Biomedical Research Center, Louisiana State University System, Baton Rouge, Louisiana

MANDEEP R. MEHRA, MD
Co-Director, BWH Cardiovascular, Executive Director, Center for Advanced Heart Disease, Brigham and Women's Hospital, Professor of Medicine, Harvard Medical School, Boston, Massachusetts

ROBERT J. MENTZ, MD
Duke University Medical Center, Duke Clinical Research Institute, Durham, North Carolina

RICHARD V. MILANI, MD
Department of Cardiovascular Diseases, John Ochsner Heart and Vascular Institute, Ochsner Clinical School, University of Queensland School of Medicine, New Orleans, Louisiana

DANIEL P. MORIN, MD, MPH, FHRS
Department of Cardiology, Ochsner Medical Center; Associate Professor of Cardiology, Ochsner Clinical School, Queensland University School of Medicine, New Orleans, Louisiana

AMY NEWHOUSE, MD
PGY-3, Combined Internal Medicine and Psychiatry Residency, Departments of Medicine and Psychiatry, Duke University Medical Center, Durham, North Carolina

CLAUDIO RONCO, MD, PhD
International Renal Research Institute, S. Bortolo Hospital, Vicenza, Italy

SUDARONE THIHALOLIPAVAN, MD
Department of Cardiology, Ochsner Medical Center, New Orleans, Louisiana

HECTOR O. VENTURA, MD, FACC, FAHA, FRCPE, FACCP
Professor of Medicine, Department of Cardiovascular Diseases, Head of Heart Failure and Heart Transplant, John Ochsner Heart and Vascular Institute, Ochsner Clinical School, University of Queensland School of Medicine, New Orleans, Louisiana

THOMAS G. VON LUEDER, MD, PhD
Department of Cardiology, Oslo University Hospital Ullevål; Institute of Clinical Sciences, University of Oslo, Oslo, Norway

CHRISTOPHER J. WHITE, MD
Professor and Chairman, Department of Cardiology, Ochsner Clinic Foundation, Ochsner Clinical School, University of Queensland, New Orleans, Louisiana

KERRY WRIGHT, MBBS
Instructor in Medicine, Division of Rheumatology, Department of Medicine, Mayo Clinic, Rochester, Minnesota

Contents

> Hypertensive heart disease (HHD) has been considered the adaptive hypertrophy of the left ventricle wall to increased blood pressure. Recent findings in hypertensive animals and patients now challenge this paradigm by showing that HHD also results from pathologic structural remodeling of the myocardium in response to hemodynamic and nonhemodynamic factors that are altered in arterial hypertension. The possibility that hypertensive patients predisposed to develop heart failure may be detected before the appearance of clinical manifestations provides a new way to prevent this major arterial complication.

> Sleep-disordered breathing (SDB) is prevalent in patients with heart failure, and is associated with increased morbidity and mortality. SDB is proinflammatory, with nocturnal oxygen desaturations and hypercapnia appearing to play a pivotal role in the development of oxidative stress and sympathetic activation. Preliminary data suggest that attention to the diagnosis and management of SDB in patients with heart failure may improve outcomes. Ongoing research into the roles of comorbidities such as SDB as a treatment target may lead to better clinical outcomes and improved quality of life for patients with heart failure.

> Cardiorenal syndrome (CRS) includes a broad spectrum of diseases within which both the heart and kidneys are involved, acutely or chronically. An effective classification of CRS in 2008 essentially divides CRS in two main groups, cardiorenal and renocardiac CRS, based on primum movens of disease (cardiac or renal); both cardiorenal and renocardiac CRS are then divided into acute and chronic, according to onset of disease. The fifth type of CRS integrates all cardiorenal involvement induced by systemic disease. This article addresses the pathophysiology, diagnosis, treatment, and outcomes of the 5 distinct types of CRS.

Anemia is a common comorbidity in patients with heart failure (HF) and is associated with poor prognosis. Iron deficiency, with or without anemia, confers increased risk of mortality and morbidity. Along with the altered iron metabolism in HF patients, inflammation creates challenges in the interpretation of laboratory parameters used to diagnose anemia in HF. Since the RED-HF trial failed to demonstrate any benefit from the use of erythropoiesis-stimulating agents (ESAs) on mortality or morbidity in HF patients, ESAs are no longer considered a treatment option, although intravenous iron has potential as therapy for anemic and nonanemic HF patients.

Depression frequently accompanies heart failure and has been linked with increased morbidity and mortality. Patients with heart failure who have depression have more somatic symptoms, hospitalizations, increased financial burden, and poorer quality of life. Furthermore, depression has been shown to be an independent predictor of future cardiac events in patients with heart failure, regardless of disease severity, making it worthwhile to consider among other cardiac risk factors, such as diabetes and smoking. This article summarizes the trials assessing the treatment of depression in heart failure and provides an algorithm for approaching these patients.

Heart failure (HF) and atrial fibrillation (AF) commonly coexist and adversely affect mortality when found together. AF begets HF and HF begets AF. Rhythm restoration with antiarrhythmic drugs failed to show a mortality benefit but can be effective in improving symptoms. Nonpharmacologic treatment of AF may be of value in the HF population.

Overweight and obesity adversely affect cardiovascular (CV) risk factors and CV structure and function, and lead to a marked increase in the risk of developing heart failure (HF). Despite this, an obesity paradox exists, wherein those who are overweight and obese with HF have a better prognosis than their leaner counterparts, and the underweight, frail, and cachectic have a particularly poor prognosis. In light of this, the potential benefits of exercise training and efforts to improve cardiorespiratory fitness, as well as the potential for weight reduction, especially in severely obese patients with HF, are discussed.

Congestive heart failure (CHF) is a prevalent disease with many comorbidities and is associated with high health care expenditures. Peripheral arterial disease (PAD) is a known comorbidity of CHF and is associated with worse morbidity and mortality. CHF and PAD share risk factors, pathophysiology, treatment strategies, and prognostic features. We review the impact of PAD on patients with CHF using several studies to support PAD's influence on outcomes in CHF. Based on the evidence and current guidelines, patients with heart failure who are smokers, and those who have known coronary artery disease and/or diabetes should be screened for PAD.

Rheumatic diseases are associated with an increased risk of cardiovascular (CV) mortality attributed to a higher incidence of heart failure (HF) and ischemic heart disease. Although traditional CV risk factors contribute to the increased incidence seen in this population, by themselves they do not account for the increased risk; in fact, obesity and hyperlipidemia may play a paradoxic role. Immune-mediated mechanisms and chronic inflammation likely play a role in the pathogenesis of CV disease in patients with rheumatic diseases. The usual clinical features of ischemic heart disease and HF are less likely to be seen in this patient population.

Enhanced survival following acute myocardial infarction and the declining prevalence of hypertension and valvular heart disease as contributors to incident heart failure (HF) have fueled the emergence of coronary artery disease (CAD) as the primary risk factor for HF development. Despite the acknowledged role of CAD in the development of HF, the role of coronary revascularization in reducing HF-associated morbidity and mortality remains controversial. The authors review key features of the epidemiology and pathophysiology of CAD in patients with HF as well as the emerging data from recent clinical trials that inform the modern approach to management.

Heart failure (HF) is predominantly a disease that affects the elderly population, a cohort in which comorbidities are common. The majority of comorbidities and the degree of their severity have prognostic implications in HF. Polypharmacy in HF is common, has increased throughout the past 2 decades, and may pose a risk for adverse drug interactions, accidental overdosing, or medication nonadherence. Polypharmacy, in particular in the elderly, is rarely assessed in traditional clinical trials, highlighting a need for entirely novel HF research strategies.

HEART FAILURE CLINICS

DOWNLOAD
Free App!

Review Articles
THE CLINICS

NOW AVAILABLE FOR YOUR iPhone and iPad

Foreword
Comorbid Conditions in Heart Failure: An Unhappy Marriage

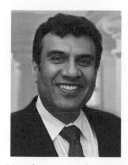 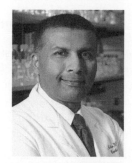

Mandeep R. Mehra, MD   Javed Butler, MD, MPH
Consulting Editors

The general issue of comorbidity is of major clinical importance for patients, health care providers, and society as a whole. A principal manifestation of aging, multimorbidity poses many challenges on the overall health of an individual and to the health care system in heart failure. Polypharmacy in heart failure patients with multiple morbidities influences their prognosis, adds a disease burden, and challenges adherence to medical management while increasing overall cost of care. Heart failure has special bidirectional relationships with cardiac and noncardiac comorbidity that are pathophysiologically intertwined. Examples of such intertwined comorbidities include arrhythmias, valvular disease, renal dysfunction, pulmonary dysfunction (both obstructive and restrictive pulmonary physiology), pulmonary hypertension, sleep apnea, liver dysfunction, diabetes mellitus, anemia, stroke, and skeletal myopathy. Such limitations are not just in the physical domain; mental diseases such as depression can also perpetuate a negative self-fulfilling cycle of clinical decline in heart failure. Beyond the direct organ system interactions and their confounding factors, more insight is now being developed to appreciate common system pathophysiologic mechanisms like inflammation and oxidative stress that are operative in a unifying manner to influence the partnership of disease-disease interaction.

In this unique issue of *Heart Failure Clinics*, Drs Zannad and Ventura have assembled 11 highly experienced teams of clinicians and researchers to provide a commentary on issues pertinent to heart failure and various cardiovascular and noncardiovascular comorbidities, and additional topics of grave importance, such as polypharmacy and frailty. It is a testament to the exquisite experience of these editors that they have brought together, in a single issue, a focus on dealing with the most relevant clinical questions to the care of heart failure patients that are difficult for most health care providers to grapple with. In this regard, we believe that this incremental knowledge bundled together is aptly designed to achieve our collective goal—to improve the care of our growing aged-patient population with heart failure.

Mandeep R. Mehra, MD
BWH Heart and Vascular Center and
Harvard Medical School
Brigham and Womens Hospital
75 Francis Street, A Building
3rd Floor, Room AB324
Boston, MA 02115, USA

Javed Butler, MD, MPH
Heart Failure Research
Emory Clinical Cardiovascular Research Institute
Emory University
1462 Clifton Road Northeast, Suite 504
Atlanta, GA 30322, USA

E-mail addresses:
MMEHRA@partners.org (M.R. Mehra)
javed.butler@emory.edu (J. Butler)

Preface

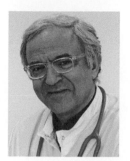

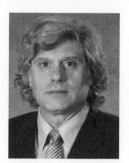

Faiez Zannad, MD, PhD, FESC   Hector O. Ventura, MD, FACC, FAHA, FRCPE, FACCP

Editors

Heart failure is a major public health problem worldwide and its prevalence and incidence continue to grow in part because of the increasing age of the population. Thus, heart failure is the leading diagnosis at hospital discharge for patients 65 years or older and the cost of managing these patients is also increasing.

In most patients and particularly in elderly patients, heart failure is accompanied by a range of comorbidities that play an integral role in its progression and response to treatment. Comorbidity is defined as a chronic condition that coexists in an individual with another condition that is being described. The objective of this issue of *Heart Failure Clinics* is to review several comorbidities, either cardiac or noncardiac, that can clinically impact the management of patients with heart failure. The authors of the individual articles give an overview of the importance of the comorbidity in patients with heart failure and also discuss the management of these patients. All authors are clinicians and investigators that have a broad interest in the topic and manage patients with heart failure and the specific comorbidity.

The prevalence of comorbidities in patients with heart failure continues to grow and diagnosis and treatment options will continue to rise. We hope that the perspectives in this issue will help the clinicians in the field of heart failure to best understand and manage these difficult patients.

Faiez Zannad, MD, PhD, FESC
Division of Hypertension and Heart Failure
Institut Lorrain du Coeur et des Vaisseaux
Center Hospitalier Universitaire of Nancy
CHU Brabois
54500 Vandoeuvre Les Nancy
France

Clinical Investigation Centre, Inserm
University of Lorraine
Nancy, France

Hector O. Ventura, MD, FACC, FAHA,
FRCPE, FACCP
The Ochsner Clinical School
University of Queensland Section
John Ochsner Heart and Vascular Institute
1514 Jefferson Highway
New Orleans, LA 70121, USA

E-mail addresses:
f.zannad@chu-nancy.fr (F. Zannad)
hventura@ochsner.org (H.O. Ventura)

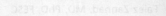

Erratum

An error was made in an article published in the January 2014 Supplement to *Heart Failure Clinics* (Volume 10, 1S) on page S1. "A History of Devices as an Alternative to Heart Transplantation" by Garrick C. Stewart, MD, and Mandeep R. Mehra, MD, should have included the following disclosure:

MRM is a consultant with Thoratec, chair of the REVIVE-IT DSMB (a National Heart, Lung, and Blood Institute-sponsored trial with Thoratec as the device sponsor) and editor of the *Journal of Heart and Lung Transplantation*. In addition he consults for Boston Scientific, Medtronic, St. Jude Medical, Baxter, the American Board of Internal Medicine, and the National Institutes of Health.

Heart Failure Clin 10 (2014) xiii
http://dx.doi.org/10.1016/j.hfc.2014.01.001
1551-7136/14/$ – see front matter © 2014 Published by Elsevier Inc.

Erratum

An error was made in an article published in the January 2014 Supplement to Heart Failure Clinics (Volume 10, 1S) on page 6. "A History of Devices as an Alternative to Heart Transplantation," by Gerald C. Stewart, MD, and Mandeep R. Mehra, MD, should have included the following disclosure:

MRM is a consultant with Thoratec, chair of the REVIVE-IT DSMB (a National Heart, Lung, and Blood Institute-sponsored trial with Thoratec as the device sponsor and editor of the Journal of Heart and Lung Transplantation. In addition he consults for Boston Scientific, Medtronic, St. Jude Medical, Baxter, the American Board of Internal Medicine, and the National Institutes of Health.

Arterial Hypertension in Patients with Heart Failure

Javier Díez, MD, PhD[a,b,c],*

KEYWORDS

- Arterial hypertension • Ejection fraction • Heart failure • Left ventricular hypertrophy
- Myocardial remodeling

KEY POINTS

- Hypertension carries the highest population-attributable risk for heart failure together with coronary heart disease, and as a comorbidity is present in most patients with heart failure.
- There is interindividual variability in the progression from hypertension to heart failure in both the geometry of left ventricular growth and the level of ejection fraction.
- The assessment of the hypertensive failing heart must combine imaging and biochemical markers of the structural and function alterations of the myocardium.
- The prevalence of heart failure calls for prevention efforts, and arterial hypertension is a prime target for such interventions.
- Because arterial hypertension may complicate heart failure, adding further morbidity and mortality risk, its management influences the prognosis of patients with heart failure.

INTRODUCTION

Arterial hypertension remains a major public health problem associated with considerable morbidity and mortality. In general, arterial hypertension may damage the coronary subepicardial tree, the cardiac muscle, and the aortic valve (**Fig. 1**). Because increased blood pressure (BP) is one of the major risk factors that facilitates coronary atherosclerosis, the prevalence of arterial hypertension is greater than 60% in patients with ischemic heart disease.[1] In contrast, hypertensive heart disease (HHD) can be defined as the response of the myocardium to the afterload imposed by increased BP that leads to left ventricular (LV) hypertrophy (LVH).[2] In addition, the prevalence of aortic valve sclerosis is higher in hypertensive patients than in subjects with normal BP, namely in aged people.[3] Although ischemic

heart disease, HHD, and aortic valve disease may all facilitate LV dysfunction and cause heart failure (HF), and coexist in hypertensive patients, this article focuses on HHD. Therefore, different aspects of the epidemiology, pathophysiology, and clinical handling of HF related to HHD are reviewed. In addition, because arterial hypertension has been reported to be the most common comorbid condition in patients with HF, some aspects related to its impact on the clinical evolution and handling of HF are also considered.

HHD AS A CAUSE OF HF
Epidemiologic Aspects

Epidemiologic data from the Framingham Study provide insights into modifiable risk factors that promote HF.[4–6] In this regard, based on population-attributable risks, hypertension has

Disclosures: The author has no conflict of interest.
[a] Department of Cardiovascular Sciences, Centre of Applied Medical Research, Pamplona, Spain; [b] Department of Cardiology and Cardiac Surgery, University Clinic, Pamplona, Spain; [c] University of Navarra, Pamplona, Spain
* Department of Cardiovascular Sciences, Centre of Applied Medical Research, Av. Pío XII 55, Pamplona 31008, Spain.
E-mail address: jadimar@unav.es

Heart Failure Clin 10 (2014) 233–242
http://dx.doi.org/10.1016/j.hfc.2013.12.004
1551-7136/14/$ – see front matter © 2014 Elsevier Inc. All rights reserved.

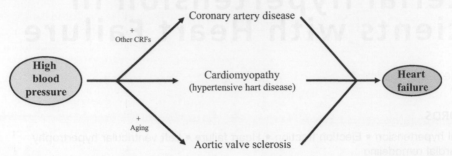

Fig. 1. Pathways leading to heart failure (HF) and other clinical manifestations such as arrhythmias and ischemic syndrome in arterial hypertension. CRFs, cardiovascular risk factors.

the greatest impact, accounting for 39% of HF incidence in men and 59% in women. Hypertension increased the age-adjusted and risk-factor adjusted hazard of HF 2-fold in men and 3-fold in women, with a greater impact of the systolic than diastolic BP. Because that the pattern of HF risk factors is likely to vary across world regions based on risk factor prevalence and quality of health care, a recent systematic review and pooled analysis in 6 world regions revealed that hypertension prevalence was high in patients with HF in all regions but the highest in eastern and central Europe and sub-Saharan Africa (age and sex adjusted, 35.0% and 32.6%, respectively).[7]

The burden of HF is also high in hypertensive patients under treatment. A systematic review of 23 hypertension trials performed between 1997 and 2007 including 193,424 patients revealed a 28.9% incidence of new HF cases.[8] The development of HF was more prevalent in older, black, diabetic, and very-high-risk individuals.

Examination of the baseline characteristics of patients with HF and reduced ejection fraction (HFREF) and patients with HF and preserved ejection fraction (HFPEF) (N = 19,519) included in the Digitalis Investigation Group trials, the CHARM (Candesartan in Heart Failure: Assessment of Reduction in Mortality and Morbidity) trials, and the I-PRESERVE (Irbesartan in Heart Failure with Preserved Systolic Function Trial) trial shows that the hypertensive cause of HF was assigned to more than 20% of patients with HFPEF, but to less than 10% of patients with HFREF.[9] Therefore, the notion has emerged that arterial hypertension facilitates the development of HFPEF.

However, this notion is not always supported by epidemiologic data. Ho and colleagues[10] recently reported the findings of the study on new-onset HF cases between 1981 and 2008 in Framingham Heart Study participants, classified into HFPEF and HFREF (ejection fraction [EF] >45% vs ≤45%). The investigators used Cox multivariable regression to examine predictors of 8-year risk of

incident HF and competing-risks analysis to identify predictors that differed between HFPEF and HFREF. Among 6340 participants (aged 60 ± 12 years), 512 developed incident HF. Of 457 participants with EF evaluation at the time of HF diagnosis, 196 (43%) were classified as HFPEF and 261 (56%) as HFREF. Fourteen predictors of overall HF were identified. Older age, diabetes mellitus, and a history of valvular disease predicted both types of HF. Higher body mass index, smoking, and atrial fibrillation predicted HFPEF only, whereas male sex, higher total cholesterol, higher heart rate, arterial hypertension, LVH, previous symptomatic cardiovascular disease, and left bundle-branch block predicted HFREF only.

In combining individual patient data from 31 studies (41,972 patients), the investigators of the Meta-analysis Global Group in Chronic Heart Failure (MAGGIC) showed that patients with HFREF (N = 10,347) have higher total mortality compared with patients with HFPEF (N = 31,625).[11] However, this difference was seen regardless of whether arterial hypertension was the cause of HF or only a comorbidity. Thus, arterial hypertension did not seem to influence the prognosis of patients with HF.

Pathophysiologic Aspects

The conventional pathophysiologic view of HHD has been that initially arterial hypertension is associated with concentric LVH because the LV wall thickens in response to increased BP as a compensatory mechanism, and that subsequently, after a series of poorly characterized events, compensated LVH transitions to HF.[12] However, experimental and clinical evidence from the last decades indicates that arterial hypertension may progress to HF through several pathways (**Fig. 2**).[13] First, it is well known that patients with concentric LVH develop HFPEF. Second, concentric LVH may also progress to HFREF, most commonly via an interval myocardial infarction, although transition from concentric LVH to

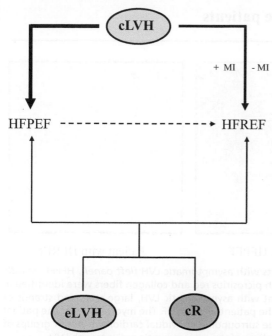

Fig. 2. Pathways leading to HF in HHD. The thickness of the continuous lines represents the importance of the pathway in terms of frequency. The dotted line represents the possibility that HFPEF may evolve to HFREF. cLVH, concentric LVH; cR, concentric remodeling; eLVH, eccentric LVH; MI, myocardial infarction.

HFREF may occur even in the absence of myocardial infarction. Third, some hypertensive patients may develop a geometric pattern of LV growth that is different from concentric hypertrophy (eg, concentric remodeling and eccentric LVH) and that may also evolve to either HFPEF or HFREF. These different possibilities of progression from arterial hypertension to HF may be the result of the influences of modulator factors (eg, genetic background, gender, aging, lifestyle factors, obesity, and diabetes mellitus) as well as of the structural changes of the myocardium that occur in response to hemodynamic and nonhemodynamic mechanisms.

Cardiomyocyte hypertrophy leading to LV wall thickening is the primary cellular mechanism by which the heart reduces stress on the LV wall imposed by the unrelenting pressure overload in arterial hypertension. However, evidence exists that blunting of cardiomyocyte hypertrophy does not result in dysfunction/failure despite pressure overload.[14] Therefore, a shift in the paradigm is occurring in the sense that genetic reprogramming associated with cardiomyocyte hypertrophy is no longer considered an entirely adaptive process. Detailed analysis of the genetic changes that accompany cardiomyocyte hypertrophy permits

the conclusion that they translate into derangements in energy metabolism, contractile cycle and excitation-contraction coupling, cytoskeleton and membrane properties, and autocrine functions, which in turn provide the basis for the cardiomyocyte malfunctioning associated with hypertensive LVH and predispose to LV dysfunction and failure.[15]

Beyond cardiomyocyte hypertrophy, complex changes in myocardial architecture develop leading to the structural remodeling of the myocardium that characterizes HHD.[16] In particular, hypertensive myocardial remodeling involves loss of viable cardiomyocytes caused by increased rates of apoptosis and death, alterations in the organization of the collagen matrix, and microcirculatory changes characterized by wall thickening of small arteries and arterioles and decreased number of capillaries. For the collagen matrix, 2 types of lesions can be identified: increased accumulation of cross-linked collagen fibers forming strands and microscars within the interstitium (ie, fibrosis), and loss of the collagen reticular network that surrounds and interconnects individual cardiomyocytes and groups of cardiomyocytes (ie, scaffold disruption) (**Fig. 3**). Although the former lesion is predominant in the stiffer and hypertrophied left ventricle of patients with HFPEF,[17] the latter is more frequently seen in the dilated left ventricle of patients with HFREF.[18]

When HF is already established, arterial hypertension may aggravate LV dysfunction. In patients with HFREF, arterial hypertension further worsens the loading conditions of the failing left ventricle, and small increases in afterload can produce large decreases in stroke volume.[19] In contrast, arterial hypertension may contribute to worsening of LV performance by slowing myocardial relaxation and increasing passive stiffness in patients with HFPEF.[19]

Diagnostic Aspects

Imaging or biochemical biomarkers are objectively measured and evaluated characteristics that may provide important information on the pathogenesis of HF, but may also be a valuable clinical tool in the identification of patients at risk for HF, in the diagnosis and risk stratification of these patients, and in monitoring their therapy.

Imaging plays a central role in the diagnosis and guiding of treatment in patients with HF, including those with arterial hypertension.[20] Echocardiography is widely available and clinically useful in the detection of LVH and the assessment of diastolic and systolic function. In addition, several studies have shown the association of echo Doppler

Hypertensive patients

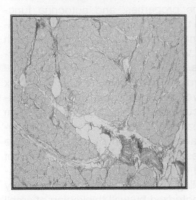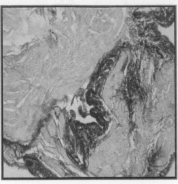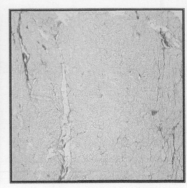

Patient with asymptomatic LVH   Patient with HFPEF   Patient with HFREF

Fig. 3. Endomyocardial tissue from 3 hypertensive patients with asymptomatic LVH (*left panel*), HFPEF (*middle panel*), and HFREF (*right panel*). Sections were stained with picrosirius red and collagen fibers were identified in red (×40). Compared with the myocardium of the patient with asymptomatic LVH, large scars and strands of collagen tissue (fibrosis) were seen in the myocardium of the patient with HFPEF. The myocardium of the patient with HFREF showed loss of the thin bands of collagen tissue surrounding individual cardiomyocytes or groups of cardiomyocytes (scaffold disruption) present in the myocardium of the asymptomatic patients with LVH.

indices with poor outcomes in patients with HFREF[21,22] and patients with HFPEF.[23]

Although echocardiography is recognized as central to management of HF, other imaging methodologies may offer some advantages for the diagnostic characterization of HHD in patients with HF. For instance, cardiac magnetic resonance (CMR) has been shown to be more reproducible than echocardiography for the estimation of LV mass and categorization of LVH.[24] In addition, CMR may facilitate the quantification of myocardial deformation and strain more accurately than it does echocardiography.[25] CMR techniques may allow the noninvasive assessment of diffuse myocardial fibrosis[26] as well as of myocardial ischemia caused by changes in the microcirculation.[27]

Although there are numerous studies investigating circulating biomarkers in HF, there are few that relate these biomarkers to HF in hypertensive patients. Gluba and colleagues[28] recently summarized data from 12 studies focused on circulating biomarkers showing potential usefulness in diagnosis of LV dysfunction and prediction of outcomes in hypertensive patients with HF (**Table 1**). Although some of these biomarkers are related to cardiomyocyte stress (eg, cardiotrophin-1),[29] others are more linked to inflammatory pathways (eg, interleukin-6 and interleukin-8, monocyte chemoattractant protein)[30] and to alterations of the myocardial collagen matrix (eg, procollagen-derived peptides and matrix metalloproteinases).[18,31]

Most studies on the role of biochemical biomarkers in HF have included patients with HFREF, but studies on the value of biomarkers, other than brain natriuretic peptide (BNP) and NT-proBNP, in HFPEF are scarce or lacking. Cheng and colleagues[32] recently reported the results of a systematic review of 26 epidemiologic studies (including 2546 patients, 79% of them with arterial hypertension) on the association of circulating biomarkers with HFPEF. Again, biomarkers of cardiomyocyte stress, inflammation, and extracellular matrix remodeling, as well as biomarkers of renal damage and dysfunction, were associated with both development of HFPEF and clinical outcomes of patients with HFPEF (see **Table 1**).

The complexity of HF pathophysiology suggests that a single imaging or circulating biomarker cannot reflect all the features of this syndrome, whereas the combined use of several biomarkers (multimarker approach) would better characterize patients with HF and create personalized options for their management, helping identify which patients (eg, patients with HF with arterial hypertension) to follow with a specific protocol.

Preventive and Therapeutic Aspects

HF is one of the major health care problems worldwide. Thus, it is necessary to optimize strategies for preventing HF, especially in the presence of risk factors such as arterial hypertension. Placebo-controlled studies have consistently

Table 1
Principal circulating biomarkers investigated in patients with HF with arterial hypertension

Biomarker	Cardiomyocyte Stress/Injury	Cardiac (Systemic) Inflammation	Cardiac (Other End-organ) Fibrosis	Renal Injury/ Dysfunction
Cardiac troponins	+	—	—	—
Soluble ST2	+	—	—	—
Cardiotrophin-1	+	—	—	—
BNPs	+	—	—	—
Adrenomedullin	+	—	—	—
Interleukins	—	+	—	—
TNF-α	—	+	—	—
MCP-1	—	+	—	—
CRP	—	+	—	—
Collagen peptides	—	—	+	—
MMPs/TIMPs	—	—	+	—
Galectin-3	—	—	+	—
Cystatin C	—	—	—	+
Creatinine	—	—	—	+

Soluble ST2 is also known as interleukin-1 receptorlike 1.
Abbreviations: BNPs, brain natriuretic peptides; CRP, C-reactive protein; MCP-1, monocyte chemoattractant protein-1; MMPs, matrix metalloproteinases; TIMPs, tissue inhibitors of MMPs; TNF-α, tumor necrosis factor-alpha.
Data from Gluba A, Bielecka-Dabrowa A, Mikhailidis DP, et al. An update on biomarkers of heart failure in hypertensive patients. J Hypertens 2012;30:1683; and Cheng JM, Akkerhuis KM, Battes LC, et al. Biomarkers of heart failure with normal ejection fraction: a systematic review. Eur J Heart Fail 2013;15(12):1355–58.

shown that all principal antihypertensive agents reduce the incidence of HF, thus confirming that BP reduction is a fundamental strategy to prevent HF in patients with arterial hypertension.[33] For instance, a meta-analysis of 12 hypertension trials that included development of HF showed significant treatment benefits.[34] In particular, the incidence of HF was decreased by 52% (95% confidence interval [CI], 41–62) compared with placebo recipients (**Fig. 4**).[34]

It is still debated whether there are differences among the various antihypertensive pharmacologic

classes in HF prevention. A recent network meta-analysis designed to investigate this issue was performed on 26 randomized controlled trials in hypertension published from 1997 to 2009 and including 223,313 patients. Diuretics, angiotensin-converting enzyme (ACE) inhibitors, and angiotensin II receptor blockers (ARBs) represented the most efficient classes of drugs to reduce the HF onset compared with placebo.[35] In contrast, calcium channel blockers, together with β-blockers and α-blockers, were among the least effective first-line agents in HF prevention.[35] These findings

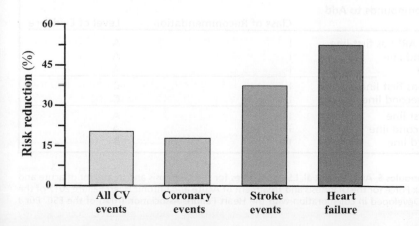

Fig. 4. Impact of hypertension treatment on the risk of different types of cardiovascular (CV) events. (*Data from* Moser M, Hebert PR. Prevention of disease progression, left ventricular heart hypertrophy and congestive heart failure in hypertension treatment trials. J Am Coll Cardiol 1996;27:1215.)

support the notion that there are differences among antihypertensive agents to prevent HF in patients with arterial hypertension.

Because HF may complicate the treatment of arterial hypertension, the choice of antihypertensive drugs to reduce increased BP in patients with HF requires some special considerations. In patients with HFREF and arterial hypertension, therapy is intended predominantly to treat vascular impedance and myocardial remodeling and not at the pressure per se.[36,37] Furthermore, in a meta-analysis of 10 prospective observational studies of patients with HF with a mean EF of 28.3%, a higher systolic BP was associated with better outcomes.[38] In particular, the decrease in mortality associated with a 10 mm Hg higher systolic BP was 13.0% (95% CI, 10.6%–15.4%) in this HF population. This finding was not related to cause, ACE inhibitor, or β-blocker use. On the contrary, in patients with HFPEF and arterial hypertension, the target BP level should be less than 130/80 mm Hg or the lowest level that can be achieved without side effects, according to the current recommendations by the Heart Failure Society of America.[39]

A wealth of data indicate that ACE inhibitors reduce mortality and hospitalization rates in patients with HFREF, thus these agents are first-line therapy in these patients and should be used as the basis of antihypertensive treatment if they present increased BP levels.[40,41] Treatment with β-blockers, because of their significant survival benefit, is essential to HF management and should be used for controlling arterial hypertension in patients with HFREF.[42,43] Mineralocorticoid receptor antagonists (MRA) not only exert a significant

survival benefit in these patients but also significantly decrease BP levels compared with placebo; thus, they could be of incremental value in arterial hypertension management of HFREF.[44,45] In recent guidelines by the European Society of Cardiology, diuretics (thiazides or loop diuretics) and calcium channel blockers (amlodipine or felodipine) are recommended as third and fourth steps, respectively, to treat hypertension in patients with HFREF when hypertension persists despite treatment with a combination of as many as possible of an ACE inhibitor (or an ARB), a β-blocker, and an MRA (**Table 2**).[46]

In patients with HFPEF, because reduced relaxation and increased stiffness of myocardium are key factors for impaired LV performance in these patients, agents that can reverse LVH are preferred for hypertension management. The available clinical evidence suggests that inhibition of the renin-angiotensin system may be the most effective approach for LV mass reduction,[47] although data on outcomes provide no significant evidence of benefit for ACE inhibitors[48] or ARBs.[49] MRA in small studies seem to be promising in reducing BP and improving LV function,[50] but results from recent large studies do not support a major beneficial role of these agents in patients with HFPEF.[51,52] However, definitive results will be available when the multicenter Treatment of Preserved Cardiac Function Heart Failure with Aldosterone Antagonist (TOPCAT) trial is published.[53] In patients with HFPEF, β-blockers are not associated with reduced mortality.[54] However, β-blockers can effectively reduce blood pressure, increase LV diastolic filling time, and thus enhance LV filling and coronary perfusion.[55,56]

Table 2
Protocol of stepped antihypertensive treatment recommended by the European Society of Cardiology Guidelines in patients with HF and reduced ejection fraction

Step	Pharmacologic Compounds to Add Progressively[a]	Class of Recommendation	Level of Evidence
1	ACE inhibitor (or ARB) as first line	I	A
	β-Blocker as second line	I	A
	MRA as third line	I	A
2	Thiazide diuretic as first line	I	C
	Loop diuretic as second line	I	C
3	Amlodipine as first line	I	A
	Hydralazine as second line	I	A
	Felodipine as third line	IIa	B

[a] In case high BP persists.

Data from McMurray JJ, Adamopoulos S, Anker SD, et al. ESC guidelines for the diagnosis and treatment of acute and chronic heart failure 2012: The Task Force for the Diagnosis and Treatment of Acute and Chronic Heart Failure 2012 of the European Society of Cardiology. Developed in collaboration with the Heart Failure Association (HFA) of the ESC. Eur J Heart Fail 2012;14:839.

ARTERIAL HYPERTENSION AS A COMORBIDITY OF HF

A broad spectrum of concomitant cardiovascular and noncardiovascular disorders may complicate HF, adding further morbidity and mortality risk.[57] In this regard, arterial hypertension is a frequent finding in the HF population. In a study in elderly patients with HF the prevalence of essential hypertension was 55% with an additional 11% contribution from patients with complicated and secondary hypertension.[58] The prevalence of hypertension in intervention trials ranges from 42% in the SOLVD (Studies of Left Ventricular Dysfunction) trial, including patients with systolic dysfunction,[41] to 64% in the recent I-PRESERVE trial, including patients with HFPEF.[49] Compared with patients with HFREF, patients with HFPEF have a higher prevalence of arterial hypertension as comorbidity.[59,60] Arterial hypertension was also reported to be the most common comorbid condition (73%) in the Acute Decompensated Heart Failure National Registry (ADHERE) including 105,388 patients hospitalized with acute decompensated HF in the United States.[61]

In the setting of arterial hypertension, factors such as lack of vasodilator reserve and reduced arterial compliance further affect cardiac output, particularly on exercise.[19] These factors are common to both HFPEF and HFREF.

The prognostic significance of BP in patients with HF varies depending on the patients' conditions. In patients with normal LV systolic function, hypertension is a risk factor for symptomatic HF and, often, for acute HF. In contrast, in patients with LV systolic dysfunction, hypotension rather than hypertension is a risk factor of increased mortality and morbidity.[62]

Drugs for the treatment of arterial hypertension are also indicated for the treatment of HF, with the only exceptions being calcium antagonists and alpha-antagonists. Dihydropyridine calcium antagonists can be added in patients with concomitant HF and hypertension resistant to other therapies, particularly if angina is associated.[46,63] Aggressive treatment of hypertension is reasonable in patients with HFPEF. Renin-angiotensin-aldosterone inhibitors seem particularly effective in these patients. However, there is a lack of evidence of efficacy on outcomes for any treatment, including ARBs, in patients with HFPEF.[46,49]

SUMMARY

HHD has classically been considered as the adaptive hypertrophy of LV wall to increased BP. Recent findings in hypertensive animals and patients now challenge this paradigm by showing that HHD also results from pathologic structural remodeling of the myocardium in response to a mosaic of hemodynamic and nonhemodynamic factors that are altered in arterial hypertension. The potential clinical relevance of this shift in paradigm is strengthened because it entails a new approach to the cardiac impact of arterial hypertension in terms of more precise diagnosis and more demanding treatment, particularly in those hypertensive patients with HF. This novel view of HHD may also have epidemiologic importance. The possibility that hypertensive patients predisposed to develop HF may be detected before the appearance of clinical manifestations provides a new way to prevent this major arterial complication. This new paradigm of HHD will benefit from the application of integrated omic technologies designed to reveal critical genes, pathways, metabolites, and networks for LV dysfunction/failure in arterial hypertension.[64] In addition, arterial hypertension may complicate HF, adding further morbidity and mortality risk. Therefore, advances in the treatment of HF must be attended by improving the management of arterial hypertension.

REFERENCES

1. Yusuf PS, Hawken S, Ôunpuu S, et al. Effect of potentially modifiable risk factors associated with myocardial infarction in 52 countries (the INTERHEART study): case-control study. Lancet 2004;364:937–52.
2. Frohlich ED, Apstein C, Chobanian AV, et al. The heart in hypertension. N Engl J Med 1992;327: 998–1008.
3. Agno FS, Chinali M, Bella JN, et al. Aortic valve sclerosis is associated with preclinical cardiovascular disease in hypertensive adults: the HyperGen study. J Hypertens 2005;23:867–73.
4. Kannel WB. Incidence and epidemiology of heart failure. Heart Fail Rev 2000;5:167–73.
5. Kenchaiah S, Narula J, Vasan RS. Risk factors for heart failure. Med Clin North Am 2004;88: 1145–72.
6. Mahmood SS, Wang TJ. The epidemiology of congestive heart failure: the Framingham Heart Study perspective. Glob Heart 2013;8:77–82.
7. Khatibzadeh S, Farzadfar F, Oliver J, et al. Worldwide risk factors for heart failure: a systematic review and pooled analysis. Int J Cardiol 2012; 168:1186–94.
8. Tocci G, Sciarretta S, Volpe M. Development of heart failure in recent development trials. J Hypertens 2008;26:1477–86.

9. Campbell RT, Jhund PS, Castagno D, et al. What have we learned about patients with heart failure and preserved ejection fraction from DIG-PEF, CHARM-preserved, and I-PRESERVE? J Am Coll Cardiol 2012;60:2349–56.

10. Ho JE, Lyass A, Lee DS, et al. Predictors of new-onset heart failure: differences in preserved versus reduced ejection fraction. Circ Heart Fail 2013;6: 279–86.

11. Meta-analysis Global Group in Chronic Heart Failure (MAGGIC). The survival of patients with heart failure with preserved or reduced left ventricular ejection fraction: an individual patient data meta-analysis. Eur Heart J 2012;33:1750–7.

12. Meerson FZ. Compensatory hyperfunction of the heart and cardiac insufficiency. Circ Res 1962;10: 250–8.

13. Drazner MH. The progression of hypertensive heart disease. Circulation 2011;123:327–34.

14. Giampietri C, Petrungaro S, Musumeci M, et al. c-Flip overexpression reduces cardiac hypertrophy in response to pressure overload. J Hypertens 2008;26:1008–16.

15. Frohlich ED, González A, Díez J. Hypertensive left ventricular hypertrophy risk: beyond adaptive cardiomyocyte hypertrophy. J Hypertens 2010;29: 17–26.

16. Díez J, González A, López B, et al. Mechanisms of disease: pathologic structural remodeling is more than adaptive hypertrophy in hypertensive heart disease. Nat Clin Pract Cardiovasc Med 2005;2: 209–16.

17. López B, Querejeta R, González A, et al. Collagen cross-linking but not collagen amount associates with elevated filling pressures in hypertensive patients with stage C heart failure: potential role of lysyl oxidase. Hypertension 2012;60:677–83.

18. López B, González A, Querejeta R, et al. Alterations in the pattern of collagen deposition may contribute to the deterioration of systolic function in hypertensive patients with heart failure. J Am Coll Cardiol 2006;48:89–96.

19. Yip GW, Fung JW, Tan YT, et al. Hypertension and heart failure: a dysfunction of systole, diastole or both? J Hum Hypertens 2009;23:295–306.

20. Steeds RP. Multimodality imaging in heart failure patients. Curr Opin Cardiol 2013;28:209–15.

21. Pozzoli M, Traversi E, Cioffi G, et al. Loading manipulations improve the prognostic value of Doppler evaluation of mitral flow in patients with chronic heart failure. Circulation 1997;95:1222–30.

22. Giannuzzi P, Temporelli PL, Bosimini E, et al. Independent and incremental prognostic value of Doppler-derived mitral deceleration time of early filling in both symptomatic and asymptomatic patients with left ventricular dysfunction. J Am Coll Cardiol 1996;28:383–90.

23. Ohtani T, Mohammed SF, Yamamoto K, et al. Diastolic stiffness as assessed by diastolic wall strain is associated with adverse remodelling and poor outcomes in heart failure with preserved ejection fraction. Eur Heart J 2012;33:1742–9.

24. Armstrong AC, Gidding S, Gjesdal O, et al. LV mass assessed by echocardiography and CMR, cardiovascular outcomes, and medical practice. JACC Cardiovasc Imaging 2012;5:837–48.

25. Piella G, De Craene M, Bijnens BH, et al. Characterizing myocardial deformation in patients with left ventricular hypertrophy of different etiologies using the strain distribution obtained by magnetic resonance imaging. Rev Esp Cardiol 2010;63: 1281–91.

26. Miller CA, Naish JH, Bishop P, et al. Comprehensive validation of cardiovascular magnetic resonance techniques for the assessment of myocardial extracellular volume. Circ Cardiovasc Imaging 2013;6:373–83.

27. Schwitter J, DeMarco T, Kneifel S, et al. Magnetic resonance-based assessment of global coronary flow and flow reserve and its relation to left ventricular functional parameters: a comparison with positron emission tomography. Circulation 2000;101: 2696–702.

28. Gluba A, Bielecka-Dabrowa A, Mikhailidis DP, et al. An update on biomarkers of heart failure in hypertensive patients. J Hypertens 2012;30:1681–9.

29. López B, González A, Querejeta R, et al. Association of plasma cardiotrophin-1 with stage C heart failure in hypertensive patients: potential diagnostic implications. J Hypertens 2009;27:418–24.

30. Collier P, Watson CJ, Voon V, et al. Can emerging biomarkers of myocardial remodelling identify asymptomatic hypertensive patients at risk for diastolic dysfunction and diastolic heart failure? Eur J Heart Fail 2011;13:1087–95.

31. Querejeta R, López B, González A, et al. Increased collagen type I synthesis in patients with heart failure of hypertensive origin: relation to myocardial fibrosis. Circulation 2004;110:1263–8.

32. Cheng JM, Akkerhuis KM, Battes LC, et al. Biomarkers of heart failure with normal ejection fraction: a systematic review. Eur J Heart Fail 2013; 15(12):1350–62.

33. Georgiopoulou VV, Kalogeropulos AP, Butler J. Heart failure in hypertension. Prevention and treatment. Drugs 2012;72:1373–98.

34. Moser M, Hebert PR. Prevention of disease prevention, left ventricular heart hypertrophy and congestive heart failure in hypertension treatment trials. J Am Coll Cardiol 1996;27:1214–8.

35. Sciarretta S, Palano F, Tocci G, et al. Antihypertensive treatment and development of heart failure in hypertension: a Bayesian network meta-analysis of studies in patients with hypertension and high

cardiovascular risk. Arch Intern Med 2011;171: 384–94.

36. Muiesan ML, Salvetti M, Rizzoni D, et al. Association of change in left ventricular mass with prognosis during long-term antihypertensive treatment. J Hypertens 1995;13:1091–5.

37. Schlaich MP, Schmieder RE. Left ventricular hypertrophy and its regression: pathophysiology and therapeutic approach: focus on treatment by antihypertensive agents. Am J Hypertens 1998; 11(11 Pt 1):1394–404.

38. Whinnett ZI, Davies JE, Fontana M, et al. Quantifying the paradoxical effect of higher systolic blood pressure on mortality in chronic heart failure. Heart 2009;95:56–62.

39. Lindenfeld J, Albert NM, Boehmer JP, et al. HFSA 2010 comprehensive heart failure practice guideline. J Card Fail 2010;16:e1–194.

40. Effects of enalapril on mortality in severe congestive heart failure: results of the Cooperative North Scandinavian Enalapril Survival Study (CONSENSUS). The CONSENSUS Trial Study Group. N Engl J Med 1987;316:1429–35.

41. Effect of enalapril on survival in patients with reduced left ventricular ejection fractions and congestive heart failure. The SOLVD Investigators. N Engl J Med 1991;325:293–302.

42. Packer M, Bristow MR, Cohn JN, et al. The effect of carvedilol on morbidity and mortality in patients with chronic heart failure. US Carvedilol Heart Failure Study Group. N Engl J Med 1996;334:1349–55.

43. Brophy JM, Joseph L, Rouleau JL. Beta-blockers in congestive heart failure: a Bayesian meta-analysis. Ann Intern Med 2001;134:550–60.

44. Effectiveness of spironolactone added to an angiotensin converting enzyme inhibitor and a loop diuretic for severe chronic congestive heart failure (the Randomized Aldactone Evaluation Study [RALES]). Am J Cardiol 1996;78:902–7.

45. Pitt B, White H, Nicolau J, et al. Eplerenone reduces mortality 30 days after randomization following acute myocardial infarction in patients with left ventricular systolic dysfunction and heart failure. J Am Coll Cardiol 2005;46:425–31.

46. McMurray JJ, Adamopoulos S, Anker SD, et al. ESC guidelines for the diagnosis and treatment of acute and chronic heart failure 2012: the Task Force for the Diagnosis and Treatment of Acute and Chronic Heart Failure 2012 of the European Society of Cardiology. Developed in collaboration with the Heart Failure Association (HFA) of the ESC. Eur J Heart Fail 2012;14:803–69.

47. Lang CC, Struthers AD. Targeting the renin-angiotensin-aldosterone system in heart failure. Nat Rev Cardiol 2013;10:125–34.

48. Fonarow GC, Stough WG, Abraham WT, et al. Characteristics, treatments, and outcomes of patients with preserved systolic function hospitalized for heart failure: a report from the OPTIMIZE-HF Registry. J Am Coll Cardiol 2007;50:768–77.

49. Massie BM, Carson PE, McMurray JJ, et al. Irbesartan in patients with heart failure and preserved ejection fraction. N Engl J Med 2008;359:2456–67.

50. Mottram PM, Haluska B, Leano R, et al. Effect of aldosterone antagonism on myocardial dysfunction in hypertensive patients with diastolic heart failure. Circulation 2004;110:558–65.

51. Edelmann F, Wachter R, Schmidt AG, et al. Effect of spironolactone on diastolic function and exercise capacity in patients with heart failure with preserved ejection fraction: the Aldo-DHF randomized controlled trial. JAMA 2013;309:781–91.

52. Patel K, Fonarow GC, Kitzman DW, et al. Aldosterone antagonists and outcomes in real-world older patients with heart failure and preserved ejection fraction. JACC Heart Fail 2013;1:40–7.

53. Treatment of preserved cardiac function heart failure with an Aldosterone anTagonist (TOPCAT) [online]. Available at: http://www.topcatstudy.com/index.asp. Accessed November 30, 2011.

54. Hernandez AF, Hammill BG, O'Connor CM, et al. Clinical effectiveness of beta-blockers in heart failure: findings from the OPTIMIZE-HF (Organized Program to Initiate Lifesaving Treatment in Hospitalized Patients with Heart Failure) Registry. J Am Coll Cardiol 2009;53:184–92.

55. Bergstrom A, Andersson B, Edner M, et al. Effect of carvedilol on diastolic function in patients with diastolic heart failure and preserved systolic function. Results of the Swedish Doppler-echocardiographic study (SWEDIC). Eur J Heart Fail 2004;6:453–61.

56. Capomolla S, Febo O, Gnemmi M, et al. Beta-blockade therapy in chronic heart failure: diastolic function and mitral regurgitation improvement by carvedilol. Am Heart J 2000;139:596–608.

57. Metra M, Zacà V, Parati G, et al. Cardiovascular and noncardiovascular comorbidities in patients with chronic heart failure. J Cardiovasc Med (Hagerstown) 2011;12:76–84.

58. Braunstein JB, Anderson GF, Gerstenblith G, et al. Noncardiac comorbidity increases preventable hospitalizations and mortality among Medicare beneficiaries with chronic heart failure. J Am Coll Cardiol 2003;42:1226–33.

59. Lenzen MJ, Scholte OP, Reimer WJ, et al. Differences between patients with a preserved and a depressed left ventricular function: a report from the EuroHeart Failure Survey. Eur Heart J 2004; 25:1214–20.

60. Brouwers FP, Hillege HL, van Gilst WH, et al. Comparing new onset heart failure with reduced ejection fraction and new onset heart failure with preserved ejection fraction: an epidemiologic perspective. Curr Heart Fail Rep 2012;9:363–8.

61. Adams KF Jr, Fonarow GC, Emerman CL, et al. Characteristics and outcomes of patients hospitalized for heart failure in the United States: rationale, design, and preliminary observations from the first 100,000 cases in the Acute Decompensated Heart Failure National Registry (ADHERE). Am Heart J 2005;149:209–16.

62. Kalantar-Zadeh K, Block G, Horwich T, et al. Reverse epidemiology of conventional cardiovascular risk factors in patients with chronic heart failure. J Am Coll Cardiol 2004;43:1439–44.

63. Hunt SA, Abraham WT, Chin MH, et al. 2009 Focused update incorporated into the ACC/AHA 2005 guidelines for the diagnosis and management of heart failure in adults a report of the American College of Cardiology Foundation/American Heart Association Task Force on Practice Guidelines developed in collaboration with the International Society for Heart and Lung Transplantation. J Am Coll Cardiol 2009;53:e1–90.

64. Díez J, Frohlich ED. A translational approach to hypertensive heart disease. Hypertension 2010;55:1–8.

Sleep-Disordered Breathing in Patients with Heart Failure

Robert J. Mentz, MD*, Mona Fiuzat, PharmD

KEYWORDS

- Comorbidities • Sleep apnea • Heart failure • Clinical trials • Outcomes • Adaptive servoventilation
- Positive airway pressure

KEY POINTS

- Sleep-disordered breathing is prevalent in patients with heart failure, and is associated with increased morbidity and mortality.
- Sleep-disordered breathing is proinflammatory, with nocturnal oxygen desaturations and hypercapnia playing a role in the development of oxidative stress and sympathetic activation.
- Attention to the diagnosis and management of sleep-disordered breathing in patients with heart failure may improve outcomes.

INTRODUCTION

Although there have been important successes in the development of therapies for chronic heart failure (HF) in recent decades, most recent HF trials have failed to show added benefit from new therapies,[1–3] and rates of adverse events remain high. In particular, there has been little progress in the development of new therapies for acute HF.[4] This lack of progress suggests the need for a critical reappraisal of treatment strategies in HF, including the treatment of comorbidities.

The presence of comorbidities in HF patients has been associated with significantly increased morbidity and mortality.[5] The risk of hospitalization markedly increases with the number of noncardiovascular chronic conditions.[6] Rehospitalization rates following acute HF are nearly as high for noncardiovascular causes as for HF.[7] Comorbid pulmonary and renal dysfunction, along with sleep-disordered breathing (SDB), complicates the management of HF patients. This article summarizes the impact of SDB on the characteristics, treatment, and outcomes of HF patients. Data investigating the treatment of SDB in HF patients are reviewed, and areas for future research identified.

EPIDEMIOLOGY AND DEFINITIONS

SDB is common in patients with HF.[8] It occurs in up to 50% to 80% of HF patients[9] and is highly prevalent in both those with preserved ejection fraction (EF) and reduced EF. Two primary types of SDB occur in HF patients: obstructive sleep apnea (OSA) and central sleep apnea/Cheyne-Stokes respiration (CSA/CSR). The prevalence of SDB in HF patients is substantially higher than in the general community, where approximately 18% of subjects have OSA (2:1 male predominance) and less than 1% have CSA.[10]

OSA involves repeated collapse of the pharynx that triggers apneas during sleep (**Box 1**).[9,11] Apnea is defined as a greater than 90% reduction in tidal volume lasting 10 seconds or longer, and hypopnea is a reduction in tidal volume of 50% to 90% lasting 10 seconds or longer, accompanied by a 3% or greater decrease in oxyhemoglobin

Funding: Funded by NIH, Grant number(s): T32GM086330-03.
Disclosures: Research funding and consulting from ResMed Corporation (M. Fiuzat). No relevant disclosures (R.J. Mentz).
Duke University Medical Center, Duke Clinical Research Institute, 2301 Erwin Road, Durham, NC 27710, USA
* Corresponding author. Duke University Medical Center, 2301 Erwin Road, Durham, NC 27710.
E-mail address: robert.mentz@duke.edu

Box 1
Definitions of sleep-disordered breathing

Apnea

- A greater than 90% reduction in tidal volume lasting 10 seconds or longer

Hypopnea

- A reduction in tidal volume of 50% to 90% that lasts 10 seconds or longer
- Accompanied by a 3% or more decrease in oxyhemoglobin saturation (Sao_2) or termination by arousal from sleep

Sleep Breathing Disorder

- Five or more episodes of apnea or hypopnea per hour of sleep
- Accompanied by either hypersomnolence or at least 2 episodes of choking or gasping during sleep, recurrent awakenings, unrefreshing sleep, daytime fatigue, or impaired concentration or memory

Obstructive Sleep Apnea

- Repeated collapse of the pharynx that triggers apneas during sleep
- Reduction in the tidal volume with apneas and/or hypopneas in the setting of typical breathing efforts

Central Sleep Apnea

- Apneas for 10 seconds or longer without typical breathing efforts

saturation or termination by arousal from sleep. A sleep breathing disorder is defined as the presence of 5 or more episodes of apnea or hypopnea per hour of sleep (ie, apnea-hypopnea index [AHI]), which is accompanied by either hypersomnolence or at least 2 episodes of choking or gasping during sleep, recurrent awakenings, unrefreshing sleep, daytime fatigue, or impaired concentration or memory. The AHI is used to grade severity as mild (6–14 episodes/h), moderate (15–29 episodes/h), or severe (≥30 episodes/h). OSA involves reduction in the tidal volume in the setting

of typical breathing efforts, whereas CSA involves apnea for 10 seconds or longer without typical efforts as diagnosed on polysomnography. CSA and OSA rarely occur together in normal subjects, but commonly coexist in HF patients, although one pattern usually predominates.[12]

One study of 700 stable HF outpatients with reduced EF (HFrEF) and symptoms of New York Heart Association (NYHA) functional class II and higher demonstrated that 76% of patients exhibited SDB with a breakdown of CSA and OSA in 40% and 36% of patients, respectively.[13] In particular, CSA seemed to be a marker of HF severity given the association with worse NYHA functional class and lower EF. However, the prevalence of SDB is high even in those with milder HF symptoms.[14] SDB has been shown to be at least as common in acute HF patients as in chronic HF patients.[15] Strikingly in one study of acute HF patients nearly all hospitalized patients had evidence of SDB with a mean AHI of 41 and approximately 50% of total sleep time in CSR.[16] Acute treatment of HF also did not appear to consistently improve SDB. Women with HF may be less likely than men to have SDB, and the severity of SDB may be lower.[17] HF with preserved EF (HFpEF) patients have a similarly high prevalence of SDB compared with those with HFrEF.[18,19] However, the breakdown between the predominant type of SDB in HFpEF may favor OSA rather than CSA, as in HFrEF patients.[20]

Risk factors for the development of SDB in HF patients include male sex and increased age for both types of SDB (**Table 1**).[21,22] Elevated body mass index (BMI) is an additional risk factor for OSA (perhaps only in men), while atrial fibrillation, hypocapnia during wakefulness (partial pressure of carbon dioxide <38 mm Hg), and severe left ventricular impairment increase the likelihood of CSA.[8,21]

OSA has been associated with increased morbidity and mortality in the general population.[23–25] In acute HF patients, SDB is an independent predictor of cardiac readmission.[26] In chronic HF patients, untreated moderate to severe OSA was associated with increased mortality on multivariable analysis in a small study of 164 patients

Table 1
Risk factors for sleep-disordered breathing

Both Obstructive and Central Sleep Apnea	Obstructive Sleep Apnea	Central Sleep Apnea
Male sex Increased age	Elevated body mass index (possibly males only)	Atrial fibrillation Hypocapnia during wakefulness Severe left ventricular impairment

(Fig. 1).[27] CSA has also been shown to be a predictor of mortality in HFrEF,[28] with increased risk at higher AHI values.[29] Another study found that the risk associated with SDB was confined to those with ischemic causes of HF.[30] By contrast, Roebuck and colleagues[31] did not find increased long-term mortality associated with OSA in patients with HF. Thus, the question of independent risk conferred by SDB in HF requires further study.

PATHOPHYSIOLOGIC INTERACTIONS

The pathophysiology of OSA and CSA are distinct. OSA is primarily a failure to maintain airway patency, although abnormal respiratory feedback loops may play a role in HF patients.[32,33] In the general population, OSA patients tend to have a smaller upper airway, which may be exacerbated by the nocturnal response of the pharyngeal dilator muscles to negative pressure and increasing carbon dioxide. Unfavorable upper airway anatomy may be due to acquired conditions such as obesity or intrinsic structural abnormalities, which may be further compromised by poor sleep posture. However, in HF patients, the AHI has a much weaker correlation with BMI.[34] Thus it has been suggested that factors other than obesity may play a prominent role in the development of OSA in HF patients. These mechanisms may include nocturnal rostral fluid movement with increased pharyngeal

obstruction.[35] In fact, the type and severity of apnea vary according to fluctuations in volume status and the degree of cardiac dysfunction.[36] With greater fluid accumulation, patients transition from predominantly OSA to CSA.[35] During a given night, the proportion of OSA events may decrease over time with a concomitant increase in the proportion of CSA events.[12]

CSA is mainly due to the instability of the ventilatory control systems.[33] Breathing is controlled by a feedback loop whereby an increase in the arterial partial pressure of carbon dioxide ($Paco_2$) stimulates breathing and a decrease inhibits it. In healthy individuals, this maintains the $Paco_2$ within a narrow range. However, HF patients have enhanced central chemoreceptor sensitivity, which results in a significantly larger ventilatory response to carbon dioxide.[37,38] This hyperventilatory response, which is further exacerbated in the setting of an elevated pulmonary capillary wedge pressure, may lower the CO_2 value below the apneic threshold, with resultant central apnea.[39] Circulation time is also increased in HF as a result of reduced cardiac output, which delays the sensing of alterations in $Paco_2$ by the central chemoreceptors. The enhanced response to carbon dioxide and hyperventilation in response to pulmonary congestion appear to be instrumental in the development of CSA, while the circulation time influences the resultant breathing pattern.[33]

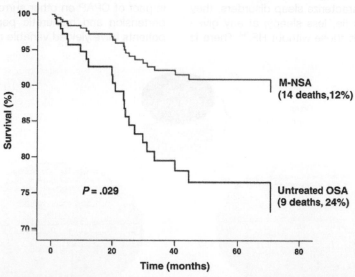

Fig. 1. Multivariable Cox proportional hazards survival plots for patients with mild or no sleep apnea versus untreated obstructive sleep apnea. Multivariable plots show worse survival of patients with heart failure with untreated obstructive sleep apnea (OSA) compared with those with mild or no sleep apnea (M-NSA) (hazard ratio = 2.81, P = .029) after adjusting for significant confounders (left ventricular ejection fraction, New York Heart Association functional class, and age). The adjusted survival curves are shown at the average values of these confounders. (From Wang H, Parker JD, Newton GE, et al. Influence of obstructive sleep apnea on mortality in patients with heart failure. J Am Coll Cardiol 2007;49(15):1628; with permission.)

Chronic SDB causes a series of derangements that may lead to the development or exacerbation of HF (**Fig. 2**). SDB is proinflammatory, with nocturnal oxygen desaturations and hypercapnia appearing to play a pivotal role in the development of oxidative stress and sympathetic activation.[9] Patients with ischemic cardiomyopathy may be more susceptible than those with nonischemic etiology to these adverse consequences.[30] Hypertension, diabetes, coronary artery disease, and atrial fibrillation, all well-established HF risk factors, are also adversely affected by SDB.[40–43] Thus the pathophysiology of HF and SDB are intertwined, with each contributing to the development and progression of the other.

DIAGNOSTIC ISSUES

SDB cannot be diagnosed in HF patients by symptoms or by routine cardiac assessment.[14] SDB is diagnosed by overnight polysomnography in a sleep laboratory with documentation of sleep architecture, cardiac rhythm, oxygenation, airflow, and thoracoabdominal movements. Portable monitoring devices may be used as an alternative, if diagnosis via polysomnography is inaccessible or unfeasible.[44] Despite the high prevalence of SDB in HF patients, it is underdiagnosed because SDB symptoms are less common than in the general population.[33] For instance, HF patients with SDB have less subjective daytime sleepiness. On the Epworth Sleepiness Scale (ESS), a common metric used to characterize sleep disorders, they have lower scores (ie, less sleepy) at any given AHI compared with those without HF.[34] There is

also no significant relationship between the ESS and increasing AHI in the HF population. For any given AHI, patients with HF have longer sleep-onset latency and less sleep than the general population, despite reporting less sleepiness. Thus, a clinician's level of suspicion for SDB based on a patient's symptom complex or scores on standard sleep metrics may be lower for HF patients than for the general population, despite the potential severity of the underlying disorder. Diagnosis is further hampered by the absence of a simple and accurate screening tool, and limited access to sleep facilities in the large numbers of patients with HF.

THERAPEUTIC ISSUES

As OSA and CSA have different causes, therapy may differ for the disorders. At present, the primary treatment for OSA is continuous positive airway pressure (CPAP). Several small, short-duration studies demonstrated that CPAP therapy in HF patients with OSA reduced sympathetic activity with associated decreases in blood pressure and heart rate,[45,46] and also increased daytime heart-rate variability, suggesting improved vagal modulation.[47] Most studies exploring the impact of CPAP on cardiac function and symptoms have demonstrated a beneficial effect. For instance, CPAP has been shown to reduce left ventricular dimensions and improve EF, cardiac efficiency, and quality of life.[46,48,49] By contrast, studies of the impact of CPAP on other surrogates such as hypertension and natriuretic peptide levels in HF patients have yielded variable results.[46,48,50]

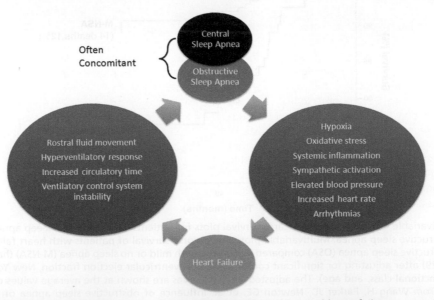

Fig. 2. Interaction of the pathophysiology of sleep-disordered breathing and heart failure.

While conventional CPAP has been shown to improve morbidity and, possibly, mortality in the general population,[23,51–53] its influence on outcomes in HF patients has been less clear. Observational studies assessing the efficacy of CPAP on morbidity and mortality in chronic HF patients with OSA have suggested potential benefits.[9] Two small studies in HF patients with more than 2 years of follow-up suggested lower death or rehospitalization risk[54] and a trend for reduced mortality in the CPAP treatment groups.[27] Large-scale, appropriately powered, randomized trials are needed to empirically demonstrate the benefit of CPAP in OSA patients with HF.

Because CSA may be related to the severity of HF, optimization of HF therapy may improve CSA. Observational studies suggest that diuretics, β-blockers, and biventricular pacing may reduce the severity of CSA.[55] For instance, small, uncontrolled studies of the impact of biventricular pacing have suggested a potential benefit on SDB,[56] yet results have been conflicting[57] and further study is required.

In contrast to OSA, the mechanism by which CPAP may benefit the underlying pathophysiology of CSA is less clear, given the lack of upper airway obstruction. However, CPAP may provide a hemodynamic benefit by reducing left ventricular afterload and cardiac filling pressures.[58] In a small study of 66 patients, Sin and colleagues[59] reported an improvement in EF and transplant-free survival in HF patients with CSA randomized to CPAP if they complied with treatment. The largest randomized, prospective study was the CANPAP study (CANadian continuous Positive Airway Pressure for patients with heart failure and central sleep apnea) (N = 258), which found no difference in 2-year survival with CPAP despite improvements in EF, norepinephrine levels, and 6-minute walk distance.[60] However, the mean duration of nightly CPAP therapy was approximately 4 hours over 3 months and less than 4 hours at the 12-month follow-up. Furthermore, CPAP reduced the mean AHI only to 19. A post hoc analysis suggested that responders to CPAP (ie, improvement in AHI to <15 at 3 months) had a significant improvement in EF and transplant-free survival in comparison with nonresponders or controls.[61] The investigators concluded that CPAP might improve outcomes if CSA is suppressed soon after its initiation. However, these results must be viewed as hypothesis-generating, given the limitations of subgroup analyses.

Minute ventilation-targeted adaptive servoventilation (ASV) is a distinct form of noninvasive ventilation that automatically adjusts the degree of pressure support in response to the patient's breathing efforts. ASV may treat both CSA and OSA with improved tolerability compared with CPAP devices. Previous HF studies have demonstrated benefits regarding quality of life, natriuretic peptide levels, and left ventricular function with ASV.[62,63] A recent randomized trial of 23 HF patients with CSA unsuppressed despite at least 3 months of CPAP (defined as AHI ≥15) demonstrated that ASV treatment was more effective at suppressing the AHI, with a greater improvement in EF and better compliance than continued CPAP.[64] However, survival benefits from autotitration devices in HF patients have not been demonstrated, and randomized trials of ASV in HF are ongoing. The Serve-HF trial (Treatment of Predominant Central Sleep Apnoea by Adaptive Servo Ventilation in Patients With Heart Failure) is an ongoing European trial in HF patients with reduced EF (target enrollment N = 1313), which will evaluate the long-term morbidity/mortality and cost-effectiveness of ASV (ClinicalTrials.gov Identifier: NCT00733343). The Cardiovascular Improvements with MV-ASV Therapy in Heart Failure (CAT-HF) trial will investigate ASV therapy initiated during a hospitalization for acute HF (target enrollment N = 215) with a 6 month global rank endpoint of survival free from cardiovascular hospitalization and improvement in functional capacity measured by 6-minute walk distance (ClinicalTrials.gov Identifier: NCT01953874).

CLINICAL PERSPECTIVE

For patients with HF, there is a paucity of data from prospective, randomized controlled trials addressing the potential benefits of treatment for either OSA or CSA. As such, there are no consensus guidelines endorsed by either sleep medicine or HF specialists on management strategies for SDB associated with HF. Nonetheless, observational data and preliminary randomized data suggest a role for the treatment of SDB in HF patients through optimization of standard guideline-based HF management and consideration of the use of noninvasive ventilation devices. The International Collaboration of Sleep Apnea Cardiovascular Trialists has recently summarized the current status of research in the field, and has highlighted future steps.[65]

SUMMARY

This article highlights the high prevalence and implications of SDB in HF patients, and reviews preliminary data suggesting that careful attention to the diagnosis and management of SDB may help to improve patient outcomes. The lack of recent progress in reducing the exceedingly high event rate in HF patients suggests the need for a reappraisal of treatment strategies, including the treatment of comorbidities. A focus on SDB represents a logical consideration in the holistic management of HF patients, given the closely interrelated nature of these conditions.

REFERENCES

1. Massie BM, O'Connor CM, Metra M, et al. Rolofylline, an adenosine A1-receptor antagonist, in acute heart failure. N Engl J Med 2010;363(15):1419–28.

2. Gheorghiade M, Bohm M, Greene SJ, et al. Effect of aliskiren on postdischarge mortality and heart failure readmissions among patients hospitalized for heart failure: the ASTRONAUT randomized trial. JAMA 2013;309(11):1125–35.

3. Swedberg K, Young JB, Anand IS, et al. Treatment of anemia with darbepoetin alfa in systolic heart failure. N Engl J Med 2013;368(13):1210–9.

4. Felker GM, Pang PS, Adams KF, et al. Clinical trials of pharmacological therapies in acute heart failure syndromes: lessons learned and directions forward. Circ Heart Fail 2010;3(2):314–25.

5. Mentz RJ, Felker GM. Noncardiac comorbidities and acute heart failure patients. Heart Fail Clin 2013;9(3):359–67.

6. Braunstein JB, Anderson GF, Gerstenblith G, et al. Noncardiac comorbidity increases preventable hospitalizations and mortality among Medicare beneficiaries with chronic heart failure. J Am Coll Cardiol 2003;42(7):1226–33.

7. O'Connor CM, Miller AB, Blair JE, et al. Causes of death and rehospitalization in patients hospitalized with worsening heart failure and reduced ventricular ejection fraction: results from efficacy of vasopressin antagonism in heart failure outcome study with tolvaptan (EVEREST) program. Am Heart J 2010;159(5):841–9.e1.

8. Ferrier K, Campbell A, Yee B, et al. Sleep-disordered breathing occurs frequently in stable outpatients with congestive heart failure. Chest 2005;128(4):2116–22.

9. Kasai T, Bradley TD. Obstructive sleep apnea and heart failure: pathophysiologic and therapeutic implications. J Am Coll Cardiol 2011;57(2):119–27.

10. Young T, Shahar E, Nieto FJ, et al. Predictors of sleep-disordered breathing in community-dwelling adults: the sleep heart health study. Arch Intern Med 2002;162(8):893–900.

11. Sleep-related breathing disorders in adults: recommendations for syndrome definition and measurement techniques in clinical research. The report of an American Academy of Sleep Medicine Task Force. Sleep 1999;22(5):667–89.

12. Tkacova R, Niroumand M, Lorenzi-Filho G, et al. Overnight shift from obstructive to central apneas in patients with heart failure: role of PCO_2 and circulatory delay. Circulation 2001;103(2):238–43.

13. Oldenburg O, Lamp B, Faber L, et al. Sleep-disordered breathing in patients with symptomatic heart failure: a contemporary study of prevalence in and characteristics of 700 patients. Eur J Heart Fail 2007;9(3):251–7.

14. Vazir A, Hastings PC, Dayer M, et al. A high prevalence of sleep disordered breathing in men with mild symptomatic chronic heart failure due to left ventricular systolic dysfunction. Eur J Heart Fail 2007;9(3):243–50.

15. Khayat RN, Jarjoura D, Patt B, et al. In-hospital testing for sleep-disordered breathing in hospitalized patients with decompensated heart failure: report of prevalence and patient characteristics. J Card Fail 2009;15(9):739–46.

16. Padeletti M, Green P, Mooney AM, et al. Sleep disordered breathing in patients with acutely decompensated heart failure. Sleep Med 2009;10(3):353–60.

17. Paulino A, Damy T, Margarit L, et al. Prevalence of sleep-disordered breathing in a 316-patient French cohort of stable congestive heart failure. Arch Cardiovasc Dis 2009;102(3):169–75.

18. Bitter T, Faber L, Hering D, et al. Sleep-disordered breathing in heart failure with normal left ventricular ejection fraction. Eur J Heart Fail 2009;11(6):602–8.

19. Chan J, Sanderson J, Chan W, et al. Prevalence of sleep-disordered breathing in diastolic heart failure. Chest 1997;111(6):1488–93.

20. Herrscher TE, Akre H, Overland B, et al. High prevalence of sleep apnea in heart failure outpatients: even in patients with preserved systolic function. J Card Fail 2011;17(5):420–5.

21. Sin DD, Fitzgerald F, Parker JD, et al. Risk factors for central and obstructive sleep apnea in 450 men and women with congestive heart failure. Am J Respir Crit Care Med 1999;160(4):1101–6.

22. Bradley TD, Floras JS. Sleep apnea and heart failure: part I: obstructive sleep apnea. Circulation 2003;107(12):1671–8.

23. Marin JM, Carrizo SJ, Vicente E, et al. Long-term cardiovascular outcomes in men with obstructive sleep apnoea-hypopnoea with or without treatment with continuous positive airway pressure: an observational study. Lancet 2005;365(9464):1046–53.

24. Punjabi NM, Caffo BS, Goodwin JL, et al. Sleep-disordered breathing and mortality: a prospective cohort study. PLoS Med 2009;6(8):e1000132.

25. Gami AS, Olson EJ, Shen WK, et al. Obstructive sleep apnea and the risk of sudden cardiac death: a longitudinal study of 10,701 adults. J Am Coll Cardiol 2013;62(7):610–6.

26. Khayat R, Abraham W, Patt B, et al. Central sleep apnea is a predictor of cardiac readmission in hospitalized patients with systolic heart failure. J Card Fail 2012;18(7):534–40.

27. Wang H, Parker JD, Newton GE, et al. Influence of obstructive sleep apnea on mortality in patients with heart failure. J Am Coll Cardiol 2007;49(15): 1625–31.

28. Javaheri S, Shukla R, Zeigler H, et al. Central sleep apnea, right ventricular dysfunction, and low diastolic blood pressure are predictors of mortality in systolic heart failure. J Am Coll Cardiol 2007;49(20):2028–34.

29. Lanfranchi PA, Braghiroli A, Bosimini E, et al. Prognostic value of nocturnal Cheyne-Stokes respiration in chronic heart failure. Circulation 1999; 99(11):1435–40.

30. Yumino D, Wang H, Floras JS, et al. Relationship between sleep apnoea and mortality in patients with ischaemic heart failure. Heart 2009;95(10): 819–24.

31. Roebuck T, Solin P, Kaye DM, et al. Increased long-term mortality in heart failure due to sleep apnoea is not yet proven. Eur Respir J 2004;23(5):735–40.

32. White DP. Pathogenesis of obstructive and central sleep apnea. Am J Respir Crit Care Med 2005; 172(11):1363–70.

33. Ng AC, Freedman SB. Sleep disordered breathing in chronic heart failure. Heart Fail Rev 2009;14(2): 89–99.

34. Arzt M, Young T, Finn L, et al. Sleepiness and sleep in patients with both systolic heart failure and obstructive sleep apnea. Arch Intern Med 2006; 166(16):1716–22.

35. Yumino D, Redolfi S, Ruttanaumpawan P, et al. Nocturnal rostral fluid shift: a unifying concept for the pathogenesis of obstructive and central sleep apnea in men with heart failure. Circulation 2010; 121(14):1598–605.

36. Ryan CM, Floras JS, Logan AG, et al. Shift in sleep apnoea type in heart failure patients in the CANPAP trial. Eur Respir J 2010;35(3):592–7.

37. Javaheri S. A mechanism of central sleep apnea in patients with heart failure. N Engl J Med 1999; 341(13):949–54.

38. Dempsey JA. Crossing the apnoeic threshold: causes and consequences. Exp Physiol 2005; 90(1):13–24.

39. Solin P, Bergin P, Richardson M, et al. Influence of pulmonary capillary wedge pressure on central apnea in heart failure. Circulation 1999;99(12):1574–9.

40. Punjabi NM, Beamer BA. Alterations in glucose disposal in sleep-disordered breathing. Am J Respir Crit Care Med 2009;179(3):235–40.

41. Lavie P, Herer P, Hoffstein V. Obstructive sleep apnoea syndrome as a risk factor for hypertension: population study. BMJ 2000;320(7233):479–82.

42. Gami AS, Pressman G, Caples SM, et al. Association of atrial fibrillation and obstructive sleep apnea. Circulation 2004;110(4):364–7.

43. Peker Y, Carlson J, Hedner J. Increased incidence of coronary artery disease in sleep apnoea: a long-term follow-up. Eur Respir J 2006;28(3):596–602.

44. Erman MK, Stewart D, Einhorn D, et al. Validation of the ApneaLink for the screening of sleep apnea: a novel and simple single-channel recording device. J Clin Sleep Med 2007;3(4):387–92.

45. Usui K, Bradley TD, Spaak J, et al. Inhibition of awake sympathetic nerve activity of heart failure patients with obstructive sleep apnea by nocturnal continuous positive airway pressure. J Am Coll Cardiol 2005;45(12):2008–11.

46. Mansfield DR, Gollogly NC, Kaye DM, et al. Controlled trial of continuous positive airway pressure in obstructive sleep apnea and heart failure. Am J Respir Crit Care Med 2004;169(3):361–6.

47. Gilman MP, Floras JS, Usui K, et al. Continuous positive airway pressure increases heart rate variability in heart failure patients with obstructive sleep apnoea. Clin Sci (Lond) 2008;114(3):243–9.

48. Kaneko Y, Floras JS, Usui K, et al. Cardiovascular effects of continuous positive airway pressure in patients with heart failure and obstructive sleep apnea. N Engl J Med 2003;348(13):1233–41.

49. Yoshinaga K, Burwash IG, Leech JA, et al. The effects of continuous positive airway pressure on myocardial energetics in patients with heart failure and obstructive sleep apnea. J Am Coll Cardiol 2007;49(4):450–8.

50. Smith LA, Vennelle M, Gardner RS, et al. Auto-titrating continuous positive airway pressure therapy in patients with chronic heart failure and obstructive sleep apnoea: a randomized placebo-controlled trial. Eur Heart J 2007;28(10):1221–7.

51. Doherty LS, Kiely JL, Swan V, et al. Long-term effects of nasal continuous positive airway pressure therapy on cardiovascular outcomes in sleep apnea syndrome. Chest 2005;127(6):2076–84.

52. Campos-Rodriguez F, Pena-Grinan N, Reyes-Nunez N, et al. Mortality in obstructive sleep apnea-hypopnea patients treated with positive airway pressure. Chest 2005;128(2):624–33.

53. Campos-Rodriguez F, Martinez-Garcia MA, de la Cruz-Moron I, et al. Cardiovascular mortality in women with obstructive sleep apnea with or without continuous positive airway pressure treatment: a cohort study. Ann Intern Med 2012;156(2):115–22.

54. Kasai T, Narui K, Dohi T, et al. Prognosis of patients with heart failure and obstructive sleep apnea treated with continuous positive airway pressure. Chest 2008;133(3):690–6.

55. Olson LJ, Somers VK. Treating central sleep apnea in heart failure: outcomes revisited. Circulation 2007;115(25):3140–2.

56. Stanchina ML, Ellison K, Malhotra A, et al. The impact of cardiac resynchronization therapy on obstructive sleep apnea in heart failure patients: a pilot study. Chest 2007;132(2):433–9.

57. Oldenburg O, Faber L, Vogt J, et al. Influence of cardiac resynchronisation therapy on different types of sleep disordered breathing. Eur J Heart Fail 2007;9(8):820–6.

58. Bradley TD, Floras JS. Sleep apnea and heart failure: part II: central sleep apnea. Circulation 2003; 107(13):1822–6.

59. Sin DD, Logan AG, Fitzgerald FS, et al. Effects of continuous positive airway pressure on cardiovascular outcomes in heart failure patients with and without Cheyne-Stokes respiration. Circulation 2000;102(1):61–6.

60. Bradley TD, Logan AG, Kimoff RJ, et al. Continuous positive airway pressure for central sleep apnea and heart failure. N Engl J Med 2005;353(19): 2025–33.

61. Arzt M, Floras JS, Logan AG, et al. Suppression of central sleep apnea by continuous positive airway pressure and transplant-free survival in heart failure: a post hoc analysis of the Canadian Continuous Positive Airway Pressure for Patients with Central Sleep Apnea and Heart Failure trial (CANPAP). Circulation 2007;115(25):3173–80.

62. Sharma BK, Bakker JP, McSharry DG, et al. Adaptive servoventilation for treatment of sleep-disordered breathing in heart failure: a systematic review and meta-analysis. Chest 2012;142(5): 1211–21.

63. Pepperell JC, Maskell NA, Jones DR, et al. A randomized controlled trial of adaptive ventilation for Cheyne-Stokes breathing in heart failure. Am J Respir Crit Care Med 2003;168(9):1109–14.

64. Kasai T, Kasagi S, Maeno K, et al. Adaptive servo-ventilation in cardiac function and neurohormonal status in patients with heart failure and central sleep apnea nonresponsive to continuous positive airway pressure. JACC: Heart Fail 2013;1(1):58–63.

65. Gottlieb DJ, Craig SE, Lorenzi-Filho G, et al. Sleep apnea cardiovascular clinical trials—current status and steps forward: the International Collaboration of Sleep Apnea Cardiovascular Trialists. Sleep 2013;36(7):975–80.

Cardiorenal Syndrome

Claudio Ronco, MD, PhD[a], Luca Di Lullo, MD, PhD[b],*

KEYWORDS

- Cardiorenal syndrome • Acute kidney disease • Acute decompensated heart failure
- Chronic heart failure • Chronic kidney disease • Sepsis

KEY POINTS

- Diagnosis of type-1 cardiorenal syndrome (CRS) focuses on laboratory findings and ultrasonography and/or second-level radiologic assays.
- Type-2 CRS is characterized by onset of chronic kidney disease (CKD) in patients with heart failure, but coexistence of cardiovascular disease and CKD is not enough to propose a type-2 CRS diagnosis.
- Type-3 CRS represents a typical scenario after cardiovascular surgery or contrast exposure; prevention is a key point in managing this kind of CRS.
- Because type-4 CRS is characterized by chronic cardiovascular involvement in CKD patients, correction of traditional and nontraditional cardiovascular risk factors is crucial.
- Once diagnosis of type-5 CRS is made, every organ and tissue involved must be investigated evaluate for risk prediction and protect from further and irreversible alterations in organ function.

INTRODUCTION

The term cardiorenal syndrome (CRS) includes a broad spectrum of diseases within which both the heart and kidneys are involved, acutely or chronically. According to a recent definition proposed by the Consensus Conference of Acute Dialysis Quality Initiative Group,[1] CRS has been used to define different clinical conditions in which heart and kidney dysfunction overlap. The heart and kidney are both involved in basic physiology, and their functions are strictly linked; while the heart provides nourishing and oxygen-rich fluids to all body areas, the kidney is responsible for providing fluid, electrolytes, and acid-base homeostasis, together with erythropoietin synthesis and vitamin D activation.

CRS complexity needs to be explained firstly by examining its pathogenesis and epidemiology, then by analyzing diagnostic, clinical, and therapeutic pathways.

A clear classification of CRS is crucial because an extensive and correct application is required, presenting an important challenge for nephrologists and cardiologists whereby they must widen their own fields of expertise. This integration might create common frontiers of cardiology and nephrology, providing with a more holistic and complete clinical presentation of patients.

An effective classification of CRS was proposed in a Consensus Conference by the Acute Dialysis Quality Group[1] in 2008 (**Table 1**). This classification essentially divides CRS in two main groups, cardiorenal and renocardiac CRS, based on primum movens of disease (cardiac or renal); both cardiorenal and renocardiac CRS are then divided into acute and chronic, according to onset of disease. The fifth type of CRS integrates all cardiorenal involvement induced by systemic disease.

TYPE-1 CRS

Type-1 CRS occurs in about 25% of patients hospitalized for acute decompensated heart failure (ADHF)[2,3]; among these patients preexistent chronic kidney disease (CKD) is common, and

[a] International Renal Research Institute, S. Bortolo Hospital, Viale F. Ridolfi 37, Vicenza 36100, Italy; [b] Department of Nephrology and Dialysis, L. Parodi-Delfino Hospital, Piazza A. Moro, Colleferro, Roma 1-00034, Italy
* Corresponding author.
E-mail address: dilullo.luca@inwind.it

Heart Failure Clin 10 (2014) 251–280
http://dx.doi.org/10.1016/j.hfc.2013.12.003
1551-7136/14/$ – see front matter © 2014 Elsevier Inc. All rights reserved

Table 1
Classification of cardiorenal syndrome

Type	Denomination	Description	Example
1	Acute cardiorenal	Heart failure leading to acute kidney disease (AKD)	Acute coronary syndrome leading to acute heart and kidney failure
2	Chronic cardiorenal	Chronic heart failure leading to kidney failure	Chronic heart failure
3	Acute nephrocardiac	AKD leading to acute heart failure	Uremic cardiomyopathy, AKD-related
4	Chronic nephrocardiac	Chronic kidney disease leading to heart failure	Left ventricular hypertrophy and diastolic heart failure due to kidney failure
5	Secondary	Systemic disease leading to heart and kidney failure	Sepsis, vasculitis, diabetes mellitus

contributes to acute kidney injury (AKI) in 60% of all cases studied. AKI can be considered an independent mortality risk factor in patients with ADHF, including those with ST-elevated myocardial infarction and/or reduced left ventricular ejection fraction (LVEF).[4]

Pathophysiology

Type-1 CRS (acute cardiorenal) is characterized by acute worsening of cardiac function leading to AKI.[5,6] It usually presents in the setting of an acute cardiac disease such as ADHF, and can follow an ischemic (acute coronary syndrome, cardiac surgery complications) or nonischemic heart disease (valvular disease, pulmonary embolism).

AKI is a well-known complication in patients hospitalized for ADHF; up to 45% of patients require more complex management because of higher mortality rates. Preliminary observations indicate the importance of timing in the development of AKI and its early diagnosis (**Fig. 1**).

Hemodynamic mechanisms probably play a major role in CRS type 1 in presence of an ADHF, leading to decreased renal arterial flow and a consequent decrease in glomerular filtration rate (GFR). Once hemodynamics is restored, renal and cardiac parameters return to normal (**Fig. 2**).[7] ADHF patients present with a wide spectrum of clinical features, and different hemodynamic profiles have been proposed depending on patients' hemodynamics (adequacy of perfusion and decreased effective circulation fluid volume [ECFV]) and extent of pulmonary congestion (increase in central venous pressure [CVP]). Four distinct profiles will result, termed wet or dry and warm or cold. Type-1 CRS can develop in every class of patients described.[8]

In the cold pattern, reduction in patients' carbon monoxide (CO) and ECFV represent the main

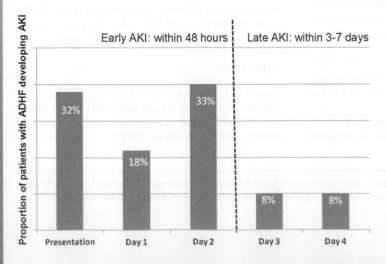

Y-axis: Proportion of patients with ADHF developing AKI

Early AKI: within 48 hours | Late AKI: within 3-7 days

Presentation: 32%
Day 1: 18%
Day 2: 33%
Day 3: 8%
Day 4: 8%

Fig. 1. Timing of acute kidney injury (AKI) in the setting of acute decompensated heart failure (ADHF).

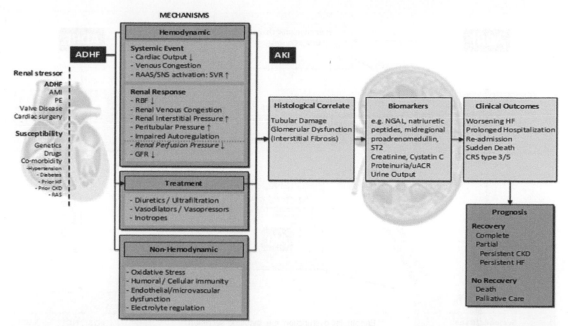

Fig. 2. Overview on mechanisms, histologic correlates, biomarkers, and outcomes in cardiorenal syndrome (CRS) type 1 in the setting of acute decompensated heart failure. ADHF, acute decompensated heart failure; AKI, acute kidney injury (the term AKI also covers the term WRF [worsening renal function], which is usually defined as a doubling of serum creatinine); AMI, acute myocardial infarction; CKD, chronic kidney disease; GFR, glomerular filtration rate; HF, heart failure; IL-18, interleukin-18; KIM-1, kidney injury molecule 1; L-FABP, liver-type fatty acid binding protein; NAG, N-acetylglucosamine; NGAL; neutrophil gelatinase–associated lipocalin; PE, pulmonary embolism; RAS, renal artery stenosis; SVR, systemic vascular resistance; uACR, urinary albumin:creatinine ratio. (*From* Cruz DN, Schmidt-Ott KM, Vescovo G, et al. Pathophysiology of cardiorenal syndrome type 2 in stable chronic heart failure: workgroup statements from the eleventh consensus conference of the Acute Dialysis Quality Initiative (ADQI). Contrib Nephrol 2013;182:117–36; with permission.)

hemodynamic change, whereas there is a marked increase in CVP in wet-pattern patients.

Cold-pattern patients also present with a decrease in renal blood flow, but its relationship with CO variations remains unclear; it is probably related to activation of the renin-angiotensin system and systemic nervous system (SNS), causing afferent vasoconstriction, decreased renal blood flow, and a decrease in renal perfusion pressure.

Other patients present with a wet patter caused by increased pulmonary and/or systemic congestion; in these patients high CVP directly affects renal vein and kidney perfusion pressure.[9,10] An increase in CVP also results in increased interstitial pressure, with collapse of tubules and progressive lack of renal function.[11]

Warm-profile patients present with reduction in cardiac output and ECFV, but not to the extent of cold-pattern patients. In these patients the main pathophysiologic feature is represented by disproportionate decreased renal blood flow in respect of CO; renal artery stenosis, which could be present in up to 40% patients with chronic heart failure (HF), may be accountable for this

situation.[12] Warm-pattern patients usually undergo chronic therapy with renin-angiotensin aldosterone system (RAAS) inhibitors, potentially limiting the response to ECFV reductions.

"Warm and wet" patients represent the most frequent profile in acute and chronic advanced HF.[13] Mechanisms of increased CVP are similar to those in cold-profile patients, but renal perfusion pressure is less affected because of higher arterial blood pressures.[9]

Apart from hemodynamic pathophysiologic pathways, other nonhemodynamic mechanisms have been proposed as being involved in type-1 CRS, including SNS and RAAS activation, chronic inflammatory status, and impairment of reactive oxygen species/nitric oxide (NO) production (**Fig. 3**). In patients with HF, a decrease in cardiac output and ECFV of renal arteries leads to activation of SNS and RAAS. Therefore, paraventricular nucleus–mediated increased stimulation of SNS (increased angiotensin II, decreased NO, and increased afferent renal sympathetic activity) can contribute to alterations in GFR and renal blood flow (**Figs. 2 and 3**).[11]

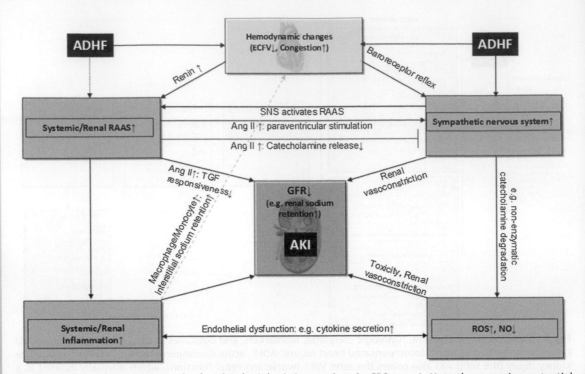

Fig. 3. Nonhemodynamic network of pathophysiologic interactions in CRS type 1. Note the emerging potential role of macrophages/monocytes as mediators of sodium and fluid retention. ADHF, acute decompensated heart failure; AKI, acute kidney injury; Ang II, angiotensin II; ECFV, effective circulation fluid volume; GFR, glomerular filtration rate; NO, nitric oxide; RAAS, renin-angiotensin-aldosterone system; ROS, reactive oxygen species; SNS, sympathetic nervous system; TGF, transforming growth factor. (*From* Cruz DN, Schmidt-Ott KM, Vescovo G, et al. Pathophysiology of cardiorenal syndrome type 2 in stable chronic heart failure: workgroup statements from the eleventh consensus conference of the Acute Dialysis Quality Initiative (ADQI). Contrib Nephrol 2013;182:117–36; with permission.)

Recently a potential role for mononuclear cells system in the regulation of blood pressure was suggested.[14] Macrophages are thought to play a protective role against the development of arterial hypertension; impairment of macrophage activity could lead to volume overload and congestion, even in the absence of any hemodynamic cardiovascular event. Patients with ADHF show more frequent defective regulation of monocyte apoptosis and activation of inflammatory pathways relative to healthy subjects.[15]

Gut underperfusion and endotoxin release in HF patients have been proposed as pathophysiologic mechanisms in progression of HF and CRS. HF patients present an ischemia of intestinal villi with local production of lipopolysaccharide, and consequent systemic endotoxemia.[16]

Finally, iatrogenesis should be considered in the pathophysiology of type-1 CRS. Pharmacologic treatment of diabetes mellitus, oncologic diseases, and HF itself can contribute to starting or worsening a type-1 CRS. Metformin, among the most widely used antidiabetic drugs, can provide a negative inotropic effect because of lactic acid production.[17,18] Chemotherapeutic agents lead to abnormal production of uric acid, with direct inhibitory effects on myocardium and tubulointerstitial components of the kidney.[19] Antibiotics may cause interstitial nephritis and tubular dysfunction, contributing to end-stage kidney disease.[20] Combined therapy with angiotensin-converting enzyme (ACE) inhibitors and angiotensin II receptor blockers (ARBs) can worsen renal function, especially in patients with a GFR of less than 40 mL/min.[21] Misuse of nonsteroidal anti-inflammatory agents abuse, inhibiting cyclooxygenases 1 and 2, impairs prostaglandin synthesis and provides salt and water retention, with poor outcomes in HF patients.[22]

Diagnosis

The diagnosis of type-1 CRS focuses on laboratory findings, and ultrasonography and/or second-level radiologic assays.

Because morbidity and mortality rates of type-1 CRS remain high, an early diagnosis is required. Neutrophil gelatinase-associated lipocalin (NGAL) is involved in cardiomyocyte apoptosis by increasing intracellular iron accumulation.[19] Administration of recombinant NGAL to mice induced an acute inflammatory response with compensatory changes in cardiac functional parameters, reflecting its potential role as a cardiorenal biomarker.[19] These findings agree with those reported in human myocarditis whereby NGAL was strongly induced in affected myocardiocytes, vascular wall cells, fibroblasts, and neutrophils.[23] NGAL levels increase with inflammatory stage and decrease with recovery.[23] Regarding the potential role of NGAL in CRS, available data show its involvement in fluid-status regulation; mineralocorticoid receptor activation leads to raised levels of NGAL and upregulation of NGAL expression.[23]

Neurohormonal involvement is underlined by incretion of natriuretic peptides, mid-regional proadrenomedullin, and copeptin.[24,25] Available data show how type-1 CRS is more frequent in patients with higher levels of natriuretic peptides together with signs and symptoms of pulmonary congestion, right heart dysfunction, and increased CVP.[26] Patients with type-1 CRS present with abnormalities in cell-signaling pathways: soluble ST2, new predictor of risk for hospitalization and death in HF patients,[27,28] seems to be similar in nature to natriuretic peptides, reflecting the degree of immune cell activation and signaling during progressive HF.[29]

ST2 is the receptor for interleukin (IL)-33, an angiohypertrophic and antifibrotic cytokine with myocardial effects[30]; soluble ST is a circulating inhibitor of the ST2 receptor, and counteracts the regenerative effects of IL-33. As already noted, it is clear how systemic cell signaling could manage negative tubuloglomerular feedback and consequent transient reduction in renal filtration.[31,32]

Cystatin C, a 25-kDa glomerular-filtration protein secreted by all nucleated cells, represents a valid surrogate with which to test renal function, and has been recognized as more predictive of long-term mortality and rehospitalization for ADHF than both serum creatinine and serum B-type natriuretic peptide (BNP).[33,34]

Because of its biochemical characteristics, serum cystatin C may be helpful in obtaining an earlier diagnosis of AKI in patients with CRS type 1.

Other tubular injury biomarkers are represented by kidney injury molecule 1 (KIM-1), liver-type fatty acid binding protein (L-FABP), and interleukin-18 (IL-18), while NGAL has provided the most comprehensive experimental and clinical data in ADHF patients, showing that it strongly correlates with renal function markers[35] and adverse cardiovascular outcomes or death.[36] Serum NGAL level was found to be a stronger predictor than BNP of 30-day all-cause death and ADHF readmissions.[37] On this basis, acute tubular damage in type-1 CRS probably accounts for the future development of CRS type 3. Preliminary data suggest how NGAL levels could predict AKI in patients with ADHF to a greater extent than levels of serum cystatin C and serum creatinine.[38–40] Other potential helpful biomarkers to be tested for the early diagnosis of AKI in HF patients include osteopontin, N-acetyl-β-D-glucosaminidase, stromal cell-derived factor 1, endoglin, galectin-3, and exosomes, although currently there are insufficient data available to warrant their use in routine diagnosis.[41]

Together with laboratory diagnosis, type-1 CRS can be diagnosed by bioelectrical devices, especially regarding fluid assessment in such patients. Several clinical studies showed an association between decreased impedance values (increased body fluid volume) and adverse events such as rehospitalization and death; bioimpedance measurement also helped to distinguish cardiogenic dyspnea from noncardiogenic dyspnea.[42,43] High sensitivity and specificity of reduced bioimpedance values were confirmed by radiographic findings consistent with pulmonary edema.[44] Results of bioimpedance testing represent a potential criterion for discharge readiness and the readmission ratio.[45]

Bioimpedance measurement may provide an early diagnosis of ADHF, differential diagnosis of dyspnea, and therapeutic management of CRS type 1, although further clinical data are needed.

Ultrasonography can provide further elements for the diagnosis type-1 CRS. Typical echocardiographic include abnormal myocardial kinetics (indicating an ischemic condition) and left ventricular hypertrophy (LVH), valvular stenosis and insufficiency (particularly in case of rapid deterioration, such as valvular endocarditis or valvular rupture), pericardial effusion, normal inspiratory collapse of the inferior vena cava (excluding severe hypervolemia), and aortic aneurysm or dissection.[46]

Ultrasonographic evaluation of the kidneys usually show normal or larger dimensions with preserved corticomedullary ratio; color Doppler evaluation shows regular intraparenchymal blood flow, often associated with an increase in resistance index (>0.8 cm/s).[46]

Outcomes and Treatment

Renal function often improves in response to standard therapy aimed at reducing filling pressures with loop diuretics and nitrates in warm and wet ADHF patients with AKI at presentation; this observation suggests that increased renal venous congestion may be the predominant mechanism underlying AKI.

The Pre-RELAX-AHF study found that a drop in systolic blood pressure within the first 48 hours of vasodilator therapy was an independent predictor of AKI by day 5.[47] These data, together with clinical experience, support the idea that therapy-related reduction in renal perfusion pressure and/or ECFV are the predominant mechanisms underlying AKI that develops within the first days of hospitalization.

Usually ACE inhibitors are slowly titrated up during the course of hospitalization. The hemodynamic effect of ACE inhibitors (vasodilation of the efferens glomerular vessel) and its associated drop in filtration pressure, as well as "prerenal" kidney dysfunction caused by the reduction in ECFV associated with intensified therapy with loop diuretics, may be the predominant mechanism underlying AKI that develops late during hospitalization.

Finally, the severity and duration of AKI seem to be related to long-term patient outcome; early diagnosis and treatment is therefore recommended.[48]

TYPE-2 CRS

CRS type 2 is characterized by chronic abnormalities in cardiac function leading to kidney injury or dysfunction; the temporal relationship between heart and kidney disease is an epidemiologic and pathophysiologic aspect of the definition itself. Literature data show that chronic heart and kidney disease often coexist, but large cohort studies have assessed the onset of one disease (eg, chronic HF), subsequently describing the prevalence of the other (CKD).[49,50] It is difficult to establish which of these two diseases is primary and which is secondary. CKD has been observed in 45% to 63% of patients with chronic HF,[49–51] but it is unclear as to how to classify these patients, which often include those shifting from a condition of type-1 CRS. Moreover, it is not easy to distinguish these patients from those with type-4 CRS (chronic renocardiac syndrome).[2]

Pathophysiology

By definition type-2 CRS is characterized by CKD onset in HF patients, but coexistence of cardiovascular disease and CKD is not enough to propose a diagnosis of type-2 CRS. Two fundamental features are proposed for such a diagnosis: chronic HF and CKD are simultaneously present, and chronic HF causally underlies occurrence or progression of CKD.[52] Examples of type-2 CRS can be provided by cyanotic nephropathy, occurring in patients with congenital heart disease when heart disease clearly precedes kidney involvement or acute coronary syndrome, leading to left ventricular dysfunction and onset or progression of coexisting CKD.

Although multiple and complex mechanisms have been proposed to explain the pathophysiology of type-2 CRS, neurohormonal activation, kidney hypoperfusion and venous congestion, inflammation, atherosclerosis, and oxidative stress represent the most important.

On the other hand, recurrent episodes of acute heart and/or kidney decompensation can be associated with HF and CKD progression, such as demonstrated by data showing how previous hospitalizations for HF are mortality predictors after other HF risk factors have been controlled for.[53] Reoccurrence of HF admissions is independently associated with development of CKD (estimated GFR [eGFR] <60 mL/min).[54]

In HF experimental studies, a reduction in glomerular plasma flow together with elevated GFR (efferent arteriolar constriction) is observed; if these changes persist (up to 6 months in experimental models), podocyte injury and focal and segmental glomerulosclerosis can occur. Many of these histologic changes can be inferred from a local renal increase in SNS and RAAS activation.[55]

Kidneys of HF patients seems to release large amounts of circulating renin with consequent abnormal production of angiotensin II,[56] causing efferent arteriolar constriction and an increase in oncotic pressure of peritubular capillaries. High venous pressure is described as an alternative worsening GFR factor in HF patients, especially in those with preserved ejection fraction. Patients with HF and venous congestion often present with signs of RAAS activation not requiring decreased circulating volume as stimulus[57]; it has been suggested that RAAS and SNS activation contribute to CKD progression in type-2 CRS. As a consequence, production of angiotensin II and aldosterone release lead to distal nephron-augmented sodium reabsorption, and subsequent pressure and volume overload. Increased aldosterone levels can contribute to glomerular fibrosis caused by upregulation of transforming growth factor (TGF)-β and increased secretion of fibronectin.[58,59]

Chronic and acute inflammation could also be accountable for CKD progression in chronic HF patients. In the presence of cardiac ischemia, myocytes can release inflammatory cytokines,[60] and venous congestion itself, increasing the absorption of endotoxin in the gut, can lead to synthesis and release of inflammatory mediators, such as tumor necrosis factor (TNF)-α, and large numbers of ILs including IL-1β, IL-18, and IL-6.[61]

Diagnosis

Assessment of kidney injury in HF patients has been previously limited to creatinine (and eGFR) and urinary protein excretion assay. Undoubtedly, decreased eGFR and increased urinary albumin excretion are independent predictors of prognosis and are associated with higher risk of death, cardiovascular death, and hospitalization in patients with preserved or reduced LVEF; moreover, eGFR and albuminuria levels are prognostic for renal outcomes in CKD patients[62–64] but not in HF patients.[65]

Recently, novel kidney biomarkers (cystatin C, NGAL, KIM-1, and N-acetylglucosamine [NAG]) have been evaluated in patients with chronic HF.[66–68]

In many clinical studies the levels of these biomarkers are slightly elevated in patients with chronic HF in comparison with the control population, even in patients with normal renal function. These data suggest that biomarker levels might have prognostic properties with regard to cardiovascular outcomes but not renal outcomes (**Table 2**).[69–71]

Cystatin C has been reported as an independent predictor of cardiac transplantation and hospitalizations for recurrent HF, and correlates with proBNP levels and left ventricular dysfunction.[67,68]

NGAL seems to be highly expressed in myocardial cells during myocarditis and acute coronary syndrome as well as in atherosclerotic plaques; in many, but not all, clinical studies blood and urine NGAL levels both correlate with eGFR and biochemical markers of HF degree, and are associated with increased mortality and hospitalization for acute HF.[72,73]

Urinary KIM-1 levels are elevated in symptomatic HF patients,[74] whereas KIM-1 and NAG levels correlate with severity of heart involvement and are predictors of mortality and hospitalization for ADHF.

Ultrasonographic diagnosis of type-2 CRS involves both renal and cardiac evaluation. The ultrasound pattern of kidneys usually reveals classic parameters of chronicity, such as reduction of cortical thickness, reduction of corticomedullary ratio, and increased parenchymal echogenicity.

Echocardiography shows high atrial volumes or areas as indices of volume overload (**Fig. 4**),

normal or decreased ejection fraction, right chamber dilation, and decreases in estimated pulmonary arterial pressure and tricuspid annulus plane systolic excursion (TAPSE index) as parameters of congestive HF, pulmonary hypertension or decreased ejection fraction, pericardial effusion (**Fig. 5**), and chronic valvular abnormality with particular regard to valvular calcifications.[46]

Outcomes and Treatment

Based on RAAS activation in type-2 CRS patients, many clinical studies have focused their attention on blocking RAAS with both ACE inhibitors and ARBs. The main drugs investigated have been the ACE inhibitors enalapril and captopril and the ARBs valsartan and candesartan. The SOLVD study showed that GFR delay was slightly greater in the enalapril group than in the placebo group; in the same study, diabetic patients showed proteinuria reduction when treated with enalapril.[75,76] In the CONSENSUS trial the enalapril group showed a mean creatinine increase of 10% to 15%.[77] The VALHEFT study demonstrated a slight decrease in GFR levels in patients on valsartan, whereas proteinuria dipstick positivity was associated with an increased (28%) mortality risk.[78] At present, literature evidence is inconclusive regarding the role of ACE inhibitors and ARBs in preventing progression of type-2 CRS.

Therapy with inhibitors of aldosterone receptors in patients with chronic HF underlines the significant improvement with regard to survival and hospitalization rates. The RALES trial, conducted with spironolactone, showed a reduction in mortality despite 17% worsening renal function in treated patients compared with 7% in the placebo group[79]; a decrease in collagen synthesis markers was also observed in patients treated with spironolactone, suggesting a protective role against fibrosis.[80]

It is crucial that a slight creatinine increase (expected in patients treated with ACE inhibitors or ARBs) does not mean a type-2 CRS progression; it is also true that serum creatinine is an inadequate biomarker for progression of disease because of difficulty in discerning true progressive CKD from hemodynamic (and probably reversible) eGFR changes resulting from RAAS inhibition.

Following the publication of the COPERNICUS and CAPRICORN trials, β-blockers have become the first-choice treatment for HF; carvedilol was associated with a transient increase in serum creatinine in CKD patients.[81]

Bisoprolol showed benefits in stage-III CKD patients in comparison with a placebo group, with no

Table 2
Selected studies on novel renal biomarkers in chronic heart failure

Authors, Ref. Year	Study Population	Specimen	Biomarker	HF vs Control Subjects	Biomarker Correlates with (in HF Patients Only)			
					Renal Function	Clinical HF Severity	Natriuretic Peptides	Renal Outcomes
Tang et al,[67] 2008	Clinically stable CHF outpatients (n = 139)	Plasma	Cystatin C	No controls	Yes	Yes	Yes	NS
Damman et al,[68,69] 2008, 2010	Clinically stable CHF outpatients (n = 90)	Urine	NGAL	HF > controls	No	NS	No	NS
			NAG	HF > controls	Yes	NS	Yes	NS
			KIM-1	HF > controls	No	NS	Yes	NS
Jungbauer et al,[74] 2011	CHF (n = 173)	Urine	NGAL	HF = controls	Yes, with albuminuria; No, with Cr/eGFR	No	No	No association with diuretic dose
			NAG	HF = controls	Yes	Yes	Yes	Elevated in patients on higher (vs lower) diuretic doses
			KIM-1	HF > controls	Yes, with albuminuria; No, with Cr/eGFR	Yes	Yes	Elevated in patients on higher (vs lower) diuretic doses
Malyszko et al,[70] 2009	CHF due to CAD (n = 150)	Serum	NGAL	No controls	Yes	Yes	NS	NS
			Cystatin C		Yes	NS	NS	NS
		Urine	NGAL		Yes	Yes	NS	NS
			Cystatin C		NS	NS	NS	NS
Bolignano et al,[72] 2009	CHF (elderly, age >65 y) (n = 46)	Serum	NGAL	HF > controls	No	Yes	NS	NS
Yndestad et al,[71] 2009	CHF (n = 150)	Serum	NGAL	HF > controls	NS	Yes	Yes	NS
Shrestha et al,[73] 2011	CHF (LVEF ≤35%) (n = 130)	Plasma	NGAL	No controls	Yes	Yes	Yes	NS

Abbreviations: CAD, coronary artery disease; CHF, chronic heart failure; Cr, creatinine; eGFR, estimated glomerular filtration rate; HF, heart failure; LVEF, left ventricular ejection fraction; NS, not stated.
Data from Refs.[67–74]

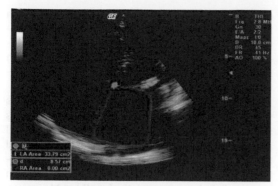

Fig. 4. Left atrial dilation in a patient with CRS type 2.

increase in serum creatinine levels,[82] and nebivolol treatment did not modify GFR levels.[83]

Because chronic inflammation has been postulated as a risk factor in progression of type-2 CRS, some investigators used TNF-α inhibitors in the treatment of HF; trials with infliximab or etanercept showed a decrease in C-reactive protein and IL-6 levels, but there are no reports on renal function.[84]

Cardiac resynchronization (CRT) or left ventricular assist devices (LVAD) can improve hypoperfusion in HF patients; one study showed how CRT increased GFR in a subgroup of patients with CKD stage II to IIIa.[85]

TYPE-3 CRS

Type-3 CRS, also defined as acute renocardiac syndrome, occurs when AKI contributes to and/or precipitates the development of acute cardiac injury. Many pathophysiologic causes of AKI can predispose to development of CRS type 3 (**Boxes 1** and **2**).

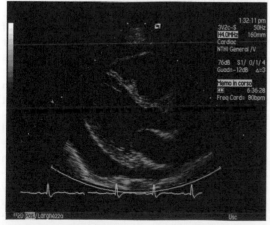

Fig. 5. Pericardial effusion in a patient with chronic kidney disease stage V.

Box 1
Summary of potential contributing causes for AKI contributing to CRS type 3

Prototypical Condition

    Contrast-induced AKI

    Drug-induced AKI

    Major surgery

    Cardiac surgery

    Postinflammatory glomerulonephritis

    Rhabdomyolysis

    Acute pyelonephritis

    Postobstructive uropathy

AKI may directly or indirectly produce an acute cardiac event; many experimental data suggest that cardiac damage con be supported by inflammatory status, oxidative stress, and secretion of neurohormones following AKI.[86,87]

AKI can be associated with volume overload, metabolic acidosis, and electrolyte disorders such as hyperkalemia and hypocalcemia; coronary artery disease (CAD), left ventricular dysfunction, and fibrosis have also been described in patients with AKI, with consequent direct negative effects on cardiac performance.[88]

AKI can affect cardiac function, contributing to alterations in drug pharmacokinetics and dynamics. Only poor epidemiologic data are available regarding the incidence and prevalence of acute cardiac events (arrhythmia, CAD, HF)

Box 2
Summary of susceptibilities for CRS type 3

Risk-Modifying Factors

    Age

    Sex

    Coronary artery disease

    Hypertension

    Hypercholesterolemia

    Diabetes mellitus

    Congestive heart failure

    Pulmonary disease

    Chronic kidney disease

    Systemic vascular disease

    Systemic immune disease

    Infection/sepsis

following AKI, as well as the length of time between AKI onset and cardiac events.[89]

Pathophysiology

Direct and indirect pathophysiologic mechanisms can produce acute cardiac events and injuries during or after an AKI episode.

Direct mechanisms

AKI is always characterized by nonhemodynamic events originating in the kidney with long-distance effects, including heart and cardiovascular factors.[90]

Pathophysiologic interactions between the kidney and heart during AKI has been referred to as cardio-renal connectors,[55] such as activation of the immune system (ie, pro- and anti-inflammatory release of cytokines and chemokines) and SNS, hyperactivity of RAAS, and the coagulation cascade; unfortunately there are no widespread data suggesting a pathophysiologic role in type-3 CRS onset.

Most of the experimental available data are focused on immune cardiorenal connectors and, especially on renal ischemia and reperfusion injury; animal models show that AKI encourages an immune response characterized by secretion of pro- and anti-inflammatory mediators, such as structural and functional changes in immune cell responsiveness; leukocyte function is also affected by alterations in adhesion. It is well known that leukocytes play an important role in cardiac dysfunction following acute coronary disease; blocking leukocyte activity can protect against myocardial damage.[91]

Circulating levels of TNF-α, IL-1, and IL-6 seem to increase immediately after renal experimental ischemia and, together with other cytokines as well as and interferon-α, they have direct cardiodepressant effects underlined by reduction in LVEF and elevation of left ventricular end-diastolic and end-systolic volumes and areas.[92]

Cytokine release can affect myocardial cells directly, on their contractility or by close interactions with the extracellular matrix, leading to negative inotropic effects; the complete cellular mechanism is still unclear but probably involves secondary mediators such as sphingolipids, arachidonic acid, and intracellular Ca^{2+} alterations.[87]

In animal models, infusion of TNF-α results in a decrease in left ventricular diastolic pressure with secondary coronary vasoconstriction; more infusions cause time-dependent dysfunction (regional contractility alterations) of the left ventricle and its dilation, lasting up to 10 days.[93] Together with left ventricular systolic dysfunction, several diastolic abnormalities are observed, including slow relaxation of left ventricle and raised left atrium filling pressure, indicating an increase in left ventricular diastolic stiffness. Acute infusion of TNF-α directly increases oxygen consumption through myocardial cells affecting contractility and excitation contraction coupling.[94]

In the presence of renal ischemia, rat hearts show increased expression of adhesion molecules such as ICAM-1, together with myocardial apoptosis (this is not true in the case of bilateral nephrectomy), proving that systemic inflammation, and not AKI, plays an immediate role in myocardial damage and dysfunction. Moreover, patients with chronic HF show increased levels of proinflammatory cytokines associated with higher rates of impaired left ventricular remodeling, chronic cachexia, and mortality.[95]

In an AKI rat model, administration of cyclosporine A (1–5 mg/kg) attenuated the development of AKI, IL-6 expression, and cellular apoptosis in comparison with a control population.[96] On the other hand, an incomplete or milder form of renal ischemia can provide a protective effect on the heart. In a rat model, a 15-minute renal artery occlusion at 30°C induced marked reductions in total infarcted areas relative to a control population; this effect can be partially explained by alterations in SNS and upregulation of anti-inflammatory and antiapoptotic mediators.[97]

Although only limited data describing neuroendocrine activation (SNS and RAAS) in type-3 CRS have been published, SNS activation is a key point in the development of both AKI and HF.[98]

During AKI, hyperactivity of SNS with abnormal secretion of norepinephrine occurs, impairing myocardial activity in several ways: direct norepinephrine effect, impairment of Ca^{2+} metabolism, increase in myocardial oxygen demand with potential evolution to myocardial ischemia, myocardial cell β1-adrenergic–mediated apoptosis, stimulation of α1 receptors, and activation of RAAS. β1-Adrenergic stimulus of juxtaglomerular cells reduces renal blood flow and stimulates further renin secretion by RAAS.

Abnormal and uncontrolled RAAS activation leads to release of angiotensin II with consequent systemic vasoconstriction and elevation of vascular resistance; on the other hand, angiotensin II itself directly modifies myocardial structure, promoting cellular hypertrophy and apoptosis.[99] In an experimental model of renal ischemia, investigators postulated how increased RAAS activity may be accountable for diminished coronary response to adenosine, bradykinin, and L-arginine.[88] These data probably underline that AKI could directly account for impaired coronary vasoreactivity, and increased susceptibility to ischemia and other major cardiovascular events.

Other animal models have shown how AKI can contribute to altered permeability of lung vessels, with resultant interstitial edema and bleeding, mediated by inflammatory mediators, altered expression of epithelial sodium channel, and aquiporin-5 expression.[100]

As mentioned earlier, myocardial cell apoptosis and neutrophil activation greatly contribute to the pathophysiologic pathways of coronary arteries following AKI, leading to lethal major cardiac events, as can be seen in rat transgenic models[101]: in these models kidney ischemia, not uremia, induces apoptosis in myocardial cells. It seems that an apoptotic rate of 23 cardiomyocytes per 10^5 nuclei is sufficient to develop a lethal dilated cardiomyopathy.[102]

The best evidence for a cardiorenal link between AKI and cardiac fibrosis is the β-galactoside–binding lectin galectin-3, whose mRNA expression is upregulated after renal ischemia; it is also implicated in the development of myocardial fibrosis and HF in AKI, and its inhibition can delay the progression of myocardial fibrosis.[103]

Indirect mechanisms

Indirect pathophysiologic mechanisms during AKI development, such as volume overload, hypertension, acidemia, hyperkalemia, hypophosphatemia, and uremic toxins, can also affect cardiac function and outcome.

In critical care patients, volume overload is associated with poor outcomes, and fluid restriction, rather than a liberal fluid regimen, is significantly associated with improved lung function.[104] Several studies show a strong association between fluid overload and less favorable outcomes in critical care patients with AKI[105]; fluid retention can also lead to fatal arrhythmias and contribute to LVH and fibrosis.[106]

Hypertension is particularly prevalent in critically ill patients with AKI, probably because of the cause itself (ie, sepsis, cardiogenic shock), but is also related to several mechanisms contributing to systemic and pulmonary hypertension, such as elevated preload (due to volume overload), and activation of SNS and RAAS. In critical care patients, these modifications can easily lead to myocardial ischemia and ventricular failure.[107]

Metabolic acidosis is a common feature of CKD and AKI, and is the reason for most renal replacement therapy in critical care units.[108] Acidemia can directly affect myocardial contractility by acting on β-receptor expression and altered intracellular calcium balance.[109]

Strictly linked to acid-base impairment, hyperkalemia represents a potentially lethal complication in subjects presenting with AKI, and requires immediate renal replacement therapy. Hyperkalemia is closely linked to the development of arrhythmias.[110]

CKD and AKI are often characterized by the presence of hyperphosphatemia; however, once renal replacement therapy is started hypophosphatemia often occurs, leading to left systolic ventricular dysfunction.[111]

Finally, uremic toxins, including β2-microglobulin and fibroblast growth factor (FGF)-23, are associated with cardiovascular injury in CKD patients, although with different pathways in respect of CKD[112]; the final result is development of LVH and cardiac fibrosis.[112]

All the aforementioned pathophysiologic findings determine the various effects on cardiac functions.

Electrophysiologic effects

Electrolyte alterations directly affect cellular membrane potentials, with development of potential fatal arrhythmias. The classic electrocardiogram (ECG) of hyperkalemic patients is represented by tenting of the T wave owing to rapid and consistent changes in extracellular potassium levels, leading to increased activity of the potassium channel (and inactivation of sodium channel) with faster repolarization and inclination to arrhythmias.

Thus, hyperkalemia reduces resting membrane potentials (both atrial and ventricular) and induces ST-T segment abnormalities (ie, elevations in V1 and V2), simulating an ischemic pattern. In some patients, hyperkalemia can simulate a Brugada-like pattern, characterized by right bundle branch block and persistent ST-T segment elevation in at least 2 precordial leads.

Hypermagnesemia is often related to atrioventricular nodal and intraventricular conduction impairment up to the time of cardiac arrest.

Hypercalcemia is accountable for the short duration of ventricular action potential during phase 2, and the ECG shows shortening of the QT interval. Hypercalcemia can also produce ST-T segment abnormalities that simulate an ischemic pattern, as Ca^{2+} plays a central role in the regulation of the cardiac cycle (contraction and relaxation).[113]

Ischemic effects

Acidemia, neurohormonal activation, and abnormal production and accumulation of uremic toxins and cytokines are linked to myocardial ischemia that occurs during AKI.[93] Sympathetic activation leads to vasoconstriction and increased oxygen requested by myocardial tissue; when oxygen delivery is restricted, ischemia can occur. TNF-α, endothelin, and bradykinin induce coronary vasoconstriction leading to vessel stenosis.

Higher levels of oxygen demand can produce subendocardial ischemia resulting from oxygen redistribution; evidence demonstrates how, during AKI, coronary autoregulation is imbalanced and coronary vascular reserve and coronary vascular conductance are markedly diminished.[93]

Recent data have pointed to a potential link between NGAL and CRS.[114] NGAL expression rapidly increases in kidneys after acute inflammation and/or tubular injury (ie, renal ischemia), and has also been involved in the pathophysiologic pathways of HF, myocarditis, and coronary atherosclerotic disease.[115]

KIM-1, a marker of kidney tubular damage, is also involved in HF risk during AKI, acting on myocardial inflammation, modifications of atherosclerotic plaques, and susceptibility to ischemic events.[115]

Myocardial effects

Animal models of renal ischemia showed functional changes in myocardium, including left ventricular eccentric hypertrophy, increased left ventricular end-diastolic and end-systolic volumes, and decreased fractional shortening and ejection fraction. Pathophysiologic pathways are ascribable to accumulation of inflammatory mediators, acute fluid retention, metabolic acidosis, and accumulation of uremic toxins.[87]

Diagnosis

Regarding laboratory findings, creatinine and GFR assessment still remains crucial in the evaluation, together with electrolytes and acid-base patterns.

Other crucial biomarkers, as mentioned earlier, are represented by NGAL and KIM-1, markers of kidney tubular damage that are able to predict the risk for HF in AKI patients.

Ultrasonographic evaluation of type-3 CRS patients shows several patterns on both kidney and heart examination. Kidney size and echogenicity provide primary features to aid in discerning between acute and chronic nephropathies, always remembering how kidney volume and longitudinal diameters correlate with patient height and body surface[116,117] and that chronic renal failure does not exclude normal or enlarged kidneys (eg, early stages of diabetic nephropathy, human immunodeficiency virus–related glomerulonephritis, or cast nephropathy).

A hyperechogenic renal cortex with a low corticomedullary ratio is predictive of chronic nephropathy (see **Figs. 4** and **5**).[116,117] Moreover, cortical hyperechogenicity can present in acute tubular necrosis (**Fig. 6**) or systemic lupus erythematosus nephritis.[116,117] In these cases, an enlarged renal parenchyma may suggest a condition of edema in the acute setting.

Doppler and color Doppler evaluation can be crucial to the diagnosis and prognosis in the acute setting, mainly with regard to evaluation of diastolic flow in interlobular arteries.[118] Renal

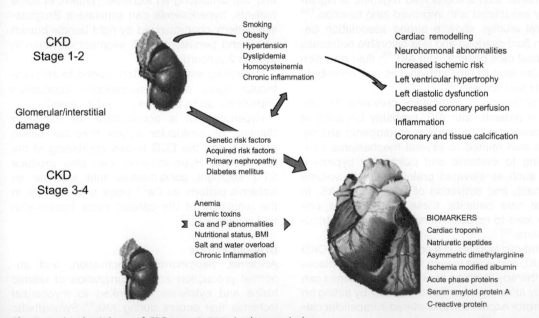

CKD Stage 1-2

Glomerular/interstitial damage

CKD Stage 3-4

Smoking
Obesity
Hypertension
Dyslipidemia
Homocysteinemia
Chronic inflammation

Genetic risk factors
Acquired risk factors
Primary nephropathy
Diabetes mellitus

Anemia
Uremic toxins
Σ Ca and P abnormalities
Nutritional status, BMI
Salt and water overload
Chronic Inflammation

Cardiac remodelling
Neurohormonal abnormalities
Increased ischemic risk
Left ventricular hypertrophy
Left diastolic dysfunction
Decreased coronary perfusion
Inflammation
Coronary and tissue calcification

BIOMARKERS
Cardiac troponin
Natriuretic peptides
Asymmetric dimethylarginine
Ischemia modified albumin
Acute phase proteins
Serum amyloid protein A
C-reactive protein

Fig. 6. Pathophysiology of CRS type 4. BMI, body mass index.

ultrasonography is also crucial in the differential diagnosis of obstructive nephropathies.

The echocardiographic pattern is not diagnostic, showing an increase in atrial volumes or areas as indices of volume overload, or pleural or pericardial effusion; it is often associated with lung comets evidenced on a thoracic ultrasonogram.[46]

Outcomes and Treatment

Only poor data on the impact of AKI on cardiac events and outcomes are available at present. In a cohort study, the association between AKI following coronary angiography (CI-AKI) and cardiovascular-related hospitalizations was evaluated.[119] Severity of CI-AKI was associated with dose response and risk of hospitalization for HF.

Other available data are from prospective evaluation of patients receiving reperfusion therapy after anterior myocardial infraction; 22% of these patients developed AKI within 48 hours, AKI was independently associated with a higher risk of HF, ventricular arrhythmias, and cardiac death.[120]

Type-3 CRS represents a typical scenario after cardiovascular surgery or contrast exposure. Prevention is a key point in managing this type of CRS. In contrast to nephropathy, available data and evidence indicate that isotonic fluids are the gold standard for prevention of kidney injury, whereas conflicting data surround the value of N-acetylcysteine.[121] More recently, a possible role for the low-osmolar, nonionic monomer iopamidol was postulated.[122]

In patients affected by left ventricular dysfunction undergoing cardiovascular surgery, nesiritide use was associated with improved postoperative renal function in a comparison with patients without nesiritide therapy, suggesting it has nephroprotective properties.[123]

TYPE-4 CRS

Type-4 CRS, also defined as chronic renocardiac syndrome, is characterized by cardiovascular involvement in patients affected by CKD at any stage according to the National Kidney Foundation (NKF) classification.

The prevalence of end-stage renal disease (ESRD) is still increasing and represents a worldwide epidemiologic problem.[124] The latest data from the United States estimate that up to 13% of the population may present with CKD at any stage of disease.

It is well established that renal dysfunction is an independent risk factor for cardiovascular disease; CKD patients show a higher mortality risk for myocardial infection and sudden death.[124]

At present, the pathophysiologic mechanisms that lead to increased cardiovascular risk in CKD patients are not completely known, but it is established that there is a firm connection between the heart and kidney.

A decline in GFR leads to activation of RAAS and SNS and, on the other hand, stimulates the calcium-parathyroid axis; this may be due to primary diseases such as diabetes or hypertension, the main causes of CKD development in Western countries.

Loss of kidney function usually leads to accumulation of sodium and water, with consequent stimulus to the production of angiotensin II and aldosterone, and the development of arterial hypertension. Hypertension, together with angiotensin and aldosterone, accelerates LVH and cardiac fibrosis.

Pathophysiology

To better understand the pathophysiologic pathways underlying type-4 CRS (see **Fig. 6**), one must consider various aspects of this CRS, from atherosclerotic damage, to development of vascular calcification, to development of LVH and cardiomyocyte remodeling. The roles of galectin-3 and FGF-23 are also discussed, based on the latest experimental evidence.

Coronary atherosclerotic heart disease

Epidemiologic and clinical evidence has proved the association between renal dysfunction and cardiovascular disease; it is well established that late stages of CKD are closely associated with higher cardiovascular morbidity. On the other hand, it is still unclear whether there is an increased incidence of cardiovascular disease in the early stages of CKD.

CKD patients present with increased rates of atherosclerotic coronary disease, acute coronary syndrome, LVH, and sudden death. The cardiovascular risk for patients with an eGFR less than 30 mL/min/1.73 m^2 is 10-fold higher than in those with eGFR greater than 60 mL/min/1.73 m^2. These higher rates are in contrast to the risk expected from typical risk factors present in CKD patients (hypertension, diabetes, dyslipidemia, and so forth); CKD is probably able to directly contribute to cardiovascular complications.[125,126]

CKD patients present, at early and late stages of disease, with a higher prevalence of CAD at angiographic evaluation; these patients also show multivessel disease and ECG evidence of previous silent ischemia.[127]

Recent data have shown that dobutamine stress echocardiography delivers the best accuracy for the screening of noninvasive CAD in renal transplant candidates.[128]

To assess CAD prevalence in early stages of CKD, an accurate review evaluated coronary catheterization in 261 patients with an eGFR between 30 and 90 mL/min; despite preserved renal function, more than half of the patients with eGFR greater than 90 mL/min had 70% stenosis in at least one coronary artery. On the other hand, more than 84% of patients in late stages of CKD (eGFR <30 mL/min) showed significant CAD with higher involvement of left coronary artery and multivessel disease.[129]

Coronary calcification, myocardial calcification, and aortic compliance

Accelerated coronary atherosclerosis is not sufficient to completely explain the higher rates of cardiovascular involvement in CKD patients. It can now be confidently stated that osteoblastic transformation of smooth muscle cells is a key factor in the pathogenesis of vascular and valvular calcification during CKD.

Impaired vitamin D synthesis, secondary hyperparathyroidism, and altered calcium phosphate metabolism contribute to vascular calcification because of their direct effects on osteoblastic cells.[130] Coronary calcifications can predict major cardiac events contributing to reduced coronary reserve in CKD patients and a higher risk of acute coronary syndromes[131,132] that increases with progression of renal disease.

Clinical studies conducted with high-resolution multislice computed tomography (CT) demonstrated early detection of coronary calcifications in CKD stage 3 according to NKF classification; data showed that 83% of patients had coronary calcification unrelated to CKD stage.[133] Calcifications were also extended to lower limb arteries, explaining the high rates of lower extremity amputation among ESRD patients, who also presented with a greater quantity and density of calcium deposits, not limited to the intima but extending to the vessels' media.[134] In other studies, an immunostaining assay of calcified areas demonstrated the presence of bone matrix proteins such as osteopontin, type I collagen, and bone sialoprotein.[135]

An autoptic evaluation showed that medial calcification was present in 16% of uremic patients but only in 3% of patients with normal renal function; medial calcification was also associated with the presence of osteocalcin, inflammatory markers (TGF-α), and activated complement elements (C3 and C4).[136]

Increased calcium content may be accountable for both reduced left ventricular compliance and the prevalence of arrhythmias. Aortic calcification is strongly associated with reduced aortic compliance and coronary artery perfusion, leading to increased central pressure and inducing subendocardial ischemia because of reduced diastolic filling.[137]

Left ventricular hypertrophy

LVH, together with left ventricular systolic and diastolic dysfunction, has always been recognized as a main cardiovascular damage marker in CKD patients. LVH prevalence undoubtedly increases with declining renal function because of traditional risk factors such as hypertension, diabetes, and volume overload. More recent data have focused on secondary hyperparathyroidism, malnutrition, and even dialysis as further risk factors in the development of LVH in CKD. LVH prevalence varies from 16% to 31% in patients with GFR greater than 30 mL/min, up to 60% to 75% in ESRD patients and 90% in persons starting renal replacement therapy.[138]

Foley and colleagues[139] found that 74% of ESRD patients had echocardiographic evidence of LVH, and 30% presented left ventricular failure. In another survey including 596 incident hemodialysis patients with no history of cardiac disease, the same group demonstrated that after 18 months of dialysis, the left ventricular mass index (LVMI) increased in 62% of patients, of whom left ventricular failure occurred in 49%.[140]

At present the mechanisms contributing to left ventricular dysfunction in CKD patients are unknown, but evidence suggests that uremia products can directly affect cardiac structure. Many of these toxins are highly protein bound and allow limited clearance by conventional dialyzers; these limitations could account for the dialysis effects on LVH and left HF.[141]

Clinical conditions leading to LVH in CKD patients are similar to those observed in other clinical patterns including hypertension, atherosclerosis, pressure overload, and RAAS activation. Atherosclerosis and hypertension directly promote myocyte hypertrophy with consequent increased left ventricular mass, increased ventricular wall thickness, secondary myocardial fibrosis, and compensatory hypertrophy.[142]

In CKD patients, aortic compliance is affected by accelerated atherosclerotic damage, but other typical CKD variables, such as hyperphosphatemia, can affect aortic compliance.[143] In the progression to middle- and end-stage CKD, progressive loss of nephrons leads to salt and water accumulation with hypertension and volume/pressure overload; these changes upregulate RAAS with release of profibrotic factors such as galectin-3, TGF-β, and endogenous cardiac steroids.[144]

As a consequence of LVH, myocytes enlarge capillary density because of increased oxygen demand; myocyte diameter and interstitial volume space are increased in CKD patients in comparison with other patient groups. Long-lasting periods of hemodynamic load promote cardiac remodeling and increase cardiac expression of interstitial myofibroblasts never present in normal myocardium.[145]

Reduction in myocardial capillary density may explain CKD patients' marked susceptibility to myocardial ischemia, LVH, and myocardial fibrosis.[145]

Uremia and cardiac fibrosis

Much evidence now suggests that CKD patients, especially in the late stages, develop a particular pattern of cardiac fibrosis. CKD and ESRD patients present with features of intermyocardial fibrosis quite different from those of hypertensive patients and patients with chronic ischemic heart disease, in which endocardial and epicardial fibrosis predominate.[146]

The mechanisms leading to CKD cardiac fibrosis are as yet not understood, but recent evidence suggests that uremic toxins such as indoxyl sulfate and p-cresol can contribute to cardiac fibrosis in renal patients. In CKD patients, indoxyl sulfate concentrations are 300-fold higher than in the control population, and directly contributes to cardiac fibrosis by synthesis of TGF-β, tissue inhibitor of metalloproteinase 1 (TIMP-1), and α-1 collagen.[147,148]

Galectin-3 and cardiac fibrosis

It is well established that diastolic dysfunction is characterized by myocardial infiltration of monocytes and macrophages. Recent evidence is consistent with an upregulation of galectin-3, a member of the β-galactoside–binding lectin family, synthesized by macrophages and able to interact with extracellular matrix proteins such as laminin, synexin, and integrins.

Galectin-3 can bind to cardiac fibroblasts and increase collagen production in myocardium.[149] Lok and colleagues[150] enrolled 232 patients with heart and kidney failure using N-terminal (NT)-proBNP and eGFR as cardiac and renal function markers, demonstrating that galectin-3 levels were independent predictors of cardiovascular mortality.

Galectin-3 levels seem to correlate with type III amino-terminal propeptide of procollagen and TIMP-1, suggesting that macrophage infiltration of myocardium plays a role in extracellular matrix protein turnover in HF patients.[151] On the other hand, other recent studies failed in demonstrating the role of macrophages in galectin-3 synthesis and consequent HF severity. A study by Gopal and colleagues[152] failed in correlating galectin-3 levels and HF (evaluated in terms of LVEF) degree, but pointed out that galectin-3 levels were affected by kidney disease: patients with an eGFR of less than 30 mL/min showed plasma galectin-3 levels 2-fold higher than that in the control population.

Fibroblast growth factor 23

Once the close linkage between eGFR decline and changes in cardiovascular structure is verified, further biomarkers must be investigated, one of which is FGF-23, a member of the fibroblast growth factor family (implicated in regulation, growth, and differentiation of cardiac myocytes) holding paracrine functions in the kidneys because of its phosphaturic properties; it blocks vitamin D_3 synthesis and inhibits proximal nephron reabsorption.[153]

During CKD progression, accumulation of phosphate leads to an increase in FGF-23 incretion, whose prolonged high levels can contribute to LVH and cardiac remodeling.

New data have shown that modest reduction in GFR can stimulate FGF-23 production. Echocardiographic assays demonstrated a 5% increase in LVMI for every log increase in plasma FGF-23 level. Patients included in the highest tertile of FGF-23 also have a 2.4-fold higher risk for coronary artery calcifications.[154]

Diagnosis

The diagnosis of type-4 CRS is based on the serologic and instrumental diagnosis of both chronic heart disease and CKD. Cardiac function is more widely assessed by NT-proBNP serum levels, whereas eGFR represents the most widely used biochemical test for the evaluation of kidney function. Based on recent evidence, evaluation of FGF-23 levels can be helpful in monitoring secondary hyperparathyroidism status, but is also involved in cardiac fibrotic remodeling.

Ultrasonographic diagnosis of type-4 CRS is classically based on kidney and heart evaluation. Kidney evaluation usually shows classic features of chronic nephropathy such as thin and hyperechogenic cortex with reduced corticomedullary ratio. A small dilation of urinary tract and parapyelic cysts are frequently observed.

Echocardiographic assay shows signs of volume overload, left ventricular dysfunction, and right ventricular dysfunction, especially in ESRD patients and those on hemodialysis. At echocardiographic evaluation can reveal increased atrial volumes or areas, pleural or pericardial effusion, and lung comets (all signs of volume overload).[46]

Cardiac ultrasonography also reveals the presence of valvular calcifications (related to secondary hyperparathyroidism)[46] and features of possible right heart dysfunction (high pulmonary artery pressure, low tricuspid annular plane systolic excursion, or right chamber dilation).[155]

Outcomes and Treatment

Because type-4 CRS is characterized by chronic cardiovascular involvement in CKD patients, correction of traditional and nontraditional cardiovascular risk factors is crucial.

Therapeutic interventions for traditional risk factors are less effective in patients with CKD[156] also for certain kinds of "therapeutic nihilism" for which treatments with antiplatelets, statins, β-blockers, and ACE inhibitors in CKD patients with CAD are often denied.[156]

Strategies to reduce cardiovascular risk in CKD patients must target both the traditional (hypertension, dyslipidemia, diabetes, obesity) and nontraditional (anemia, chronic inflammation, secondary hyperparathyroidism, LVH, oxidative stress, RAAS and SNS hyperactivity, renal replacement therapy complications).

Specific treatment targets are somewhat complicated, especially in hemodialysis patients, for whom considerable evidence supports the existence of a U-shaped curve associating mortality with blood-pressure levels, body mass index, dyslipidemia, and hyperphosphatemia.[157,158]

Although the role of secondary anemia correction is clearly established,[159] controversies are aroused regarding other risk-factor corrections such as secondary hyperparathyroidism, hypertension, and dyslipidemia.

Regarding secondary hyperparathyroidism, the EVOLVE study of hemodialysis patients found that cinacalcet therapy did not significantly reduce the risk of death or major cardiovascular events in patients with moderate to severe secondary hyperparathyroidism who were undergoing dialysis.[160]

The SHARP study investigated dyslipidemia treatment in CKD patients and was able to demonstrate a significant reduction in cardiovascular events, such as myocardial infarction, stroke, or need for coronary artery revascularization, with the use of a combination of ezetimibe plus simvastatin.[161]

Predialysis patients are strongly recommended to maintain blood-pressure levels below 130/80 mm Hg, hemoglobin A1c levels below 7%, hemoglobin levels between 11 and 12 g/dL, and

levels of low-density lipoprotein cholesterol below 90 mg/dL. Patients should avoid nephrotoxic drugs and follow a low protein diet (0.6 g/kg/d)[162,163]

Patients on dialysis should keep their blood pressure below 140/90 mm Hg before starting a dialysis session and below 130/80 mm Hg after a dialysis session.

Special consideration should be given to mineral bone disorders that prevent hyperphosphatemia and vascular calcifications, also in the early stages of CKD.[158,164]

Treatment of arrhythmias and sudden death is still a challenge for nephrologists and cardiologists; together with prior attention to prevention of electrolyte disorders (low potassium dialysate), the use of β-blockers seems beneficial. The efficacy of ACE inhibitors and ARBs has to be proved in more prospective trials.[165]

Implantation of cardiac defibrillators in dialysis patients is associated with an increased risk for bleeding and infection, and does not significantly affect morbidity and mortality.[165]

TYPE-5 CRS

Type-5 CRS is a recently defined clinical syndrome, and complete epidemiologic data are still lacking. Type-5 CRS occurs when the heart and kidney are involved simultaneously. Literature data underline that type-5 CRS encompasses many clinical syndromes such as sepsis, hepatorenal syndrome, and drug toxicity, in which the heart and kidney are involved secondarily to basic disease.[166] The temporal sequence that involves the heart and kidney depends on the underlying disease.

Pathophysiology

The pathophysiology of type-5 CRS depends on the underlying disease. Acute type-5 CRS results from systemic processes, including sepsis, infections, drugs, toxins, and connective tissue disorders such as lupus, Wegener granulomatosis, and sarcoidosis. The timeline from underlying condition to development of CRS is not always the same. For example, in sepsis-induced acute type-5 CRS there is a fulminant disease process with a dramatic impact on both kidney and heart, with obvious clinical manifestations. On the other hand, in patients with cirrhotic liver disease, type-5 CRS has a more insidious onset and the kidney and cardiac dysfunction may develop slowly until a crucial point is reached and full decompensation occurs. Several factors influence the course of type-5 CRS (**Table 3**). Although the mechanisms invoked in acute and chronic type-5 CRS are different (**Figs. 7** and **8**), the nature, severity, and duration of cardiorenal involvement

Table 3
Predisposing and modifying factors influencing development of sepsis-induced CRS type 5

Patient Attributes	Process of Care

Inducing event and immunologic response	Resuscitation
	  Volume effect on tissue edema and renal venous hypertension
	  Abdominal compartment syndrome
	  Glycocalyx

Underlying condition of heart and kidney	Search for primary focus Contrast use

Physiologic responses
  Peripheral vasodilation
  Compensatory hormonal response
  Increased vascular permeability
  Mitochondrial dysfunction and tissue hypoxia
  Cardiac filling
  Renal hypoperfusion
	Drug dosing
	  Antibiotics
	  Sedatives
	  Vasopressors and inotropes

	General supportive care Fluids Inotropes, pressors
	Specific interventions Ventilator Surgery Renal replacement therapy

is strictly linked to the therapeutic approach (see **Table 3**).

Acute type-5 CRS develops into the following steps: hyperacute (0–72 hours after diagnosis), acute (3–7 days), subacute (7–30 days), and chronic (beyond 30 days) (**Fig. 9, Table 4**).

The literature usually concerns the hyperacute phase because most of studies have focused on CRS during sepsis.

Chronic type-5 CRS (ie, CRS in cirrhotic patients) follows a variable time sequence, because in most cases there is an underlying condition and related precipitating event leading to recognition. For instance, cirrhotic patients are subject to infections, and an acute type-5 CRS can overlap a chronic process (**Fig. 10**).

Pathophysiologic changes in sepsis-related CRS can derive from systemic effects of sepsis itself, from direct sepsis effects in systemic metabolic pathways or, not least, from direct cross-talk between damaged heart and kidney. In the early stages of sepsis the microcirculation is often initially involved, in contrast with normal systemic hemodynamics,[167,168] and strongly correlates with morbidity and mortality rates.

Sepsis occurring with heart involvement (septic cardiomyopathy) represents one of main predictors of mortality in septic patients and is diagnosed in almost half of all patients.[169] Both the left and right ventricles can be injured, with dilation and decreased ejection fraction often unresponsive to fluid and catecholamine therapy.[170]

Septic cardiomyopathy, when severe, can mimic cardiogenic shock, but it is usually reversible within 7 to 10 days[171]; myocardial blood flow and oxygen consumption do not seem to be involved in the pathophysiology of septic cardiomyopathy.[172] On the other hand, proinflammatory mediators and complement factors have been proposed as crucial factors in the development of cardiac involvement during sepsis.[173,174]

Concerning sepsis-related kidney involvement, there are clear alterations in intraparenchymal blood flow independent of systemic hemodynamic changes linked to the septic process.[175,176] Mechanisms underlying these intraparenchymal vascular changes are not totally understood. Recent experimental surveys have compared 2 different sepsis models in pigs in which, irrespective of systemic hemodynamics, only pigs developing septic AKI demonstrated increased renal vascular resistance and early rises in proinflammatory cytokines (IL-6) and oxidative stress markers.[176]

Sepsis, therefore, is able to affect the autonomic nervous system (ANS), RAAS, and hypothalamic-pituitary-adrenal axis (HPA) which can affect, in several and distinctive steps, cardiac and/or renal function.

Severity of ANS dysfunction correlates with morbidity and mortality[177,178]; autonomic dysfunction can be assessed by observing decreased heart rate variability (HRV), often associated with release of inflammatory biomarkers such as IL-6, IL-10, and C-reactive protein. Data on kidney-related ANS changes are only available in animal models, where changes in renal sympathetic activity do not affect renal blood flow.[179]

Sepsis also activates RAAS in an attempt to restore and maintain blood pressure. Blockade of RAAS might be beneficial because RAAS activation has also been involved in endothelial dysfunction and mortality during severe sepsis.[180,181] Experimental data suggest negative RAAS-activation effects on renal function during sepsis.[182]

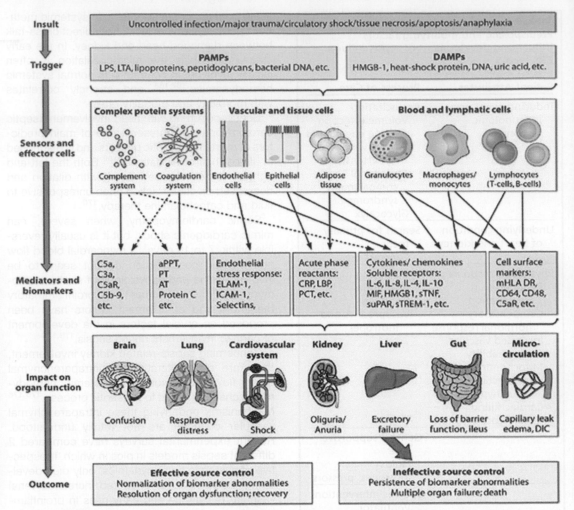

Fig. 7. Pathophysiology of sepsis-induced organ dysfunction. DAMPs, damage-associated molecular patterns; LPS, lipopolysaccharide; LTA, lipoteichoic acid; PAMPs, pathogen-associated molecular patterns.

Administration of ACE inhibitors improves GFR and diuresis, and ARBs improve renal blood flow during experimental endotoxemia.[183]

Sepsis is also involved in causing severe alteration in the HPA, leading to adrenal insufficiency[184] and increased production of proinflammatory biomarkers, free radicals, and prostaglandins. Therefore, inhibition of chemotaxis and expression of adhesion molecules can occur; administration of low-dose glucocorticoids can help reduce the need for vasopressors and the length of stay in the critical care unit.[185]

It is not easy to determine the role of sepsis in heart and kidney dysfunction, but some effects of heart and kidney cross-talk can be deduced by sepsis pathophysiology. During sepsis there is reduced cardiac output, leading to reduced renal perfusion that further worsens sepsis-induced kidney injury; therefore, AKI is characterized by fluid

overload leading to chronic HF in an already dilated heart. Ultimately, metabolic acidosis caused by AKI directly affects myocardial contractility, increases heart rate, and encourages myocardial dysfunction. Experimental data assert that AKI depresses cardiac function inducing proinflammatory and proapoptotic pathophysiologic mechanisms.[101]

Together with the hemodynamic effects of the decompensated heart on renal blood flow, there are cardiac metabolic changes resulting from reduced fluid removal by kidneys. In an experimental model AKI led to cardiac apoptosis, partially limited by anti-TNF therapy,[101] hypertrophy,[186] and an increase in cardiac macrophages.[187]

It is clear that during combined dysfunction of the heart and kidney, as occurs during sepsis, several cellular and molecular changes take place in both organs. Activation and induction of

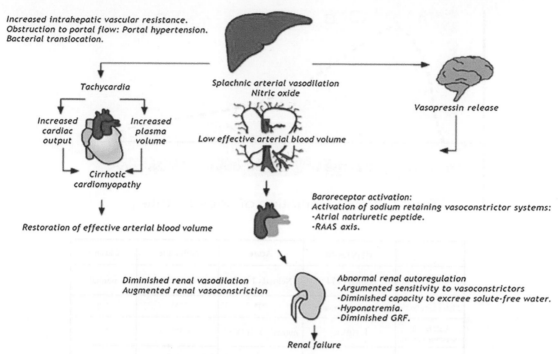

Increased intrahepatic vascular resistance.
Obstruction to portal flow: Portal hypertension.
Bacterial translocation.

Tachycardia

Splachnic arterial vasodilation
Nitric oxide

Vasopressin release

Increased cardiac output

Increased plasma volume

Low effective arterial blood volume

Cirrhotic cardiomyopathy

Restoration of effective arterial blood volume

Baroreceptor activation:
Activation of sodium retaining vasoconstrictor systems:
-Atrial natriuretic peptide.
-RAAS axis.

Diminished renal vasodilation
Augmented renal vasoconstriction

Abnormal renal autoregulation
-Argumented sensitivity to vasoconstrictors
-Diminished capacity to excreee solute-free water.
-Hyponatremia.
-Diminished GRF.

Renal failure

Fig. 8. Pathophysiology of cirrhosis-induced CRS type 5.

cytokines (TNF-α and IL-6) and leukocytes (macrophages, neutrophils, and lymphocytes) are well documented in both the heart and kidney during sepsis. Abnormalities in oxidative stress are also found, from mitochondrial dysfunction to alteration in antioxidant stress enzymes.[188,189]

Contractile heart function is mainly affected in sepsis, and muscle protein expression (actin and myosin) is abnormal as well as membrane-associated proteins such as dystrophin, which normally regulate cell shape, mechanical strength, and myocardial cell contractility. The mean amount of dystrophin and other similar glycoproteins is reduced in septic myocardium.[190]

Cardiomyocytes are connected to each other at intercalated discs whose components include connexin-43 and N-cadherin, which are reduced during sepsis, thus explaining electrical impairment.[191]

Sepsis induces tubular damage in kidneys affected by increased secretion of lipopolysaccharide, which alters HCO_3 transport and leads to abnormalities in urine acidification.[192] Lipopolysaccharide also modifies megalin, a glomerular protein involved in increasing albuminuria.[193]

Diagnosis

Regarding the diagnostic approach to sepsis-related type-5 CRS, initial emphasis has to be on the setting of severe sepsis and septic shock, then on assessment of heart and kidney, and finally on risk evaluation, before starting appropriate treatment.

Systemic inflammation, like sepsis, should be suspected when body temperature is less than 36°C (96.8°F) or greater than 38°C (100.4°F), the heart rate is greater than 90 beats/min, and tachypnea is already present (>20 breaths/min). The white blood cell count can be less than 4 × 100 cells/L or greater than 12 × 100 cells/L.

A recent review has pointed out some characteristic biomarkers whose elevation is typical during the septic process: lipopolysaccharide-binding protein, procalcitonin, C-reactive protein, and proinflammatory cytokines (IL-6, TGF-β).[194]

Assessment of cardiac function in type-5 CRS is similar to that for other clinical situations in which myocardial dysfunction is present. Natriuretic peptides and troponin-level assays provide information about cardiac chambers (especially left cardiac chambers) and damage to myocardial cells. Leukocytosis and C-reactive protein are not specific for the diagnosis of myocardial injury, and imaging devices are preferred by clinicians.

Sepsis cardiomyopathy presents a complex clinical picture, and its pathophysiology is not well understood. In the early stages of the septic process there is low-output myocardial involvement. After beginning fluid therapy the clinical

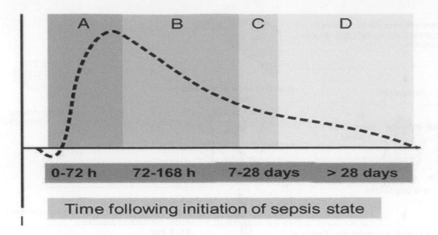

	Hyperacute	Acute	Subacute	Chronic
Systemic Hemodynamics	normal - ↑↑↑*	Normal - ↑ or ↓*	Normal*	normal
Microcirculation	Maldistribution#	???	???	???
Autonomic Nervous system	↓ HRV# *	normal - ↓ HRV# *	???	???
RAAS	↑↑↑# *	↑ - normal# *	???	???
HPA	↓↓↓*	↓↓ - ↓*	???	???

Fig. 9. Pathophysiologic changes in sepsis-induced acute CRS type 5. Organ dysfunction in sepsis can be considered in several different phases that reflect the severity of the disease. The underlying pathophysiologic mechanisms are different in each phase, and thus provide specific opportunities for targeted diagnostic and therapeutic strategies. Phase A: 0 to 72 hours = hyperacute phase; Phase B: 72 to 168 hours = acute phase; Phase C: 7 to 28 days = subacute phase; Phase D: beyond 28 days = chronic phase. Asterisks indicate clinical evidence, hash marks indicate experimental evidence. HPA, hypothalamic-pituitary-adrenal axis; HRV, heart rate variability; RAAS, renin-angiotensin-aldosterone system.

Table 4
Temporal considerations in the pathophysiology of CRS type 5

Attribute	Type-5 CRS, Acute (Sepsis) (see Fig. 1)	Type-5 CRS, Chronic (Cirrhosis) (see Fig. 2)
Time for organ dysfunction	Short: hours to days	Long: weeks to months
Underlying organ function	May be superimposed on underlying cardiac and kidney disease	Heart and kidney have adaptive responses that fail over time
Sequence of organ involvement	Generally simultaneous or in close proximity to each other	One organ precedes the other; eg, cardiac dysfunction precedes renal in cirrhosis
Underlying disease	Systemic event contributes to type-5 CRS	Precipitating events can transition to an acute deterioration in type-5 CRS; eg, gastrointestinal bleed can precipitate hepatorenal syndrome
Pathophysiology	Direct effects on organs	Failure of adaptive responses over time
Mechanisms	Determined by underlying disease	Determined by adaptive changes
Reversibility	Possible with control of sepsis and organ support	Limited unless there is replacement of diseased organ; eg, liver transplant

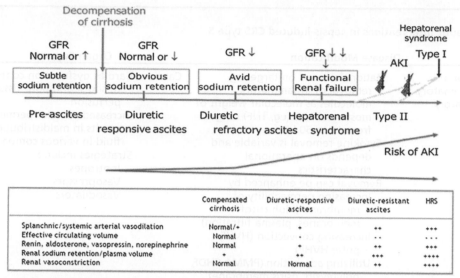

Fig. 10. Hemodynamic changes in chronic type-5 CRS during different stages of cirrhosis. HRS, hepatorenal syndrome.

picture shifts to typical distributive shock characterized by increased cardiac output and systemic vasodilation.[195] Echocardiographic assay confirms high-output cardiomyopathy with abnormalities in left ventricular regional contractility together with dilation of left heart chambers.[196]

Diagnosis of kidney involvement in sepsis-related type-5 CRS overlaps with other forms of AKI, with acute changes in serum creatinine levels according to RIFLE, AKIN, and KDIGO criteria.[197–199]

Several other biomarkers are currently being proposed, such as cystatin C (the only new biomarker approved in the United States), KIM-1, NGAL, and NAG, but the RIFLE, KDIGO, and AKIN criteria still recommend serum creatinine levels and urine output for the diagnosis and monitoring of AKI in type-5 CRS.

Outcomes and Treatment

Once the diagnosis of type 5-CRS is made, every organ and tissue involved must be investigated to evaluate risk prediction and prevent further and irreversible alterations in organ function.

Preliminary data (not published at present) seem to indicate that biomarkers of cell-cycle regulation may be able to predict which patients will develop severe AKI in few days.

Regarding cardiac risk, patients who survived septic shock were shown to have lower ejection fractions and higher left ventricular end-diastolic volumes, suggesting a protective role in myocardial depression.[200]

Treatment of type-5 CRS is mainly based on the management of underlying disease and kidney and heart complications (Table 5). Essentially, maintaining hemodynamic stability and guaranteeing tissue perfusion are key points in preventing type-5 CRS in the hyperacute phase of sepsis, together with fluid control and correct antibiotic treatment. Fluid therapy must be carefully managed to avoid fluid overload and other iatrogenic complications.[201,202]

Because inflammation and immune disorders play an important role in the pathogenesis of sepsis, removal of cytokines and immunomodulation are 2 approaches based on extracorporeal techniques using convection, high-volume hemofiltration, and high-permeability membranes.[203–205] The best results have been obtained with high-permeability membranes and absorption.[206]

A therapeutic alternative is provided by targeting cellular elements accountable for apoptosis and neutrophil activation and removing them using polymyxin filters[207] or a citrate anticoagulant-based selective cytopheretic device.[208]

To manage heart complications, especially in the hyperacute stage, a multifaceted approach is required to maintain filling pressures with fluid therapy together with vasopressors, vasodilators, and inotropes; vasopressors should be carefully deployed because of their depressive effects on cardiac output (increased afterload), especially if there is concomitant hypovolemia. Vasodilators increase cardiac output, especially in ischemic patients, whereas phosphodiesterase inhibitors have inotropic and vasodilatory effects but

Table 5
Therapeutic interventions in sepsis-induced CRS type 5

Disease Modification		Organ Support	

Removal of inflammatory mediators	Rationale based on targeting removal of inflammatory molecules as molecular weight of most cytokines (eg, TNF) ranges from 17 to 50 kDa
	Cytokine removal is variable and depends on operational characteristics
	Removal can be enhanced by
	  Increasing permeability of membrane (high-cutoff membranes, plasma filtration)
	  Increasing convection (HVHF, pulse HVHF)
	  Utilizing adsorption (PMMA CHDF, polymyxin, osiris membrane)
		Cardiac	Cardiac dysfunction contributes to shock and poor tissue perfusion
			Increased vascular permeability results in maldistribution of fluid in various compartments
			Strategies include
			  Inotropes
			  Vasopressors
			  Vasodilators

Immunomodulation	Rationale based on targeting cellular elements of disease response
	Immunoparalysis
	Apoptosis
	Neutrophil activation
	Strategies include
	  Endotoxin removal by selective binding to polymyxin
	  Anticoagulant-based strategies (citrate-enabled SCD)
	  Plasma filtration coupled to binding to sorbents
		Renal	Renal dysfunction contributes to organ failure
			Solute clearance
			Fluid management
			Acid base and electrolyte homeostasis
			Strategies include
			  Diuretics
			  RRT

Abbreviations: CHDF, continuous diafiltration; HVHF, high-volume hemofiltration; PMMA, polymethylmethacrylate; RRT, renal replacement therapy; SCD, selective cytopheretic device; TNF, tumor necrosis factor.

attenuate the increase in myocardial oxygen requirements.

Vasopressin increases arterial pressure but has negative effects on cardiac output. Recently levosimendan has been proved to provide benefits in decompensated HF by increasing ejection fraction and diuresis[209,210]; however, its efficacy is still to be proved in the prevention of type-5 CRS.

Renal support includes removal of any nephrotoxic drug and media, maintenance of adequate perfusion pressure, and, if indicated, early intervention with dialysis therapy.[211]

There is no role for dopamine in improving renal hemodynamics[212,213] and there are limited studies with fenoldopam.[214,215] Norepinephrine decreases renal perfusion under normal conditions but increases systemic blood pressure in septic patients,[216] whereas vasopressin increases diuresis and GFR in septic patients.[217,218]

Diuretics have a limited role in managing heart and kidney involvement in septic patients,[219] and

continuous renal replacement therapy should be promptly started[211]; early ultrafiltration seems to improve renal outcomes in patients with septic shock, but these data need to be confirmed in further clinical trials.

REFERENCES

1. Ronco C. The cardiorenal syndrome: basis and common ground for a multidisciplinary patient-oriented therapy. Cardiorenal Med 2011;1:3–4.
2. Bargshaw SM, Cruz DM, Aspromonte N, et al, for the Acute Dialysis Quality Initiative (ADQI) Consensus Group. Epidemiology of cardio-renal syndromes: workgroup statements from the 7th ADQI Consensus Conference. Nephrol Dial Transplant 2010;25:1406–16.
3. Damman K, Navis G, Voors AA, et al. Worsening renal function and prognosis in heart failure: systematic review and meta-analysis. J Card Fail 2007;13:599–608.

4. McCullough PA. Cardiorenal syndromes: pathophysiology to prevention. Int J Nephrol 2010; 2010:762590.

5. Ronco C. Cardiorenal syndromes: definition and classification. Contrib Nephrol 2010;164:33–8.

6. Eren Z, Ozveren O, Buvukoner E, et al. A single-centre study of acute cardiorenal syndrome: incidence, risk factors and consequences. Cardiorenal Med 2012;2:168–76.

7. Hanada S, Takewa Y, Mizuno T, et al. Effect of the technique for assisting renal blood circulation on ischemic kidney in acute cardiorenal syndrome. J Artif Organs 2012;15:140–5.

8. Stevenson LW, Perloff JK. The limited reliability of physical signs for estimating hemodynamics in chronic heart failure. JAMA 1989;261:884–8.

9. Mullens W, Abrahams Z, Francis GS, et al. Importance of venous congestion for worsening of renal function in advanced decompensated heart failure. J Am Coll Cardiol 2009;53:589–96.

10. Uthoff H, Breidthardt T, Klima T, et al. Central venous pressure and impaired renal function in patients with acute heart failure. Eur J Heart Fail 2011; 13:432–9.

11. Braam B, Cupples WA, Joles JA, et al. Systemic arterial and venous determinants of renal hemodynamics in congestive heart failure. Heart Fail Rev 2012;17:161–75.

12. De Silva R, Loh H, Rigby AS, et al. Epidemiology, associated factors, and prognostic outcomes of renal artery stenosis in chronic heart failure assessed by magnetic resonance angiography. Am J Cardiol 2007;100:273–9.

13. Nohria A, Tsang SW, Fang JC, et al. Clinical assessment identifies hemodynamic profiles that predict outcomes in patients admitted with heart failure. J Am Coll Cardiol 2003;41:1797–804.

14. Machnik A, Neuhofer W, Jantsch J, et al. Macrophages regulate salt-dependent volume and blood pressure by a vascular endothelial growth factor-C-dependent buffering mechanism. Nat Med 2009; 15:545–52.

15. Virzì GM, Torregrossa R, Cruz DN, et al. Cardiorenal syndrome type 1 may be immunologically mediated: a pilot evaluation of monocyte apoptosis. Cardiorenal Med 2012;2:33–42.

16. Kraut EJ, Chen S, Hubbard NE, et al. Tumor necrosis factor depresses myocardial contractility in endotoxemic swine. J Trauma 1999;46: 900–6.

17. Van Sloten TT, Pijpers E, Steouwer CD, et al. Metformin-associated lactic acidosis in a patient with normal kidney function. Diabetes Res Clin Pract 2012;96:57–8.

18. Arroio D, Melero R, Panizo M, et al. Metformin-associated acute kidney injury and lactic acidosis. Int J Nephrol 2011;2011:749–63.

19. Xu G, Ahn J, Chang S, et al. Lipocalin-2 induces cardiomyocyte apoptosis by increasing intracellular iron accumulation. J Biol Chem 2012;287:4808–17.

20. Prawle JR, Liu YI, Licari E, et al. Oliguria as predictive biomarker of acute kidney injury in critically ill patients. Crit Care 2011;15:R172.

21. Mc Donagh TA, Komajda M, Maggioni AP, et al. Clinical trials in acute heart failure: simpler solution to complex problems. Consensus document arising from a European Society of Cardiology cardiovascular round-table think tank on acute heart failure. Eur J Heart Fail 2011;13:1253–60.

22. Prowle JR, Echeverri JE, Ligabo EV, et al. Fluid balance and acute kidney injury. Nat Rev Nephrol 2010;6:107–15.

23. Latouche C, El Moghrabi S, Messaoudi S, et al. Neutrophil gelatinase-associated lipocalin is a novel mineralocorticoid target in the cardiovascular system. Hypertension 2012;59:966–72.

24. Maisel A, Xue Y, Shah K, et al. Increased 90-day mortality in patients with acute heart failure with elevated copeptin: secondary results from the Biomarkers in Acute Heart Failure (BACH) study. Circ Heart Fail 2011;4:613–20.

25. Shah RV, Truong QA, Gaggin HK, et al. Mid-regional pro-atrial natriuretic peptide and pro-adrenomedullin testing for the diagnostic and prognostic evaluation of patients with acute dyspnoea. Eur Heart J 2012;33:2197–205.

26. Maisel AS, Katz N, Hillege HL, et al, Acute Dialysis Quality Initiative consensus group. Biomarkers in kidney and heart disease. Nephrol Dial Transplant 2011;26:62–74.

27. Aldous SJ, Richards AM, Troughton R, et al. ST2 has diagnostic and prognostic utility for all-cause mortality and heart failure in patients presenting to the emergency department with chest pain. J Card Fail 2012;18:304–10.

28. Boisot S, Beede J, Isakson S, et al. Serial sampling of ST2 predicts 90-day mortality following destabilized heart failure. J Card Fail 2008;14:732–8.

29. Ky B, French B, McCloskey K, et al. High-sensitivity ST2 for prediction of adverse outcomes in chronic heart failure. Circ Heart Fail 2011;4:180–7.

30. Dhillon OS, Narayan HK, Quinn PA, et al. Interleukin 33 and ST2 in non-ST-elevation myocardial infarction: comparison with Global Registry of Acute Coronary Events Risk Scoring and NT-proBNP. Am Heart J 2011;161:1163–70.

31. Tojo A, Gross SS, Zhang L, et al. Immunocytochemical localization of distinct isoforms of nitric oxide synthase in the juxtaglomerular apparatus of normal rat kidney. J Am Soc Nephrol 1994;4: 1438–47.

32. Singh P, Okusa MD. The role of tubuloglomerular feedback in the pathogenesis of acute kidney injury. Contrib Nephrol 2011;174:12–21.

33. Campbell CY, Clarke W, Park H, et al. Usefulness of cystatin C and prognosis following admission for acute heart failure. Am J Cardiol 2009;104:389–92.

34. Lassus JP, Nieminen MS, Peuhkurinen K, et al, FINN-AKVA study group. Markers of renal function and acute kidney injury in acute heart failure: definitions and impact on outcomes of the cardiorenal syndrome. Eur Heart J 2010;31:2791–8.

35. Cruz DN, Gaiao S, Maisel A, et al. Neutrophil gelatinase-associated lipocalin as a biomarker of cardiovascular disease: a systematic review. Clin Chem Lab Med 2012;50:1533–45.

36. Alvelos M, Lourenço P, Dias C, et al. Prognostic value of neutrophil gelatinase-associated lipocalin in acute heart failure. Int J Cardiol 2013;165(1): 51–5.

37. Maisel AS, Mueller C, Fitzgerald R, et al. Prognostic utility of plasma neutrophil gelatinase-associated lipocalin in patients with acute heart failure: the NGAL EvaLuation Along with B-type NaTriuretic Peptide in acutely decompensated heart failure (GALLANT) trial. Eur J Heart Fail 2011;13:846–51.

38. Alvelos M, Pimentel R, Pinho E, et al. Neutrophil gelatinase-associated lipocalin in the diagnosis of type 1 cardio-renal syndrome in the general ward. Clin J Am Soc Nephrol 2011;6:476–81.

39. Aghel A, Shrestha K, Mullens W, et al. Serum neutrophil gelatinase-associated lipocalin (NGAL) in predicting worsening renal function in acute decompensated heart failure. J Card Fail 2010; 16:49–54.

40. Collins SP, Hart KW, Lindsell CJ, et al. Elevated urinary neutrophil gelatinase-associated lipocalcin after acute heart failure treatment is associated with worsening renal function and adverse events. Eur J Heart Fail 2012;14:1020–9.

41. Valente MA, Damman K, Dunselman PH, et al. Urinary proteins in heart failure. Prog Cardiovasc Dis 2012;55:44–55.

42. Di Somma S, De Berardinis B, Bongiovanni C, et al. Use of BNP and bioimpedance to drive therapy in heart failure patients. Congest Heart Fail 2010;16: S56–61.

43. Parrinello G, Paterna S, Di Pasquale P, et al. The usefulness of bioelectrical impedance analysis in differentiating dyspnea due to decompensated heart failure. J Card Fail 2008;14:676–86.

44. Milzman D, Napoli A, Hogan C, et al. Thoracic impedance vs chest radiograph to diagnose acute pulmonary edema in the ED. Am J Emerg Med 2009;27:770–5.

45. Whellan DJ, Droogan CJ, Fitzpatrick J, et al. Change in intrathoracic impedance measures during acute decompensated heart failure admission: results from the Diagnostic Data for Discharge in Heart Failure Patients (3D-HF) Pilot Study. J Card Fail 2012;18:107–12.

46. Di Lullo L, Floccari F, Granata A, et al. Ultrasonography: Ariadne's thread in the diagnosis of cardiorenal syndrome. Cardiorenal Med 2012;2(1):11–7.

47. Voors AA, Davison BA, Felker GM, Pre-RELAX-AHF study group. Early drop in systolic blood pressure and worsening renal function in acute heart failure: renal results of Pre-RELAX-AHF. Eur J Heart Fail 2011;13:961–7.

48. Shirakabe A, Hata N, Kobayashi N, et al. Prognostic impact of acute kidney injury in patients with acute decompensated heart failure. Circ J 2013;77(3):687–96.

49. Heywood JT, Fonarow GC, Costanzo MR, et al. High prevalence of renal dysfunction and its impact on outcome in 118,465 patients hospitalized with acute decompensated heart failure: a report from the ADHERE database. J Card Fail 2007;13(6):422–30.

50. Hebert K, Dias A, Delgado MC, et al. Epidemiology and survival of the five stages of chronic kidney disease in a systolic heart failure population. Eur J Heart Fail 2010;12(8):861–5.

51. Cruz DN, Bagshaw SM. Heart-kidney interaction: epidemiology of cardiorenal syndromes. Int J Nephrol 2010;2011:351291.

52. Cruz DN, Schmidt-Ott KM, Vescovo G, et al. Pathophysiology of cardiorenal syndrome type 2 in stable chronic heart failure: workgroup statements from the eleventh consensus conference of the Acute Dialysis Quality Initiative (ADQI). Contrib Nephrol 2013;182:117–36.

53. Setoguchi S, Stevenson LW, Schneeweiss S. Repeated hospitalizations predict mortality in the community population with heart failure. Am Heart J 2007;154(2):260–6.

54. Tanaka K, Ito M, Kodama M, et al. Longitudinal change in renal function in patients with idiopathic dilated cardiomyopathy without renal insufficiency at initial diagnosis. Circ J 2007;71(12):1927–31.

55. Bongartz LG, Cramer MJ, Doevendans PA, et al. The severe cardiorenal syndrome: 'Guyton revisited'. Eur Heart J 2005;26(1):11–7.

56. Merrill AJ, Morrison JL, Branno ES. Concentration of renin in renal venous blood in patients with chronic heart failure. Am J Med 1946;1(5):468.

57. Kishimoto T, Maekawa M, Abe Y, et al. Intrarenal distribution of blood flow and renin release during renal venous pressure elevation. Kidney Int 1973; 4(4):259–66.

58. Remuzzi G, Cattaneo D, Perico N. The aggravating mechanisms of aldosterone on kidney fibrosis. J Am Soc Nephrol 2008;19(8):1459–62.

59. Onozato ML, Tojo A, Kobayashi N, et al. Dual blockade of aldosterone and angiotensin II additively suppresses TGF-beta and NADPH oxidase in the hypertensive kidney. Nephrol Dial Transplant 2007;22(5):1314–22.

60. Colombo PC, Ganda A, Lin J, et al. Inflammatory activation: cardiac, renal, and cardio-renal interactions in patients with the cardiorenal syndrome. Heart Fail Rev 2012;17(2):177–90.

61. Colombo PC, Onat D, Sabbah HN. Acute heart failure as "acute endothelitis"—interaction of fluid overload and endothelial dysfunction. Eur J Heart Fail 2008;10(2):170–5.

62. Hillege HL, Nitsch D, Pfeffer MA, et al. Renal function as a predictor of outcome in a broad spectrum of patients with heart failure. Circulation 2006; 113(5):671–8.

63. Halbesma N, Jansen DF, Heymans MW, et al. Development and validation of a general population renal risk score. Clin J Am Soc Nephrol 2011; 6(7):1731–8.

64. Tangri N, Stevens LA, Griffith J, et al. A predictive model for progression of chronic kidney disease to kidney failure. JAMA 2011; 305(15):1553–9.

65. Khan NA, Ma I, Thompson CR, et al. Kidney function and mortality among patients with left ventricular systolic dysfunction. J Am Soc Nephrol 2006; 17(1):244–53.

66. Cruz DN, Fard A, Clementi A, et al. Role of biomarkers in the diagnosis and management of cardio-renal syndromes. Semin Nephrol 2012; 32(1):79–92.

67. Tang WH, Van Lente F, Shrestha K, et al. Impact of myocardial function on cystatin C measurements in chronic systolic heart failure. J Card Fail 2008; 14(5):394–9.

68. Damman K, van Veldhuisen DJ, Navis G, et al. Urinary neutrophil gelatinase associated lipocalin (NGAL), a marker of tubular damage, is increased in patients with chronic heart failure. Eur J Heart Fail 2008;10(10):997–1000.

69. Damman K, Kalra PR, Hillege H. Pathophysiological mechanisms contributing to renal dysfunction in chronic heart failure. J Ren Care 2010;36(Suppl 1): 18–26.

70. Malyszko J, Bachorzewska-Gajewska H, Poniatowski B, et al. Urinary and serum biomarkers after cardiac catheterization in diabetic patients with stable angina and without severe chronic kidney disease. Ren Fail 2009;31(10): 910–9.

71. Yndestad A, Landrø L, Ueland T, et al. Increased systemic and myocardial expression of neutrophil gelatinase-associated lipocalin in clinical and experimental heart failure. Eur Heart J 2009; 30(10):1229–36.

72. Bolignano D, Basile G, Parisi P, et al. Increased plasma neutrophil gelatinase-associated lipocalin levels predict mortality in elderly patients with chronic heart failure. Rejuvenation Res 2009; 12(1):7–14.

73. Shrestha K, Borowski AG, Troughton RW, et al. Renal dysfunction is a stronger determinant of systemic neutrophil gelatinase-associated lipocalin levels than myocardial dysfunction in systolic heart failure. J Card Fail 2011;17(6):472–8.

74. Jungbauer CG, Birner C, Jung B, et al. Kidney injury molecule-1 and N-acetyl-beta-D-glucosaminidase in chronic heart failure: possible biomarkers of cardiorenal syndrome. Eur J Heart Fail 2011; 13(10):1104–10.

75. Testani JM, Kimmel SE, Dries DL, et al. Prognostic importance of early worsening renal function after initiation of angiotensin-converting enzyme inhibitor therapy in patients with cardiac dysfunction. Circ Heart Fail 2011;4(6):685–91.

76. Capes SE, Gerstein HC, Negassa A, et al. Enalapril prevents clinical proteinuria in diabetic patients with low ejection fraction. Diabetes Care 2000; 23(3):377–80.

77. Ljungman S, Kjekshus J, Swedberg K. Renal function in severe congestive heart failure during treatment with enalapril (the Cooperative North Scandinavian Enalapril Survival Study [CONSENSUS] Trial). Am J Cardiol 1992;70(4): 479–87.

78. Anand IS, Bishu K, Rector TS, et al. Proteinuria, chronic kidney disease, and the effect of an angiotensin receptor blocker in addition to an angiotensin-converting enzyme inhibitor in patients with moderate to severe heart failure. Circulation 2009;120(16):1577–84.

79. Pitt B, Zannad F, Remme WJ, et al. The effect of spironolactone on morbidity and mortality in patients with severe heart failure. Randomized Aldactone Evaluation Study Investigators. N Engl J Med 1999;341(10):709–17.

80. Zannad F, Dousset B, Alla F. Treatment of congestive heart failure: interfering the aldosterone-cardiac extracellular matrix relationship. Hypertension 2001;38(5):1227–32.

81. Wali RK, Iyengar M, Beck GJ, et al. Efficacy and safety of carvedilol in treatment of heart failure with chronic kidney disease: a meta-analysis of randomized trials. Circ Heart Fail 2011;4(1):18–26.

82. Castagno D, Jhund PS, McMurray JJ, et al. Improved survival with bisoprolol in patients with heart failure and renal impairment: an analysis of the cardiac insufficiency bisoprolol study II (CIBIS-II) trial. Eur J Heart Fail 2010;12(6):607–16.

83. Cohen-Solal A, Kotecha D, van Veldhuisen DJ, et al. Efficacy and safety of nebivolol in elderly heart failure patients with impaired renal function: insights from the SENIORS trial. Eur J Heart Fail 2009;11(9):872–80.

84. Mann DL, McMurray JJ, Packer M, et al. Targeted anticytokine therapy in patients with chronic heart

failure: results of the Randomized Etanercept Worldwide Evaluation (RENEWAL). Circulation 2004;109(13):1594–602.

85. Boerrigter G, Costello-Boerrigter LC, Abraham WT, et al. Cardiac resynchronization therapy improves renal function in human heart failure with reduced glomerular filtration rate. J Card Fail 2008;14(7): 539–46.

86. Yap SC, Lee HT. Acute kidney injury and extrarenal organ dysfunction: new concepts and experimental evidence. Anesthesiology 2012;116(5): 1139–48.

87. Prabhu SD. Cytokine-induced modulation of cardiac function. Circ Res 2004;95(12):1140–53.

88. Kingma JG Jr, Vincent C, Rouleau JR, et al. Influence of acute renal failure on coronary vasoregulation in dogs. J Am Soc Nephrol 2006;17(5): 1316–24.

89. Chuasuwan A, Kellum JA. Cardio-renal syndrome type 3: epidemiology, pathophysiology, and treatment. Semin Nephrol 2012;32(1):31–9.

90. Grams ME, Rabb H. The distant organ effects of acute kidney injury. Kidney Int 2012;81(10):942–8.

91. Ma XL, Lefer DJ, Lefer AM, et al. Coronary endothelial and cardiac protective effects of a monoclonal antibody to intercellular adhesion molecule-1 in myocardial ischemia and reperfusion. Circulation 1992;86(3):937–46.

92. Blake P, Hasegawa Y, Khosla MC, et al. Isolation of "myocardial depressant factor(s)" from the ultrafiltrate of heart failure patients with acute renal failure. ASAIO J 1996;42(5):M911–5.

93. Edmunds NJ, Lal H, Woodward B. Effects of tumour necrosis factor-alpha on left ventricular function in the rat isolated perfused heart: possible mechanisms for a decline in cardiac function. Br J Pharmacol 1999;126(1):189–96.

94. Miyano H, Shishido T, Kawada T, et al. Acute effect of tumor necrosis factor-alpha is minimal on mechanics but significant on energetics in blood-perfused canine left ventricles. Crit Care Med 1999;27(1):168–76.

95. Rauchhaus M, Doehner W, Francis DP, et al. Plasma cytokine parameters and mortality in patients with chronic heart failure. Circulation 2000; 102(25):3060–7.

96. Wen X, Peng Z, Li Y, et al. One dose of cyclosporine A is protective at initiation of folic acid-induced acute kidney injury in mice. Nephrol Dial Transplant 2012;27(8):3100–9.

97. Verdouw PD, Gho BC, Koning MM, et al. Cardioprotection by ischemic and nonischemic myocardial stress and ischemia in remote organs. Implications for the concept of ischemic preconditioning. Ann N Y Acad Sci 1996;793:27–42.

98. Kobuchi S, Tanaka R, Shintani T, et al. Mechanisms underlying the renoprotective effect of GABA against ischemia/reperfusion-induced renal injury in rats. J Pharmacol Exp Ther 2011;338(3):767–74.

99. Kajstura J, Cigola E, Malhotra A, et al. Angiotensin II induces apoptosis of adult ventricular myocytes in vitro. J Mol Cell Cardiol 1997;29(3):859–70.

100. Nath KA, Grande JP, Croatt AJ, et al. Transgenic sickle mice are markedly sensitive to renal ischemia-reperfusion injury. Am J Pathol 2005; 166(4):963–72.

101. Kelly KJ. Distant effects of experimental renal ischemia/reperfusion injury. J Am Soc Nephrol 2003;14(6):1549–58.

102. Wencker D, Chandra M, Nguyen K, et al. A mechanistic role for cardiac myocyte apoptosis in heart failure. J Clin Invest 2003;111(10): 1497–504.

103. Liu YH, D'Ambrosio M, Liao TD, et al. N-acetyl-seryl-aspartyl-lysyl-proline prevents cardiac remodeling and dysfunction induced by galectin-3, a mammalian adhesion/growth-regulatory lectin. Am J Physiol Heart Circ Physiol 2009;296(2): H404–12.

104. Wiedemann HP, Wheeler AP, Bernard GR, et al. Comparison of two fluid-management strategies in acute lung injury. N Engl J Med 2006;354(24): 2564–75.

105. Payen D, de Pont AC, Sakr Y, et al. A positive fluid balance is associated with a worse outcome in patients with acute renal failure. Crit Care 2008; 12(3):R74.

106. Davis KL, Laine GA, Geissler HJ. Effects of myocardial edema on the development of myocardial interstitial fibrosis. Microcirculation 2000;7: 269–80.

107. Nazar A, Guevara M, Sitges M, et al. LEFT ventricular function assessed by echocardiography in cirrhosis: relationship to systemic hemodynamics and renal dysfunction. J Hepatol 2013; 58(1):51–7.

108. Legrand M, Darmon M, Joannidis M, et al. Management of renal replacement therapy in ICU patients: an international survey. Intensive Care Med 2013;39(1):101–8.

109. Nimmo AJ, Than N, Orchard CH, et al. The effect of acidosis on beta-adrenergic receptors in ferret cardiac muscle. Exp Physiol 1993;78(1):95–103.

110. Bagshaw SM, Wald R, Barton J, et al. Clinical factors associated with initiation of renal replacement therapy in critically ill patients with acute kidney injury—a prospective multicenter observational study. J Crit Care 2012;27(3):268–75.

111. Schwenger V, Weigand MA, Hoffmann O, et al. Sustained low efficiency dialysis using a single-pass batch system in acute kidney injury—a randomized interventional trial: the REnal Replacement Therapy Study in Intensive Care Unit PatiEnts. Crit Care 2012;16(4):R140.

112. Neirynck N, Vanholder R, Schepers E, et al. An update on uremic toxins. Int Urol Nephrol 2013;45(1): 139–50.

113. Shannon TR, Pogwizd SM, Bers DM. Elevated sarcoplasmic reticulum Ca2+ leak in intact ventricular myocytes from rabbits in heart failure. Circ Res 2003;93(7):592–4.

114. Ronco C, Cruz D, Noland BW. Neutrophil gelatinase-associated lipocalin curve and neutrophil gelatinase-associated lipocalin extended-range assay: a new biomarker approach in the early diagnosis of acute kidney injury and cardiorenal syndrome. Semin Nephrol 2012;32(1):121–8.

115. Carlsson AC, Larsson A, Helmersson-Karlqvist J, et al. Urinary kidney injury molecule 1 and incidence of heart failure in elderly men. Eur J Heart Fail 2013;15(4):441–6.

116. Licurse A, Kim MC, Dziura J, et al. Renal ultrasonography in the evaluation of acute kidney injury: developing a risk stratification framework. Arch Intern Med 2010;170:1900–7.

117. Ozmen CA, Akin D, Bilek SU, et al. Ultrasound as a diagnostic tool to differentiate acute from chronic renal failure. Clin Nephrol 2010;74:46–52.

118. Darmon M, Schortgen F, Vargas F, et al. Diagnostic accuracy of Doppler renal resistive index for reversibility of acute kidney injury in critically ill patients. Intensive Care Med 2011;37(1):68–76.

119. James MT, Ghali WA, Knudtson ML, et al. Associations between acute kidney injury and cardiovascular and renal outcomes after coronary angiography. Circulation 2011;123(4):409–16.

120. Selby NM, Kolhe NV, McIntyre CW, et al. Defining the cause of death in hospitalised patients with acute kidney injury. PLoS One 2012;7(11):e48580.

121. Jasuja D, Mor MK, Hartwig KC, et al. Provider knowledge of contrast-induced acute kidney injury. Am J Med Sci 2009;338:280–6.

122. Solomon RJ, Mehran R, Natarajan MK, et al. Contrast-induced nephropathy and long-term adverse events: cause and effect? Clin J Am Soc Nephrol 2009;4:1162–9.

123. Mentzer RM Jr, Oz MC, Sladen RN, et al. Effects of perioperative nesiritide in patients with left ventricular dysfunction undergoing cardiac surgery: the NAPA trial. J Am Coll Cardiol 2007;49:716–26.

124. Redóna J, Cea-Calvob L, Lozanoc JV, et al. Kidney function and cardiovascular disease in the hypertensive population: the ERIC-HTA study. J Hypertens 2006;24:663–9.

125. Anavekar NS, McMurray JJ, Velazquez EJ, et al. Relation between renal dysfunction and cardiovascular outcomes after myocardial infarction. N Engl J Med 2004;351:1285–95.

126. Rostand SG, Kirk KA, Rutsky EA. Dialysis-associated ischemic heart disease: insights from coronary angiography. Kidney Int 1984;25:653–9.

127. Joki N, Hase H, Nakamura R. Onset of coronary artery disease prior to initiation of hemodialysis in patients with end-stage renal disease. Nephrol Dial Transplant 1997;12:718–23.

128. Whalley GA, Marwick TH, Doughty RN, et al. IDEAL effect of early initiation of dialysis on cardiac structure and function: results from the echo substudy of the IDEAL Trial. Am J Kidney Dis 2013;61(2):262–70.

129. Chonchol M, Whittle J. Desbien: chronic kidney disease is associated with angiographic coronary artery disease. Am J Nephrol 2008;28:354–60.

130. McCullough PA, Agrawal V, Danielewicz E, et al. Accelerated atherosclerotic calcification and Mönckeberg's sclerosis: a continuum of advanced vascular pathology in chronic kidney disease. Clin J Am Soc Nephrol 2008;3:1585–98.

131. Gross ML, Meyer HP, Ziebart H, et al. Calcification of coronary intima and media. Clin J Am Soc Nephrol 2007;2:121–34.

132. Ragosta M, Samady H, Isaacs RB, et al. Coronary flow reserve abnormalities in patients with diabetes mellitus who have end-stage renal disease and normal epicardial coronary arteries. Am Heart J 2004;147:1017–23.

133. Garland JS, Holden RM, Groome PA, et al. Prevalence and associations of coronary artery calcification in patients with stages 3 to 5 CKD without cardiovascular disease. Am J Kidney Dis 2008; 52:849–58.

134. Adragao T, Pires A, Branco P, et al. Ankle-brachial index, vascular calcifications and mortality in dialysis patients. Nephrol Dial Transplant 2012;27: 318–25.

135. Moe SM, O'Neill KD, Duan D, et al. Medial artery calcification in ESRD patients is associated with deposition of bone matrix proteins. Kidney Int 2002;61:638–47.

136. Campean V, Nonnast-Daniel B, Garlichs C, et al. CD40-CD154 expression in calcified and non-calcified coronary lesions of patients with chronic renal failure. Atherosclerosis 2007;190:156–66.

137. Laurent S, Cockcroft J, Van Bortel L, et al. Expert consensus document on arterial stiffness: methodological issues and clinical applications. Eur Heart J 2006;27:2588–605.

138. McGregor E, Jardine AG, Murray LS, et al. Preoperative echocardiographic abnormalities and adverse outcome following renal transplantation. Nephrol Dial Transplant 1998;13: 1499–505.

139. Foley RN, Parfey PS, Harneyf JD, et al. Clinical and echocardiographic disease in patients starting end-stage renal disease therapy. Kidney Int 1995; 47:186–92.

140. Foley RN, Curtis BM, Randell EW, et al. Left ventricular hypertrophy in new hemodialysis patients

without symptomatic cardiac disease. Clin J Am Soc Nephrol 2010;5:805–13.

141. McIntyre CW, Burton JO, Selby NM, et al. Hemodialysis-induced cardiac dysfunction is associated with an acute reduction in global and segmental myocardial blood flow. Clin J Am Soc Nephrol 2008;3:19–26.

142. Parfey PS, Harnett JD, Foley RN. Heart failure and ischemic heart disease in chronic uremia. Curr Opin Nephrol Hypertens 1995;4:105–10.

143. Blancher J, Safar ME, Guerin AP, et al. Aortic pulse wave velocity index and mortality in end-stage renal disease. Kidney Int 2003;63:1852–60.

144. Bogrov AY, Shapiro JI. Endogenous digitalis: pathophysiologic roles and therapeutic applications. Nat Clin Pract Nephrol 2008;4:378–92.

145. Amann K, Breitbach M, Ritz E, et al. Myocyte/capillary mismatch in the heart of uremic patients. J Am Soc Nephrol 1998;9:1018–22.

146. Mall G, Huther W, Schneider J, et al. Diffuse intermyocardiocytic fibrosis in uraemic patients. Nephrol Dial Transplant 1990;5:39–44.

147. Meert N, Schepers E, De Smet R, et al. Inconsistency of reported uremic toxin concentrations. Artif Organs 2007;31:600–11.

148. Miyazaki T, Ise M, Seo H, et al. Indoxyl sulfate increases the gene expressions of TGF-beta 1, TIMP-1 and pro-alpha 1(I) collagen in uremic rat kidneys. Kidney Int Suppl 1997;62:S15–22.

149. Sharma UC, Pokharel S, van Brakel TJ. Galectin-3 marks activated macrophages in failure-prone hypertrophied hearts and contribute to cardiac dysfunction. Circulation 2004;110:3121–8.

150. Lok DJ, Van Der Meer P, de la Porte PW, et al. Prognostic value of galectin-3, a novel marker of fibrosis, in patients with chronic heart failure: data from the DEAL-HF study. Clin Res Cardiol 2010; 99:323–8.

151. Lin YH, Lin LY, Wu YW, et al. The relationship between serum galectin-3 and serum markers of cardiac extracellular matrix turnover in heart failure patients. Clin Chim Acta 2009;409:96–9.

152. Gopal DM, Kommineni M, Ayalon N, et al. Relationship of plasma galectin-3 to renal function in patients with heart failure: effects of clinical status, pathophysiology of heart failure, and presence or absence of heart failure. J Am Heart Assoc 2012; 1:1–7.

153. Faul C, Amaral AP, Oskouei B, et al. FGF23 induces left ventricular hypertrophy. J Clin Invest 2011;121: 4393–408.

154. Gutiérrez OM, Januzzi JL, Isakova T, et al. Fibroblast growth factor 23 and left ventricular hypertrophy in chronic kidney disease. Circulation 2009; 119:2545–52.

155. Di Lullo L, Floccari F, Polito P. Right ventricular diastolic function in dialysis patients could be affected

by vascular access. Nephron Clin Pract 2011;118: c258–62.

156. McCullough PA. Why is chronic kidney disease the "spoiler" for cardiovascular outcomes? J Am Coll Cardiol 2003;41(5):725–8.

157. Kalantar-Zadeh K, Block G, Humphreys MH, et al. Reverse epidemiology of cardiovascular risk factors in maintenance dialysis patients. Kidney Int 2003;63(3):793–808.

158. Di Lullo L, Floccari F, Santoboni A, et al. Progression of cardiac valve calcification and decline of renal function in CKD patients. J Nephrol 2013; 26(4):739–44.

159. Dmitrieva O, de Lusignan S, Macdougall IC, et al. Association of anaemia in primary care patients with chronic kidney disease: cross sectional study of quality improvement in chronic kidney disease (QICKD) trial data. BMC Nephrol 2013;14:24.

160. EVOLVE Trial Investigators, Chertow GM, Block GA, et al. Effect of cinacalcet on cardiovascular disease in patients undergoing dialysis. N Engl J Med 2012;367(26):2482–94.

161. Baigent C, Landray MJ, Reith C, et al, SHARP Investigators. The effects of lowering LDL cholesterol with simvastatin plus ezetimibe in patients with chronic kidney disease (Study of Heart and Renal Protection): a randomised placebo-controlled trial. Lancet 2011;377(9784):2181–92.

162. Kidney Disease Outcomes Quality Initiative (K/DOQI). Clinical practice guidelines on hypertension and antihypertensive agents in chronic kidney disease. Am J Kidney Dis 2004;43(5 Suppl 1): S1–290.

163. Kidney Disease Outcomes Quality Initiative (K/DOQI). Clinical practice guidelines and clinical practice recommendations for diabetes and chronic kidney disease. Am J Kidney Dis 2007; 49(2 Suppl 2):S12–154.

164. Kidney Disease Improving Global Outcomes (KDIGO). Clinical practice guideline for the diagnosis, evaluation, prevention, and treatment of chronic kidney disease—mineral and bone disorder (CKD-MBD). Treatment of CKD-MBD targeted at lowering high serum phosphorus and maintaining serum calcium. Kidney Int 2009;76(Suppl 113): S50–69.

165. Herzog CA, Mangrum JM, Passman R. Sudden cardiac death and dialysis patients. Semin Dial 2008;21(4):300–7.

166. Ronco C, McCullough PA, Anker SD, et al, Acute Dialysis Quality Initiative (ADQI) consensus group. Cardiorenal syndromes: an executive summary from the consensus conference of the Acute Dialysis Quality Initiative (ADQI). Contrib Nephrol 2010;165:54–67.

167. Lundy DJ, Trzeciak S. Microcirculatory dysfunction in sepsis. Crit Care Clin 2009;25(4):721–31.

168. Trzeciak S, Dellinger RP, Parrillo JE, et al. Early microcirculatory perfusion derangements in patients with severe sepsis and septic shock: relationship to hemodynamics, oxygen transport, and survival. Ann Emerg Med 2007;49(1):88–98, 98.e1–2.

169. Jardin F, Brun-Ney D, Auvert B, et al. Sepsis-related cardiogenic shock. Crit Care Med 1990;18(10):1055–60.

170. Lambermont B, Ghuysen A, Kolh P, et al. Effects of endotoxic shock on right ventricular systolic function and mechanical efficiency. Cardiovasc Res 2003;59(2):412–8.

171. Parker MM, Shelhamer JH, Bacharach SL, et al. Profound but reversible myocardial depression in patients with septic shock. Ann Intern Med 1984;100(4):483–90.

172. Dhainaut JF, Huyghebaert MF, Monsallier JF, et al. Coronary hemodynamics and myocardial metabolism of lactate, free fatty acids, glucose, and ketones in patients with septic shock. Circulation 1987;75(3):533–41.

173. Kumar A, Thota V, Dee L, et al. Tumor necrosis factor alpha and interleukin 1beta are responsible for in vitro myocardial cell depression induced by human septic shock serum. J Exp Med 1996;183(3):949–58.

174. Torre-Amione G, Kapadia S, Benedict C, et al. Proinflammatory cytokine levels in patients with depressed left ventricular ejection fraction: a report from the Studies of Left Ventricular Dysfunction (SOLVD). J Am Coll Cardiol 1996;27(5):1201–6.

175. Benes J, Chvojka J, Sykora R, et al. Searching for mechanisms that matter in early septic acute kidney injury: an experimental study. Crit Care 2011;15(5):R256.

176. Bougle A, Duranteau J. Pathophysiology of sepsis-induced acute kidney injury: the role of global renal blood flow and renal vascular resistance. Contrib Nephrol 2011;174:89–97.

177. Schmidt H, Hoyer D, Hennen R, et al. Autonomic dysfunction predicts both 1- and 2-month mortality in middle-aged patients with multiple organ dysfunction syndrome. Crit Care Med 2008;36(3):967–70.

178. Tateishi Y, Oda S, Nakamura M, et al. Depressed heart rate variability is associated with high IL-6 blood level and decline in the blood pressure in septic patients. Shock 2007;28(5):549–53.

179. Ramchandra R, Wan L, Hood SG, et al. Septic shock induces distinct changes in sympathetic nerve activity to the heart and kidney in conscious sheep. Am J Physiol Regul Integr Comp Physiol 2009;297(5):R1247–53.

180. Doerschug KC, Delsing AS, Schmidt GA, et al. Renin-angiotensin system activation correlates with microvascular dysfunction in a prospective cohort study of clinical sepsis. Crit Care 2010;14(1):R24.

181. Shen L, Mo H, Cai L, et al. Losartan prevents sepsis-induced acute lung injury and decreases activation of nuclear factor kappaB and mitogen-activated protein kinases. Shock 2009;31(5):500–6.

182. Hagiwara S, Iwasaka H, Matumoto S, et al. Effects of an angiotensin-converting enzyme inhibitor on the inflammatory response in in vivo and in vitro models. Crit Care Med 2009;37(2):626–33.

183. Mortensen EM, Iwasaka H, Matumoto S, et al. Impact of previous statin and angiotensin II receptor blocker use on mortality in patients hospitalized with sepsis. Pharmacotherapy 2007;27(12):1619–26.

184. Soni A, Pepper GM, Wyrwinski PM, et al. Adrenal insufficiency occurring during septic shock: incidence, outcome, and relationship to peripheral cytokine levels. Am J Med 1995;98(3):266–71.

185. Sligl WI, Milner DA Jr, Sundar S, et al. Safety and efficacy of corticosteroids for the treatment of septic shock: a systematic review and meta-analysis. Clin Infect Dis 2009;49(1):93–101.

186. Burchill L, Velkoska E, Dean RG, et al. Acute kidney injury in the rat causes cardiac remodelling and increases angiotensin-converting enzyme 2 expression. Exp Physiol 2008;93(5):622–30.

187. Tokuyama H, Kelly DJ, Zhang Y, et al. Macrophage infiltration and cellular proliferation in the non-ischemic kidney and heart following prolonged unilateral renal ischemia. Nephron Physiol 2007;106(3):p54–62.

188. Chopra M, Golden HB, Mullapudi S, et al. Modulation of myocardial mitochondrial mechanisms during severe polymicrobial sepsis in the rat. PLoS One 2011;6(6):e21285.

189. Liu M, Grigoryev DN, Crow MT, et al. Transcription factor Nrf2 is protective during ischemic and nephrotoxic acute kidney injury in mice. Kidney Int 2009;76(3):277–85.

190. Celes MR, Prado CM, Rossi MA. Sepsis: going to the heart of the matter. Pathobiology 2013;80(2):70–86.

191. Stengl M, Bartak F, Sykora R, et al. Reduced L-type calcium current in ventricular myocytes from pigs with hyperdynamic septic shock. Crit Care Med 2010;38(2):579–87.

192. Good DW, George T, Watts BA 3rd. Toll-like receptor 2 mediates inhibition of HCO(3)(-) absorption by bacterial lipoprotein in medullary thick ascending limb. Am J Physiol Renal Physiol 2010;299(3):F536–44.

193. Schreiber A, Theilig F, Schweda F, et al. Acute endotoxemia in mice induces downregulation of megalin and cubilin in the kidney. Kidney Int 2012;82(1):53–9.

194. Reinhart K, Bauer M, Riedemann NC, et al. New approaches to sepsis: molecular diagnostics and biomarkers. Clin Microbiol Rev 2012;25(4):609–34.

195. Dellinger RP, Levy MM, Carlet JM, et al. Surviving sepsis campaign: international guidelines for management of severe sepsis and septic shock: 2008. Crit Care Med 2008;36(1):296–327.

196. Vignon P, Frank MB, Lesage J, et al. Hand-held echocardiography with Doppler capability for the assessment of critically-ill patients: is it reliable? Intensive Care Med 2004;30(4):718–23.

197. Bellomo R, Ronco C, Kellum JA, et al. Acute renal failure—definition, outcome measures, animal models, fluid therapy and information technology needs: the Second International Consensus Conference of the Acute Dialysis Quality Initiative (ADQI) Group. Crit Care 2004;8(4):R204–12.

198. Mehta RL, Kellum JA, Shah SV, et al. Acute Kidney Injury Network: report of an initiative to improve outcomes in acute kidney injury. Crit Care 2007;11(2): R31.

199. Khwaja A. KDIGO Clinical Practice Guidelines for Acute Kidney Injury. Nephron Clin Pract 2012; 120(4):179–84.

200. Calvin JE, Driedger AA, Sibbald WJ. An assessment of myocardial function in human sepsis utilizing ECG gated cardiac scintigraphy. Chest 1981; 80(5):579–86.

201. Liu KD, Thompson BT, Ancukiewicz M, et al. Acute kidney injury in patients with acute lung injury: impact of fluid accumulation on classification of acute kidney injury and associated outcomes. Crit Care Med 2011;39(12):2665–71.

202. Bellomo R, Prowle JR, Echeverri JE, et al. Fluid management in septic acute kidney injury and cardiorenal syndromes. Contrib Nephrol 2010;165: 206–18.

203. De Vriese AS, Colardyn FA, Philippé JJ, et al. Cytokine removal during continuous hemofiltration in septic patients. J Am Soc Nephrol 1999;10(4): 846–53.

204. Tapia P, Chinchón E, Morales D, et al. Effectiveness of short-term 6-hour high-volume hemofiltration during refractory severe septic shock. J Trauma Acute Care Surg 2012;72(5):1228–37 [discussion: 1237–8].

205. Matson J, Zydney A, Honore PM. Blood filtration: new opportunities and the implications of systems biology. Crit Care Resusc 2004;6(3):209–17.

206. Nakamura M, Oda S, Sadahiro T, et al. Treatment of severe sepsis and septic shock by CHDF using a PMMA membrane hemofilter as a cytokine modulator. Contrib Nephrol 2010;166:73–82.

207. Cruz DN, Antonelli M, Fumagalli R, et al. Early use of polymyxin B hemoperfusion in abdominal septic shock: the EUPHAS randomized controlled trial. JAMA 2009;301(23):2445–52.

208. Humes HD, Antonelli M, Fumagalli R, et al. A selective cytopheretic inhibitory device to treat the immunological dysregulation of acute and chronic renal failure. Blood Purif 2010;29(2):183–90.

209. Hou ZQ, Sun ZX, Su CY, et al. Effect of levosimendan on estimated glomerular filtration rate in hospitalized patients with decompensated heart failure and renal dysfunction. Cardiovasc Ther 2012. http://dx.doi.org/10.1111/cdr.12001.

210. Ristikankare A, Pöyhiä R, Eriksson H, et al. Effects of levosimendan on renal function in patients undergoing coronary artery surgery. J Cardiothorac Vasc Anesth 2012;26(4):591–5.

211. Chou YH, Huang TM, Wu VC, et al. Impact of timing of renal replacement therapy initiation on outcome of septic acute kidney injury. Crit Care 2011; 15(3):R134.

212. Bellomo R, Wan L, May C. Vasoactive drugs and acute kidney injury. Crit Care Med 2008;36(Suppl 4): S179–86.

213. Schmoelz M, Schelling G, Dunker M, et al. Comparison of systemic and renal effects of dopexamine and dopamine in norepinephrine-treated septic shock. J Cardiothorac Vasc Anesth 2006;20(2): 173–8.

214. Cobas M, Paparcuri G, De La Pena M, et al. Fenoldopam in critically ill patients with early renal dysfunction. A crossover study. Cardiovasc Ther 2011;29(4):280–4.

215. Landoni G, et al. Fenoldopam in cardiac surgery-associated acute kidney injury. Int J Artif Organs 2008;31(6):561.

216. Redfors B, Bragadottir G, Sellgren J, et al. Effects of norepinephrine on renal perfusion, filtration and oxygenation in vasodilatory shock and acute kidney injury. Intensive Care Med 2011;37(1):60–7.

217. Guzman JA, Rosado AE, Kruse JA. Vasopressin vs norepinephrine in endotoxic shock: systemic, renal, and splanchnic hemodynamic and oxygen transport effects. J Appl Physiol (1985) 2003; 95(2):803–9.

218. Gordon AC, Russell JA, Walley KR, et al. The effects of vasopressin on acute kidney injury in septic shock. Intensive Care Med 2010;36(1):83–91.

219. Nigwekar SU, Waikar SS. Diuretics in acute kidney injury. Semin Nephrol 2011;31(6):523–34.

Anemia and Iron Deficiency in Heart Failure

Natasha P. Arora, MD[a], Jalal K. Ghali, MD[b],*

KEYWORDS

- Anemia • Iron deficiency • Heart failure • Iron therapy • Erythropoiesis-stimulating agents

KEY POINTS

- Anemia is highly prevalent in patients with heart failure (HF), and is associated with poor prognosis.
- Among anemic HF patients, iron deficiency is the most common form of hematinic deficiency.
- Iron deficiency in HF patients, with or without anemia, confers increased risk of mortality and morbidity.
- Erythropoiesis-stimulating agents are no longer an option in the treatment in HF patients with anemia, based on the results of the RED-HF trial.
- Although intravenous iron supplementation improves functional outcomes in anemic HF patients, long-term, adequately powered, randomized, placebo-controlled trials of intravenous iron assessing morbidity and mortality are required before any firm recommendations about its use can be made.

INTRODUCTION

Anemia is a common comorbid condition in patients with heart failure (HF),[1,2] and is associated with adverse outcomes in this patient population.[3] The etiology of anemia in HF patients is multifactorial,[2,4] and in most of these patients more than one mechanism is involved. Iron deficiency is the commonest cause of anemia worldwide.[5] Even in anemic HF patients, iron deficiency is the most common form of hematinic deficiency, regardless of renal function status.[4] Iron deficiency, with or without anemia, confers increased risk of mortality and morbidity in HF patients, and iron supplementation improves functional status.[4] This article reviews current knowledge regarding anemia and iron deficiency in HF patients.

EPIDEMIOLOGIC INSIGHTS

Depending on the definition used and patient population studied, prevalence of anemia in HF patients varies from 9% to 70%.[1,2,6,7] There are no HF-specific criteria to define anemia, and definitions based on large samples from the third US National Health and Nutrition Examination Survey and the Scripps-Kaiser database propose the following: hemoglobin less than 13.7 mg/dL and less than 12.9 mg/dL in white and black men, respectively, and less than 12.2 mg/dL and less than 11.5 mg/dL in white and black women, respectively. Using the World Health Organization definition (hemoglobin <12 g/dL in women and <13 g/dL in men), a prevalence of 22% to 46% in HF patients have been reported.[3]

Anemia is associated with increased morbidity and mortality in HF patients. In a meta-analysis of HF patients, presence of anemia almost doubled the mortality risk (odds ratio 1.96; 95% confidence interval [CI] 1.74–2.21; $P<.001$).[3] In addition to increased risk of mortality, anemia in HF patients is also associated with increased risk of various morbidities such as cognitive

Conflict of Interest: Dr J.K. Ghali has received research grants from Amgen and served on the steering committee of the RED-HF trial. Dr N.P. Arora has no conflicts of interest or financial ties to disclose.
[a] Division of Cardiovascular Services, Saint John Hospital and Medical Center, 22101 Moross Road, Detroit, MI 48236, USA; [b] Division of Cardiology, School of Medicine, Mercer University, 707 Pine Street, Macon, GA 31201, USA
* Corresponding author.
E-mail address: ghali_jk@mercer.edu

impairment,[8] increased number of hospitalizations,[9] higher New York Heart Association (NYHA) functional class,[10] lower exercise capacity,[11] and worse quality of life.[12]

Iron deficiency is the most common form of hematinic deficiency among anemic HF patients.[4] Depending on the definition and diagnostic criteria used, the reported prevalence of iron deficiency in HF patients varies widely. In a study of 955 HF patients with 32% prevalence of anemia, 52% of the anemic and 17% of nonanemic patients had evidence of iron and/or ferritin deficiency, defined as iron less than 8 μmol/L and ferritin less than 30 μg/L.[13] In another prospective study of patients with decompensated advanced HF, bone marrow aspiration showed evidence of iron deficiency in 73% of patients.[14] A ferritin level of less than 100 μg/L, and a ferritin level of 100 to 300 μg/L along with transferrin saturation of less than 20%, have been used as a diagnostic criteria for iron deficiency.[15,16] Using these criteria, a prospective observational study of 546 patients identified iron deficiency in 37% of all patients with stable systolic HF; 57% of the anemic HF patients and 32% of the nonanemic HF patients.[15] Iron deficiency was more common in females and patients with advanced NYHA class, higher plasma N-terminal pro–brain natriuretic peptide (NT-proBNP) levels, and higher serum high-sensitivity C-reactive protein. In an international pooled cohort of 1506 patients with chronic HF, iron deficiency was present in 753 (50%) of the patients, 61.2% of anemic patients, and 45.6% of nonanemic patients.[16] In another study of patients with chronic HF, deranged iron homeostasis characterized by diminished circulating (decreased transferrin saturation) and functional (decreased mean cell hemoglobin concentration) iron status with adequate stores (ferritin levels) was seen in both anemic and nonanemic HF patients.[17]

From a prognostic standpoint, in HF patients both anemia and iron deficiency are associated with adverse outcomes such as reduced exercise capacity, increased rate of hospitalizations, and impaired quality of life. Many published studies have demonstrated a strong association between anemia and mortality in HF patients. A meta-analysis of 34 such studies demonstrated a significantly higher risk of mortality in anemic chronic HF patients in comparison with nonanemic patients, even after adjustment for potential confounders.[3]

Iron deficiency even without anemia is associated with an increased risk of mortality and morbidity. In a study of 157 patients with HF, patients with iron-deficiency anemia had a 4-fold increased risk of death compared with iron-replete patients with or without anemia and a 2-fold increased risk of death in comparison with those with nonanemic iron deficiency.[17] Similarly, in a prospective observational study of 546 patients, iron deficiency was associated with an increased risk of death or heart transplantations (adjusted hazard ratio 1.58; 95% CI 1.14–2.17; P<.01), independent of the presence of anemia.[15] Among the international pooled cohort of 1506 patients with chronic HF, iron deficiency (but not anemia) was a strong and independent predictor of mortality in the multivariable hazard models (hazard ratio 1.42; 95% CI 1.14–1.77; P = .002).[16] Iron deficiency also independently predicts exercise intolerance in patients with systolic chronic HF, although the strength of these associations is relatively weak.[18] Just as importantly, health-related quality of life was negatively affected in iron-deficient chronic HF patients, with demonstrable improvement after intravenous iron therapy, independent of anemia status.[19]

PATHOPHYSIOLOGIC INTERACTION

Although the pathogenesis of anemia in HF is not yet fully delineated, factors such as reduced erythropoietin (EPO) production, EPO resistance, chronic kidney disease, inflammation, diabetes, hemodilution, gastrointestinal malabsorption and blood loss, absolute and functional iron deficiency, and drugs such as angiotensin-converting enzyme (ACE) inhibitors and angiotensin receptor blockers are believed to be contributing to the development of anemia in this patient population.[2,4,20,21]

Proinflammatory Cytokines

Elevated levels of circulating proinflammatory cytokines, such as tumor necrosis factor α, interleukin (IL)-1, and IL-6 observed in HF patients cause anemia of chronic disease.[22] Proinflammatory cytokines produce changes in EPO production, proliferation of erythroid progenitor cells, iron homeostasis, and the life span of red blood cells.[22]

Decreased EPO Production/EPO Resistance

Activation of the renin-angiotensin-aldosterone system and the sympathetic nervous system in HF patients leads to renal hypoperfusion and tissue hypoxia, causing increased EPO production. Elevated angiotensin II increases EPO production by causing renal hypoperfusion and also by direct stimulation of EPO production.[23] Chronic HF is associated with elevated proinflammatory cytokines, which may not only cause decreased EPO production but also resistance to its actions on bone marrow.[24,25] EPO levels in HF patients are lower than expected, possibly attributable to the action of proinflammatory cytokines.[24,26] Chronic kidney disease or milder forms of renal dysfunction are common in HF patients, and may contribute to decreased EPO production.

ACE Inhibitors/Angiotensin Receptor Blockers

ACE inhibitors and angiotensin receptor blockers cause a decrease in the levels of angiotensin II. Angiotensin II leads to increased EPO production and also to a breakdown of an inhibitor of hematopoiesis, namely N-acetyl-seryl-aspartyl-lysyl-proline. Therefore, ACE inhibitors and angiotensin receptor blockers lead to decreased EPO production and inhibition of hematopoiesis.

Iron-Deficiency Anemia

The etiology of iron deficiency in HF patients is also multifactorial; some of the proposed etiologic factors include poor nutritional intake, intestinal malabsorption resulting from bowel wall edema, cardiac cachexia, increased gastrointestinal blood loss owing to frequent use of chronic antiplatelet and oral anticoagulation therapy, and proinflammatory cytokine activation causing disordered iron homeostasis (**Fig. 1**).[2] Iron deficiency in HF patients may be functional, due to impaired iron metabolism with normal iron stores, or absolute, due to depletion of iron stores.[27,28] Impaired iron metabolism may be secondary to inflammatory processes[26,27] as HF, like other chronic conditions, is associated with activation of proinflammatory and anti-inflammatory processes.

Although it is known that the absorption of iron from intestine is impaired in HF patients, the exact mechanism of impaired iron absorption is not fully understood. Laboratory data from rat studies indicate that abnormal intestinal iron absorption seen in HF patients might be due to the impaired expression of duodenal iron transporters.[29] Hepcidin, an iron-regulatory hormone, is known to play an important role in HF patients.[30,31] In laboratory experiments in mice, overexpression of hepcidin results in severe iron-deficiency anemia, and the mice deficient in hepcidin are protected from inflammation-related iron-deficiency anemia.[32] Hepcidin, a key regulator of iron metabolism, is also a mediator of anemia during inflammation by trapping iron in the reticuloendothelial system and making it unavailable to bone marrow erythropoiesis.[28] IL-6 and other inflammatory cytokines increase the hepatic production and release of hepcidin, which binds to the iron exporter channel, ferroportin, present on liver Kupffer cells and macrophages. The hepcidin-ferroportin complex is internalized and degraded by lysosomes, and the lack of ferroportin prevents the release of iron from these cells in the liver.[33,34] Hepcidin also blocks the uptake of dietary iron into the bloodstream through its action on the cells of the gut mucosa. Therefore, this small peptide hormone blocks iron absorption from the intestine, and also limits the release of iron for erythropoiesis by downregulating the iron-exporter protein ferroportin. Decreased intestinal iron absorption causes absolute iron deficiency, and reticuloendothelial block causes functional iron deficiency. Iron deficiency may also result from impaired iron absorption and availability caused by inflammatory cytokines including IL-6.[22]

In a small study of patients with HF, anemia, and renal failure, hepcidin levels were associated with markers of iron load but not with inflammation, and a greater decrease in hepcidin was associated with a better response to erythropoietin.[35] Furthermore, in another small study of patients with HF, hepcidin levels were found to be either decreased or similar to those of controls.[31] In a recently published study of 321 patients with chronic systolic HF, early stage of HF was characterized by elevated hepcidin levels not accompanied by anemia or inflammation.[36] With progression of HF, the circulating hepcidin level declined and iron deficiency developed. In multivariable Cox hazard models, low hepcidin was independently associated with increased 3-year mortality in HF patients ($P<.001$). Therefore, the role of hepcidin in patients with HF needs more clarification.

In addition to its key role in erythropoiesis, iron is also involved in oxygen transport (as hemoglobin), storage (as myoglobin), and utilization, and energy production (as cytochromes and iron-sulfur enzymes in electron transport of mitochondria) in skeletal and cardiac myocytes.[37] Iron-containing proteins are also involved in the metabolism of catecholamines, collagen, and tyrosine. Iron is also involved in the synthesis and degradation of lipids, carbohydrates, and nucleic acids.[38] Serving as a metal cofactor for nonheme iron-containing proteins or hemoproteins, iron is important for sustaining life. Normal iron metabolism is crucial for cells with a high turnover (eg, tumor cells and hematopoietic cells) and high energy demand (eg, skeletal myocytes and cardiomyocytes).[38–42] Iron deficiency, with or without concomitant anemia, may exacerbate several chronic diseases.[27,40,43] In addition to impairment of erythropoiesis, iron deficiency has clinical consequences deriving from impaired oxidative metabolism, cellular energy production, and immune mechanisms.[27,40,41,44,45]

Animal data suggest that chronic iron deficiency causes structural abnormalities in the heart, such as increased heart weight and size.[46] Exercise

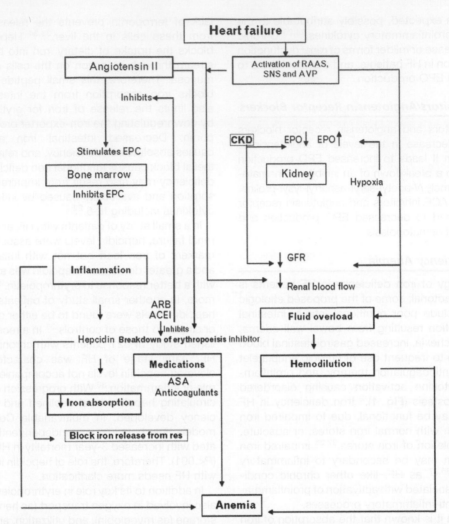

Fig. 1. Causes and mechanisms of anemia in heart failure. ACEI, angiotensin-converting enzyme inhibitor; ARB, angiotensin receptor blocker; ASA, acetylsalicylic acid; AVP, arginine vasopressin; CKD, chronic kidney disease; EPC, erythrocyte progenitor cell; EPO, erythropoietin; GFR, glomerular filtration rate; RAAS, renin-angiotensin-aldosterone system; RES, reticuloendothelial system; SNS, sympathetic nervous system.

intolerance in HF patients is mediated by reduced cardiac output reserve, and skeletal muscle changes such as impaired blood-flow regulation and abnormalities in skeletal muscle mass and metabolism.[47] These cardiac and skeletal muscle changes affect both endurance capacity and maximal performance.[37,48,49]

A study by Maeder and colleagues[50] demonstrated reduced iron content and transferrin receptor 1 (TfR1) expression in the myocardium of patients with HF, compared with controls. It has been speculated that myocardial iron depletion, perhaps caused by neurohumorally mediated TfR1 downregulation, contributes to decline in systolic function and clinical progression in patients with HF. This notion is pathophysiologically plausible, given the crucial role that iron plays in

cellular function in general and oxidative metabolism in particular, especially in metabolically active tissue.[20] Although attractive, this hypothesis needs confirmation.

DIAGNOSTIC ISSUES

In healthy subjects, iron stores and deficiency are assessed by measuring various biomarkers such as serum concentrations of iron, ferritin, and transferrin. Ferritin, which is used to define the presence of iron deficiency in healthy individuals, is an acute-phase reactant and may be falsely elevated in patients with HF. Therefore, ferritin levels in HF patients may be normal even in the presence of underlying absolute iron deficiency, making it difficult to diagnose iron-deficiency anemia in this patient population.[51] Thus, the altered iron metabolism in HF patients results in changes in the laboratory parameters used to diagnose anemia of chronic disease. In addition to the elevation in serum ferritin as an acute-phase reactant, inflammation also decreases serum iron and transferrin levels, thereby limiting the diagnostic role of their measurement as indicators of iron deficiency.[51]

Standard laboratory cutoff values for these iron parameters developed to diagnose absolute iron deficiency in healthy individuals may not be appropriate for the diagnosis of functional iron deficiency. Therefore, the overall incidence of iron deficiency may be much higher when techniques such as bone marrow aspirates are used. Although bone marrow examination is a definitive standard, its utility is limited by cost, inconvenience to the patient, and the need for resources and expertise. Moreover, its results depend on the quality of specimen obtained.[52]

The transferrin receptor is a soluble truncated form of the receptor, and can be measured in serum. Considering that soluble transferrin receptor (sTfR) increases on erythroid precursors only if they are deficient in iron regardless of iron stores, a combination of serum ferritin and sTfR concentrations can be used as an alternative to bone marrow examination for the diagnosis of functional iron deficiency.[52] As the serum concentration of sTfR is highly sensitive but not specific to marrow iron deficiency, it cannot be used as an isolated test.[52–54] Similarly, serum ferritin has high specificity, but low sensitivity, for bone marrow iron stores.[52] These 2 parameters (serum ferritin and sTfR) may be combined by calculating the ferritin index, the ratio of serum sTfR to the logarithm of serum ferritin level.[55] The ferritin index is a useful sensitive and specific indicator of the iron supply for erythropoiesis, which can be combined with a marker of functional iron deficiency, such as reticulocyte hemoglobin content, in the form of a graph or diagnostic plot.[56] This plot is a useful tool for diagnosing and differentiating different states of iron deficiency, and may help predict those patients who will respond to iron and/or erythropoiesis-stimulating agents (ESAs).[57]

In a recent attempt to assess myocardial iron load (M-Iron), ferritin (M-FR), and transferrin receptor (M-sTfR) in HF patients in relation to serum iron markers, An analysis on failing ventricular myocardium obtained from 33 consecutive patients referred to heart transplantation showed that myocardial iron load was significantly lower in the failing heart and did not correlate with serum iron level.[58] sTfR was the most reliable parameter to define iron status (a negative correlation with M-Iron) and homeostasis (negative correlation with M-FR; positive correlation with M-sTfR) in the failing myocardium. As serum sTfR correlates with myocardial iron load (M-Iron), storage capacity (M-FR), and acquisition (M-sTfR), its measurement should be strongly considered in the assessment of myocardial iron stores in HF populations, especially in those HF patients who are being considered for iron supplementation therapy (**Box 1**).

THERAPEUTIC ISSUES

The strong association between anemia and poor outcomes in patients with HF stimulated a surge of clinical studies to assess the effect of treating anemia in these patients. An extensive experience has been accumulated with the use of ESAs to raise hemoglobin, and to a lesser extent with the use of intravenous iron supplementation.

Erythropoiesis-Stimulating Agents

Several studies have assessed the potential role of ESAs in the treatment of anemia in patients with HF (**Table 1**).[59–68] Combined analysis of 3 double-blind, placebo-controlled studies[61–63] suggested an improvement in outcome.[69] A meta-analysis of 11 small, randomized controlled trials with 794 participants showed that treatment with ESAs significantly improved exercise duration, 6-minute walk distance, peak oxygen consumption, NYHA functional class, ejection fraction, BNP levels, quality of life, and HF-related hospitalizations.[70] With the limited number of events reported, there was no associated increase in adverse events or mortality (odds ratio 0.58; 95% CI 0.34–0.99; $P = .047$). This meta-analysis suggested that ESA treatment in anemic HF patients can improve exercise tolerance, reduce symptoms, and have benefits on clinical outcomes.[70] The largest multicenter, randomized, double-blind, placebo-controlled trial (N = 2278) of ESAs in HF anemic patients, known as the

---

Box 1
Recommended laboratory tests

Iron profile including: serum iron, transferrin (total iron-binding capacity), transferrin saturation, and ferritin

Vitamin B_{12} and folic acid serum levels

Thyroid function studies

Serum creatinine and estimated glomerular filtration rate

Consider measuring soluble transferrin receptor

Table 1
Studies on the use of erythropoiesis-stimulating agents in anemic patients with heart failure

Authors,[Ref.] Year	Patients Enrolled	Study Design	Follow-up Duration	ESA Used	Inclusion Criteria/Patient Characteristics	Outcomes
Silverberg et al,[59] 2001	32	Randomized, single-center	8.2 mo	EPO	LVEF ≤40% Hb 10–11.5 g/dL	Improvement in NYHA class, LVEF, need for furosemide, and length of hospital stay
Mancini et al,[60] 2003	26 enrolled 23 completed study	Randomized, single-blind, single-center	3 mo	EPO-α	NYHA III–IV Hct <35% Serum creatinine <2.5 mg/dL EPO level <100 mU/ml	Improvement in exercise capacity and quality of life
Ponikowski et al,[61] 2007	41	Randomized, double-blind, placebo-controlled, multicenter	27 wk	Darbepoetin-α	Age ≥21 y with symptomatic HF Hb ≥9 g/dL to ≤12 g/dL LVEF ≤40% Transferrin saturation >15% Serum creatinine ≤3 mg/dL BP <160/100, exercise limitation on treadmill	Improvement in health-related quality of life, trend toward improvement in exercise capacity
Van Veldhuisen et al,[62] 2007	165	Randomized, double-blind, placebo-controlled, multicenter	26 wk	Darbepoetin-α	CHF ≥3 wk LVEF ≤40% Hb 9%–12.5%	Improvement in Kansas City Cardiomyopathy Questionnaire score, no change in NYHA class, LVEF, and Minnesota Living with HF Questionnaire score, 6/110 treatment-related deaths
Ghali et al,[63] 2008 (STAMINA-HeFT Trial)	319	Randomized, double-blind, placebo-controlled, multicenter	12 mo	Darbepoetin-α	Symptomatic HF Hb ≥9 g/dL to ≤12 g/dL LVEF ≤40%	No improvement in exercise duration, NYHA class or quality of life score. Trend toward lower risk of all-cause mortality or first HF hospitalization

Study	N	Design	Duration	Agent	Inclusion Criteria	Outcomes
Parissis et al,[64] 2008	32	Randomized, single-blind, placebo-controlled, single-center	3 mo	Darbepoetin-α	NYHA II–III, LVEF <40%, Hb <12.5 g/dL, Serum creatinine <2.5 mg/dL	Improvement in LVEF, NYHA class, plasma BNP levels, and 6-min walk test score
Kourea et al,[65] 2008	41	Randomized, single-blind, placebo-controlled, single-center	3 mo	Darbepoetin-α	NYHA II–III, LVEF <40%, Hb <12.5 g/dL, Serum creatinine <2.5 mg/dL	Improvement in exercise capacity, quality of life, and psychosocial status
Parissis et al,[66] 2009	30	Randomized, single-blind, placebo-controlled, single-center	3 mo	Darbepoetin-α	NYHA II–IV, LVEF <40%, Hb <12.5 g/dL, Serum creatinine <2.5 mg/dL	Improvement in LVEF, 6-min walk distance, plasma BNP levels, and mediators of oxidative and nitrosative stress
Cosyns et al,[67] 2010	28	Randomized, placebo-controlled, single-center	2 mo	EPO	LVEF <45%, Hb <12 g/dL, Creatinine clearance <45 mL/min	Improvement in LVEF, LV volumes, mitral regurgitation severity, and hemodynamics
Swedberg et al,[68] 2013 (RED-HF Trial)	2278	Randomized, double-blind, placebo-controlled, multicenter	28 mo	Darbepoetin-α	NYHA II–IV, LVEF ≤40%, Hb 9–12 g/dL, Transferrin saturation >15%, Serum creatinine <3 mg/dL, BP <160/100	No improvement in clinical outcomes including primary outcome of death or hospitalization from worsening HF. Increase in the risk of thromboembolic events. Findings do not support the use of darbepoetin-α in patients with systolic HF and mild to moderate anemia

Abbreviations: BNP, brain natriuretic peptide; BP, blood pressure (mm Hg); CHF, congestive heart failure; EPO, erythropoietin; ESA, erythropoiesis-stimulating agent; Hb, hemoglobin; Hct, hematocrit; HF, heart failure; LV, left ventricular; LVEF, left ventricular ejection fraction; NYHA, New York Heart Association functional class.

Data from Refs.[59–68]

Table 2
Studies on the use of intravenous iron supplementation in patients with heart failure

Authors, Ref. Year	Study Design	No. of Patients	Disease Severity	Follow-up Time	Pretreatment Hemoglobin g/dL (mean ± SD)	Posttreatment Hemoglobin g/dL (mean ± SD)	Results/Conclusions	Safety
Bolger et al,[71] 2006	Prospective, uncontrolled study	16	NYHA functional class II or III	92 ± 6 d	11.2 ± 0.7	12.6 ± 1.2 (*P* value for treatment effect = .0007)	Improvement in NYHA functional class (*P*<.02), MLHF score (*P* = .002), and 6-min walk distance (*P* = .01)	No adverse events reported
Toblli et al,[72] 2007	Prospective, randomized, double-blind, placebo-controlled study	Total = 40 Control group (Group A) = 20 Treatment group (Group B) = 20 2:1 Randomization	NYHA functional class II, III, or IV Ejection fraction ≤35%	6 mo	Group A: 10.2 ± 0.5 Group B: 10.3 ± 0.6	Group A: 9.8 ± 0.6 Group B: 11.8 ± 0.7 (*P* value for treatment effect <.01)	Reduction in NT-proBNP (*P*<.01) and CRP (*P*<.01) Improvement in LVEF, NYHA functional class, exercise capacity, renal function, and quality of life (all *P*<.01), and fewer hospitalizations	No side effects reported
Okonko et al,[73] 2008 (FERRIC-HF study)	Randomized, controlled, observer-blind study	Total = 35 Control group (Group A) = 11 Treatment group (Group B) = 24 2:1 Randomization	NYHA functional class II or III Peak oxygen consumption (pVo$_2$) = 14 ± 2.7 mL/kg/min	18 wk	Group A: 12.2 ± 1 Group B: 12.6 ± 1.2	Group A: 12.6 ± 1.1 Group B: 13.2 ± 1.1 (*P* value for treatment effect <.05)	Significant increase in pVo$_2$/kg (*P* = .01) Significant improvement in NYHA class (*P* = .007) and Patient Global Assessment (0.002)	Adverse events occurred in 42% in iron group vs 64% in control group

Usmanov et al,[74] 2008	Uncontrolled, longitudinal study	32	NYHA functional class III or IV	26 wk	NYHA class III patients: 10.7 ± 0.4 NYHA class IV patients: 9.4 ± 0.6	NYHA class III patients: 13.7 ± 0.4 NYHA class IV patients: 12.7 ± 0.8 (P value for treatment effect <.05 in both groups)	Improvement in cardiac remodeling and NYHA classification in patients with baseline NYHA class III (P<.01)	No adverse effects reported
Drakos et al,[75] 2009	Randomized, unblinded	Total = 16 Group A (IV iron) = 8 Group B (IV iron + erythropoietin) = 8 1:1 Randomization	All patients had chronic HF and iron-deficiency anemia verified by bone marrow aspiration	3 mo	Group A: 10.7 ± 1.2 Group B: 10.2 ± 0.7	Group A: 13.1 ± 0.6 Group B: 13.0 ± 0.8 (P values for treatment effect <.05 for within-group comparisons)	The time course and degree of anemia correction after treatment with IV iron vs combined IV iron + erythropoietin, were similar (within-group comparison: P<.05, between-group comparison: P = nonsignificant)	No adverse effects reported
Anker et al,[76] 2009 (FAIR-HF study)	Randomized, multicenter, prospective, double-blind, placebo-controlled study	Total = 459 Control group (Group A) = 155 Treatment group (Group B) = 304 2:1 Randomization	NYHA functional class II or III	24 wk	Group A: 11.9 ± 1.4 Group B: 11.9 ± 1.3	Group A: 12.5 ± 0.1 Group B: 13.0 ± 0.1 (P value for mean treatment effect <.001)	Significant improvement in 7-Point Patient Global Assessment Scale, NYHA class, 6-min walk test, and quality of life (KCCQ) questionnaire (all P<.001) Similar effect in patients with and without anemia	Slightly more gastrointestinal disorders (16.9% vs 6.9% in iron and control groups, respectively, P = .06)

(continued on next page)

Table 2
(continued)

Authors,[Ref.] Year	Study Design	No. of Patients	Disease Severity	Follow-up Time	Pretreatment Hemoglobin g/dL (mean ± SD)	Posttreatment Hemoglobin g/dL (mean ± SD)	Results/Conclusions	Safety
Beck-da-Silva et al,[77] 2013 (IRON-HF study)	Randomized, multicenter, prospective, double-blind, placebo-controlled trial	Total = 23 Group 1 (IV iron) = 10 Group 2 (PO iron) = 7 Group 3 (placebo) = 6	NYHA functional class II–IV LVEF <40%	3 mo	Group 1: 11.2 ± 0.6 Group 2: 11.3 ± 0.5 Group 3: 10.9 ± 0.7	Not specified, no statistically significant difference between study groups	No statistically significant difference between study groups for maximal oxygen consumption (pVo₂) Correction of anemia seems to be similar between PO iron and IV iron supplementation	Three deaths during study follow-up (2 in IV iron and 1 in placebo group)

Abbreviations: CRP, C-reactive protein; IV, intravenous; KCCQ, Kansas City Cardiomyopathy Questionnaire; MLHF, Minnesota Living with Heart Failure questionnaire; NT-proBNP, N-terminal prohormone of brain natriuretic peptide; NYHA, New York Heart Association; PO, by mouth; pVo_2, peak oxygen consumption.
Modified from Arora NP, Ghali JK. Iron deficiency anemia in heart failure. Heart Fail Rev 2013;18(4):485–501, with permission of Springer; and *Data from Refs.*[71–77]

survival study or Reduction of Events by Darbepoetin Alfa in Heart Failure (RED-HF) trial, was recently published.[68] In this trial conducted at 453 sites across 33 countries, patients with systolic heart failure (ejection fraction $\leq$40%, NYHA class II–IV) and anemia (hemoglobin between 9.0 and 12.0 g/dL) were randomized to darbepoetin-α (n = 1136) or placebo (n = 1142). The study failed to demonstrate any benefit on mortality or morbidity, and the use of darbepoetin-α was associated with increased ischemic cerebral events and embolic/thrombotic events.[68] The results of this large trial do not support the use of darbepoetin-α in patients with systolic HF and mild to moderate anemia.

Intravenous Iron

Several studies have assessed the potential role of intravenous iron in the treatment of anemia or iron deficiency in HF patients (**Table 2**).[71–77] Iron supplementation has been associated with improvement in quality-of-life measures, possible reduction in hospitalizations, and increased 6 minute walk distance.[78] The meta-analysis of the trials of iron supplementation in HF patients demonstrated that treatment with intravenous iron leads to a significant reduction in hospitalizations (odds ratio 0.26; 95% CI 0.08–0.80) and adverse events (odds ratio 0.35; 95% CI 0.21–0.60), and improvements in NYHA functional class (mean improvement 1.2 classes; 95% CI 0.69–1.78) and left ventricular ejection fraction (mean improvement 5.0%; 95% CI 0.13–9.80).[78] However, there was no effect on mortality (odds ratio 0.66; 95% CI 0.30–1.44).

The long-term effect of intravenous iron on outcomes has not been assessed. Although intravenous iron supplementation may improve exercise capacity and quality of life in HF patients, it may also lead to elevated body iron stores, which could potentially confer an increased risk of cardiovascular events.[69] In a randomized trial to assess the risks and benefits of achieving normal hematocrit in patients with cardiac and end-stage renal disease on hemodialysis, patients who received intravenous iron treatment had a higher risk of death in comparison with the patients who did not receive intravenous iron (relative risk: 2.4; P<.001).[79]

Although intravenous iron may play an important role in the treatment of a large proportion of anemic and nonanemic HF patients, because of the concerns of adverse effects from chronic iron overload, long-term, adequately powered, randomized, placebo-controlled trials of intravenous iron in HF patients to assess morbidity and

mortality are required before any firm recommendations about its use in these patients may be made.

In summary, correcting hematinic deficiencies (iron, vitamin B_{12}, and folic acid) should be pursued in all patients with HF. The use of ESAs has been abandoned, and iron replacement could be provided by oral supplementation or intravenously by one of various preparations. Oral iron may be associated with constipation, diarrhea, nausea, vomiting, or abdominal discomfort. Intravenous iron is a promising approach, although the impact of intravenous iron on morbidity and mortality has not been established.

TREATING COMORBIDITIES

Three studies[80,81,82] have raised concerns about increasing morbidity and mortality associated with raising hemoglobin levels in patients with anemia and chronic kidney disease, necessitating revision of the Food and Drug Administration recommendations for initiating ESA to hemoglobin less than 10 g/dL, with new warnings of serious cardiovascular events if hemoglobin is raised to greater than 11 g/dL.

Similarly, in patients with chronic kidney disease, diabetes mellitus, and anemia, the Trial to Reduce Cardiovascular Events with Darbepoetin Alfa Therapy showed an increased risk of stroke associated with treatment with darbepoetin-α.[82] These findings, along with the results of the RED-HF trial, clearly indicate the futility of raising hemoglobin with ESA in patients with HF.

SUMMARY

Anemia is highly prevalent in patients with HF and is associated with poor prognosis. Laboratory testing is needed to establish its presence and to identify hematinic deficiencies that should be corrected. The available evidence indicates that anemia in HF should be considered a marker and not a mediator, and further effort needs to be directed toward establishing the long-term effect of iron supplementation in patients with HF.

REFERENCES

1. Lindenfeld J. Prevalence of anemia and effects on mortality in patients with heart failure. Am Heart J 2005;149(3):391–401.
2. Ghali JK. Anemia and heart failure. Curr Opin Cardiol 2009;24(2):172–8.
3. Groenveld HF, Januzzi JL, Damman K, et al. Anemia and mortality in heart failure patients a systematic review and meta-analysis. J Am Coll Cardiol 2008;52(10):818–27.

4. Arora NP, Ghali JK. Iron deficiency anemia in heart failure. Heart Fail Rev 2013;18(4):485–501.

5. Duffy TP. Microcytic and hypochromic anemias. In: Goldman L, Ausiello D, editors. Cecil textbook of medicine. Philadelphia: Saunders; 2004. p. 1003–8.

6. Caira C, Ansalone G, Mancone M, et al. Heart failure and iron deficiency anemia in Italy: results from CARMES-1 registry. Future Cardiol 2013; 9(3):437–44.

7. Beutler E, Waalen J. The definition of anemia; what is the lower limit of normal of the blood hemoglobin concentration? Blood 2006;107:1747–50.

8. Zuccala G, Marzetti E, Cesari M, et al. Correlates of cognitive impairment among patients with heart failure: results of a multicenter survey. Am J Med 2005;118(5):496–502.

9. Salisbury AC, Kosiborod M. Outcomes associated with anemia in patients with heart failure. Heart Fail Clin 2010;6(3):359–72.

10. Horwich TB, Fonarow GC, Hamilton MA, et al. Anemia is associated with worse symptoms, greater impairment in functional capacity and a significant increase in mortality in patients with advanced heart failure. J Am Coll Cardiol 2002;39(11):1780–6.

11. Kalra PR, Bolger AP, Francis DP, et al. Effect of anemia on exercise tolerance in chronic heart failure in men. Am J Cardiol 2003;91(7):888–91.

12. Adams KF Jr, Pina IL, Ghali JK, et al. Prospective evaluation of the association between hemoglobin concentration and quality of life in patients with heart failure. Am Heart J 2009;158(6):965–71.

13. de Silva R, Rigby AS, Witte KK, et al. Anemia, renal dysfunction, and their interaction in patients with chronic heart failure. Am J Cardiol 2006;98(3): 391–8.

14. Nanas JN, Matsouka C, Karageorgopoulos D, et al. Etiology of anemia in patients with advanced heart failure. J Am Coll Cardiol 2006;48(12):2485–9.

15. Jankowska EA, Rozentryt P, Witkowska A, et al. Iron deficiency: an ominous sign in patients with systolic chronic heart failure. Eur Heart J 2010; 31(15):1872–80.

16. Klip IT, Comin-Colet J, Voors AA, et al. Iron deficiency in chronic heart failure: an international pooled analysis. Am Heart J 2013;165(4):575–82.e3.

17. Okonko DO, Mandal AK, Missouris CG, et al. Disordered iron homeostasis in chronic heart failure: prevalence, predictors, and relation to anemia, exercise capacity, and survival. J Am Coll Cardiol 2011;58(12):1241–51.

18. Jankowska EA, Rozentryt P, Witkowska A, et al. Iron deficiency predicts impaired exercise capacity in patients with systolic chronic heart failure. J Card Fail 2011;17(11):899–906.

19. Comin-Colet J, Lainscak M, Dickstein K, et al. The effect of intravenous ferric carboxymaltose on health-related quality of life in patients with chronic heart failure and iron deficiency: a subanalysis of the FAIR-HF study. Eur Heart J 2013;34(1):30–8.

20. Jankowska EA, Ponikowski P. Molecular changes in myocardium in the course of anemia or iron deficiency. Heart Fail Clin 2010;6(3):295–304.

21. Le Jemtel TH, Arain S. Mediators of anemia in chronic heart failure. Heart Fail Clin 2010;6(3): 289–93.

22. Weiss G, Goodnough LT. Anemia of chronic disease. N Engl J Med 2005;352(10):1011–23.

23. Freudenthaler SM, Schreeb K, Korner T, et al. Angiotensin II increases erythropoietin production in healthy human volunteers. Eur J Clin Invest 1999;29(10):816–23.

24. Opasich C, Cazzola M, Scelsi L, et al. Blunted erythropoietin production and defective iron supply for erythropoiesis as major causes of anaemia in patients with chronic heart failure. Eur Heart J 2005;26(21):2232–7.

25. Belonje AM, Voors AA, van Gilst WH, et al. Erythropoietin in chronic heart failure. Congest Heart Fail 2007;13(5):289–92.

26. Belonje AM, Voors AA, van der Meer P, et al. Endogenous erythropoietin and outcome in heart failure. Circulation 2010;121(2):245–51.

27. Weiss G. Iron metabolism in the anemia of chronic disease. Biochim Biophys Acta 2009;1790(7):682–93.

28. Handelman GJ, Levin NW. Iron and anemia in human biology: a review of mechanisms. Heart Fail Rev 2008;13(4):393–404.

29. Naito Y, Tsujino T, Fujimori Y, et al. Impaired expression of duodenal iron transporters in Dahl salt-sensitive heart failure rats. J Hypertens 2011; 29(4):741–8.

30. Merle U, Fein E, Gehrke SG, et al. The iron regulatory peptide hepcidin is expressed in the heart and regulated by hypoxia and inflammation. Endocrinology 2007;148(6):2663–8.

31. Matsumoto M, Tsujino T, Lee-Kawabata M, et al. Iron regulatory hormone hepcidin decreases in chronic heart failure patients with anemia. Circ J 2010;74(2):301–6.

32. Nicolas G, Bennoun M, Porteu A, et al. Severe iron deficiency anemia in transgenic mice expressing liver hepcidin. Proc Natl Acad Sci U S A 2002; 99(7):4596–601.

33. Ganz T, Nemeth E. Hepcidin and disorders of iron metabolism. Annu Rev Med 2011;62:347–60.

34. Nemeth E, Tuttle MS, Powelson J, et al. Hepcidin regulates cellular iron efflux by binding to ferroportin and inducing its internalization. Science 2004; 306(5704):2090–3.

35. van der Putten K, Jie KE, van den Broek D, et al. Hepcidin-25 is a marker of the response rather than resistance to exogenous erythropoietin in chronic kidney disease/chronic heart failure patients. Eur J Heart Fail 2010;12(9):943–50.

36. Jankowska EA, Malyszko J, Ardehali H, et al. Iron status in patients with chronic heart failure. Eur Heart J 2013;34(11):827–34.

37. Haas JD, Brownlie T 4th. Iron deficiency and reduced work capacity: a critical review of the research to determine a causal relationship. J Nutr 2001;131(2S-2):676S–88S [discussion: 688S–90S].

38. Cairo G, Bernuzzi F, Recalcati S. A precious metal: iron, an essential nutrient for all cells. Genes Nutr 2006;1(1):25–39.

39. Anderson GJ, Vulpe CD. Mammalian iron transport. Cell Mol Life Sci 2009;66(20):3241–61.

40. Andrews NC. Disorders of iron metabolism. N Engl J Med 1999;341(26):1986–95.

41. Sutak R, Lesuisse E, Tachezy J, et al. Crusade for iron: iron uptake in unicellular eukaryotes and its significance for virulence. Trends Microbiol 2008; 16(6):261–8.

42. Wilson MT, Reeder BJ. Oxygen-binding haem proteins. Exp Physiol 2008;93(1):128–32.

43. Gomollon F, Gisbert JP. Anemia and inflammatory bowel diseases. World J Gastroenterol 2009; 15(37):4659–65.

44. Zimmermann MB, Hurrell RF. Nutritional iron deficiency. Lancet 2007;370(9586):511–20.

45. Anker SD, Sharma R. The syndrome of cardiac cachexia. Int J Cardiol 2002;85(1):51–66.

46. Dong F, Zhang X, Culver B, et al. Dietary iron deficiency induces ventricular dilation, mitochondrial ultrastructural aberrations and cytochrome c release: involvement of nitric oxide synthase and protein tyrosine nitration. Clin Sci (Lond) 2005; 109(3):277–86.

47. Katz SD, Zheng H. Peripheral limitations of maximal aerobic capacity in patients with chronic heart failure. J Nucl Cardiol 2002;9(2):215–25.

48. Brownlie T 4th, Utermohlen V, Hinton PS, et al. Tissue iron deficiency without anemia impairs adaptation in endurance capacity after aerobic training in previously untrained women. Am J Clin Nutr 2004; 79(3):437–43.

49. van Veldhuisen DJ, Anker SD, Ponikowski P, et al. Anemia and iron deficiency in heart failure: mechanisms and therapeutic approaches. Nat Rev Cardiol 2011;8(9):485–93.

50. Maeder MT, Khammy O, dos Remedios C, et al. Myocardial and systemic iron depletion in heart failure implications for anemia accompanying heart failure. J Am Coll Cardiol 2011;58(5):474–80.

51. Cunietti E, Chiari MM, Monti M, et al. Distortion of iron status indices by acute inflammation in older hospitalized patients. Arch Gerontol Geriatr 2004; 39(1):35–42.

52. Means RT Jr, Allen J, Sears DA, et al. Serum soluble transferrin receptor and the prediction of marrow aspirate iron results in a heterogeneous group of patients. Clin Lab Haematol 1999;21(3): 161–7.

53. Cook JD, Skikne BS, Baynes RD. Serum transferrin receptor. Annu Rev Med 1993;44:63–74.

54. Beguin Y, Clemons GK, Pootrakul P, et al. Quantitative assessment of erythropoiesis and functional classification of anemia based on measurements of serum transferrin receptor and erythropoietin. Blood 1993;81(4):1067–76.

55. Punnonen K, Irjala K, Rajamaki A. Serum transferrin receptor and its ratio to serum ferritin in the diagnosis of iron deficiency. Blood 1997;89(3): 1052–7.

56. Thomas C, Kirschbaum A, Boehm D, et al. The diagnostic plot: a concept for identifying different states of iron deficiency and monitoring the response to epoetin therapy. Med Oncol 2006; 23(1):23–36.

57. Thomas C, Thomas L. Biochemical markers and hematologic indices in the diagnosis of functional iron deficiency. Clin Chem 2002;48(7):1066–76.

58. Leszek P, Sochanowicz B, Szperl M, et al. Myocardial iron homeostasis in advanced chronic heart failure patients. Int J Cardiol 2012;159(1):47–52.

59. Silverberg DS, Wexler D, Sheps D, et al. The effect of correction of mild anemia in severe, resistant congestive heart failure using subcutaneous erythropoietin and intravenous iron: a randomized controlled study. J Am Coll Cardiol 2001;37(7): 1775–80.

60. Mancini DM, Katz SD, Lang CC, et al. Effect of erythropoietin on exercise capacity in patients with moderate to severe chronic heart failure. Circulation 2003;107(2):294–9.

61. Ponikowski P, Anker SD, Szachniewicz J, et al. Effect of darbepoetin alfa on exercise tolerance in anemic patients with symptomatic chronic heart failure: a randomized, double-blind, placebo-controlled trial. J Am Coll Cardiol 2007;49(7):753–62.

62. van Veldhuisen DJ, Dickstein K, Cohen-Solal A, et al. Randomized, double-blind, placebo-controlled study to evaluate the effect of two dosing regimens of darbepoetin alfa in patients with heart failure and anaemia. Eur Heart J 2007; 28(18):2208–16.

63. Ghali JK, Anand IS, Abraham WT, et al. Randomized double-blind trial of darbepoetin alfa in patients with symptomatic heart failure and anemia. Circulation 2008;117(4):526–35.

64. Parissis JT, Kourea K, Panou F, et al. Effects of darbepoetin alpha on right and left ventricular systolic and diastolic function in anemic patients with chronic heart failure secondary to ischemic or idiopathic dilated cardiomyopathy. Am Heart J 2008; 155(4):751.e1–7.

65. Kourea K, Parissis JT, Farmakis D, et al. Effects of darbepoetin-alpha on quality of life and emotional

stress in anemic patients with chronic heart failure. Eur J Cardiovasc Prev Rehabil 2008;15(3):365–9.

66. Parissis JT, Kourea K, Andreadou I, et al. Effects of darbepoetin alfa on plasma mediators of oxidative and nitrosative stress in anemic patients with chronic heart failure secondary to ischemic or idiopathic dilated cardiomyopathy. Am J Cardiol 2009; 103(8):1134–8.

67. Cosyns B, Velez-Roa S, Drrogmans S, et al. Effects of erythropoietin administration on mitral regurgitation and left ventricular remodeling in heart failure patients. Int J Cardiol 2010;138(3):306–7.

68. Swedberg K, Young JB, Anand IS, et al. Treatment of anemia with darbepoetin alfa in systolic heart failure. N Engl J Med 2013;368(13):1210–9.

69. Klapholz M, Abraham WT, Ghali JK, et al. The safety and tolerability of darbepoetin alfa in patients with anaemia and symptomatic heart failure. Eur J Heart Fail 2009;11:1071–7.

70. Kotecha D, Ngo K, Walters JA, et al. Erythropoietin as a treatment of anemia in heart failure: systematic review of randomized trials. Am Heart J 2011; 161(5):822–31.e2.

71. Bolger AP, Bartlett FR, Penston HS, et al. Intravenous iron alone for the treatment of anemia in patients with chronic heart failure. J Am Coll Cardiol 2006;48(6):1225–7.

72. Toblli JE, Lombrana A, Duarte P, et al. Intravenous iron reduces NT-pro-brain natriuretic peptide in anemic patients with chronic heart failure and renal insufficiency. J Am Coll Cardiol 2007;50(17):1657–65.

73. Okonko DO, Grzeslo A, Witkowski T, et al. Effect of intravenous iron sucrose on exercise tolerance in anemic and nonanemic patients with symptomatic chronic heart failure and iron deficiency FERRIC-HF: a randomized, controlled, observer-blinded trial. J Am Coll Cardiol 2008;51(2):103–12.

74. Usmanov RI, Zueva EB, Silverberg DS, et al. Intravenous iron without erythropoietin for the treatment of iron deficiency anemia in patients with moderate to severe congestive heart failure and chronic kidney insufficiency. J Nephrol 2008;21(2):236–42.

75. Drakos SG, Anastasiou-Nana MI, Malliaras KG, et al. Anemia in chronic heart failure. Congest Heart Fail 2009;15(2):87–92.

76. Anker SD, Comin Colet J, Filippatos G, et al. Ferric carboxymaltose in patients with heart failure and iron deficiency. N Engl J Med 2009;361(25): 2436–48.

77. Beck-da-Silva L, Piardi D, Soder S, et al. IRON-HF study: a randomized trial to assess the effects of iron in heart failure patients with anemia. Int J Cardiol 2013;168(4):3439–42.   http://dx.doi.org/10.1016/j.ijcard.2013.04.181 pii:S0167–5273(13)00848-6.

78. Kapoor M, Schleinitz MD, Gemignani A, et al. Outcomes of patients with chronic heart failure and iron deficiency treated with intravenous iron: a meta-analysis. Cardiovasc Hematol Disord Drug Targets 2013;13(1):35–44.

79. Besarab A, Bolton WK, Browne JK, et al. The effect of normal as compared with low hematocrit values in patients with cardiac disease who are receiving hemodialysis and epoetin. N Engl J Med 1998; 339:584–90.

80. Drueke TB, Locatelli F, Clyne N, et al. Normalization of hemoglobin level in patients with chronic kidney disease and anemia. N Engl J Med 2006;355: 2071–84.

81. Singh AK, Szczech L, Tang KL, et al. Correction of anemia with epoetin alfa in chronic kidney disease. N Engl J Med 2006;355:2085–98.

82. Pfeffer MA, Burdmann EA, Chen CY, et al. A trial of darbepoetin alfa in type 2 diabetes and chronic kidney disease. N Engl J Med 2006;355:2085–98.

Heart Failure and Depression

Amy Newhouse, MD*, Wei Jiang, MD

KEYWORDS

- Heart failure • Depression • Screening • Risk factors • Prognosis • Treatment • Pathophysiology

KEY POINTS

- In patients with heart failure, depression is associated with both increased morbidity and mortality and is an independent predictor of future cardiovascular events.
- Standard pharmacologic treatment of depression has not been shown to have a consistent beneficial effect on the treatment of both depression and prognosis of heart failure; however, evidence suggests there may be cardiovascular benefit in those whose depression does remit.
- Screening for depression (options include the PHQ-2 and PHQ-9) is recommended.
- Treatment of depression with SSRIs is generally considered to be safe.

EPIDEMIOLOGY

Depression frequently accompanies heart failure and has been linked with increased morbidity and mortality.[1] Heart failure patients who have depression have more somatic symptoms, hospitalizations, increased financial burden, and poorer quality of life.[2] Furthermore, depression has been shown to be an independent predictor of future cardiac events in patients with heart failure, regardless of disease severity, making it worthwhile to consider among other cardiac risk factors, such as diabetes and smoking.[3]

HEART FAILURE STATISTICS

The prevalence of heart failure in North America is greater than 5.7 million with an incidence of approximately 660,000 per year. The American Heart Association's Heart Disease and Stroke Statistics' data project that, by 2030, the prevalence will increase by 3 million people.[4] The mortality of heart failure remains quite high, with about 277,000 deaths per year. Approximately 20% of patients die within 1 year after diagnosis; the 5-year mortality is 59% in men and 45% in women.[5] Heart failure is the leading cause of hospitalization in Medicare patients.[6] Despite many advances in the management of heart failure, its rate of mortality has been essentially unchanged over the past decade. The economic burden has been $34.4 billion in direct and indirect costs yearly in the United States.[7]

HEART FAILURE AND DEPRESSION STATISTICS

According to the Centers for Disease Control and Prevention, the prevalence of depression in the general US population is 9.1%.[5] A meta-analysis of 27 studies reported a prevalence of 21.5% for depression in patients with heart failure.[2] More specifically, this ranges from 11% to 35% in outpatients and 35% to 70% among inpatients.[2] Patients with comorbid major depression have a 2-fold increase in mortality and a 3-fold increase in hospitalization.[3] The Cardiovascular Health Study has found that depression is an independent risk factor for cardiovascular-related death and all-cause mortality.[1]

These findings have been shown to apply to both systolic and diastolic dysfunction types of heart failure. A study from Japan compared rates of clinically significant depression between heart failure patients with preserved ejection fraction (HFpEF) and with reduced ejection fraction (HFrEF). It found comparable rates of depression

Duke University Medical Center, 2301 Erwin Road, Durham, NC 27710, USA
* Corresponding author. Duke Medical Hospital, Department of Internal Medicine, Room 8254DN, 2301 Erwin Road, Durham, NC 27710.
E-mail address: amy.newhouse@duke.edu

Heart Failure Clin 10 (2014) 295–304
http://dx.doi.org/10.1016/j.hfc.2013.10.004
1551-7136/14/$ – see front matter © 2014 Elsevier Inc. All rights reserved.

between the 2 groups: 24% in the HFrEF group and 25% in the HFpEF group. This study, like many others, demonstrated increased rates of cardiac events and cardiac mortality in patients with depressive symptoms. In the 2-year follow-up, 55% of the HFrEF group with depressive symptoms had a hospitalization for heart failure or death attributed to cardiac causes compared with 22% HFrEF in a group without significant depressive symptoms. These statistics were 35% versus 11% in the HFpEF group, respectively. These findings persisted after controlling for B-type natriuretic peptide (BNP) values and suggest that patients should be screened regardless of left ventricular ejection fraction.[8]

PATHOPHYSIOLOGY

There are multiple overlapping factors in the pathophysiology of the interface between heart failure and depression, including activation of inflammatory cascades, dysregulation of neurohormonal axes, arrhythmias, and behavioral effects. These conditions can induce positive feedback loops that actually worsen disease states.

Many studies have shown increased inflammatory markers, such as C-reactive protein (CRP), interleukin-6 (IL-6), and tumor necrosis factor-alpha (TNF-α), in both depression and heart failure as results of the chronic state of physiologic stress that occurs in both heart failure and depression.[9,10] This excess neurohormonal activation and subsequent autonomic hyperactivity can contribute to worsening of left ventricular function. Activation of the sympathetic nervous system and hypothalamic-adrenal-pituitary axis causes both vasoconstriction and volume expansion. Although this combination may be initially beneficial in low output states, it also increases afterload and decreases cardiac output, which in turn can lead to activation of the renin-angiotensin-aldosterone system and can further worsen the state of the heart disease.[11]

The effects of proinflammatory cytokines probably include direct effects on the heart as well, in addition to consequences of activation of the hypothalamic-pituitary-adrenal axis and renin-angiotensin-aldosterone system. Increases in IL-1, IL-2, IL-6, IL-10, and TNF may all be initially appropriate responses to the stresses of the disease because they enhance cardiac myocyte hypertrophy and protection from apoptosis, but, without resolution, may actually exacerbate the situation by inducing ventricular remodeling, which worsens the contractility of the left ventricle.[12] Animal studies have demonstrated a concentration-dependent association between

IL-2, IL-6, and TNF-α to negative inotropic activity.[13]

These overlaps between the pathophysiology of heart failure and depression may be relevant in choices of treatment. High neurohormonal activation with subsequent increase in norepinephrine and renin-angiotensin-aldosterone system activity and increased sympathetic nervous system activity and excess hypothalamic-pituitary-adrenal axis activity exist in both. Interestingly, treatment of patients with heart failure and major depression with tricyclic antidepressants or serotonin norepinephrine reuptake inhibitors (SNRIs) has been associated with lower serum levels of TNF-α and CRP when these patients are compared with those not on antidepressants or on selective serotonin reuptake inhibitors (SSRIs).[14] One study from Japan found that using angiotensin converting enzyme inhibitors and/or aldosterone receptor blockers was associated with fewer symptoms of depression in HFrEF. These associations were not seen in those with HFpEF,[8] consistent with previous findings that these drugs do not have a clear impact on clinical outcomes in HFpEF.[15]

Decreased heart rate variability is seen in both heart failure and depression. It is thought to be a result of an autonomic imbalance between the sympathetic and parasympathetic nervous systems.[16] Decreased heart rate variability is a marker of decreased parasympathetic tone secondary to hyperactive sympathetic signals (high levels of IL-6 and norepinephrine). This relatively unopposed sympathetic tone can provoke ventricular arrhythmias. Of the mortality in heart failure, 25% to 50% is attributed to arrhythmias,[17] and patients with depression alone have been shown to have decreased heart rate variability and increased arrhythmias as well.

In addition, low concentrations of omega-3 fatty acids have been seen in both cardiovascular diseases and in depression alone.[18,19] Low omega-3 fatty acids have also been associated with worse survival in heart failure patients with major depression independent of other common risk factors[20]; this has been attributed to its effects on cell membrane stability, inhibition of production of thromboxane A2 and inflammatory cytokines, increased heart rate variability, and improved left ventricular ejection fraction.[21–24] The mechanisms involved in depression are slightly less clear but theorized to involve neuronal cell membranes.[25] Consumption of fish oil or omega-3 fatty acids has been shown to reduce the risk of major cardiovascular events.[24]

The behavioral aspects of depression and their potential influence on heart failure cannot be ignored. Depressed patients tend to be less active and engage in more substance use (including tobacco and alcohol), and their apathy can result in worse compliance. Noncompliance is frequently a factor in heart failure–related hospitalizations. Worsening physical disease can also certainly provoke low mood and fatigue.

PROGNOSTIC IMPLICATIONS

As mentioned, multiple studies have shown that depression increases the risk of mortality, both cardiovascular and all-cause, in patients with heart failure. One study in particular quoted a hazard ratio (HR) of 2.07 for cardiovascular disease mortality and HR 1.49 for all-cause mortality.[1] The HR increases when depression is combined with amino-terminal pro-B-type natriuretic peptide (NT-proBNP) during new-onset heart failure. The presence of both depression and elevated NT-proBNP was associated with an HR of 5.42 for cardiovascular disease mortality in new-onset heart failure populations and all-cause mortality of HR 3.72. Therefore these 2 factors have additive predictive value when estimating mortality for heart failure patients.[1]

FINDINGS OF INTERVENTIONAL TRIALS

Multiple studies have investigated the ability to treat depression and the effects of doing so in patients with heart failure. Overall, they have found that the standard treatments do not have a consistent beneficial effect on depression and similarly on cardiovascular outcomes. However, there has been relevance in remission of depression, regardless of the means, because those whose depression remits tend to have decreased mortality and better quality of life.

The Sertraline Against Depression and Heart Disease in Chronic Heart Failure (SADHART-CHF) trial evaluated the effect of sertraline on both depressive symptoms and cardiovascular outcomes in patients with CHF after 12 weeks of treatment. This study was done in the wake of others that had shown improvement in mood in patients with ischemic heart disease.[26] Unfortunately, the SADHART-CHF trial did not show a significant reduction of depressive symptoms in patients receiving sertraline versus placebo. There was also no effect of treating depression on clinical outcomes of heart failure.[27] However, a substudy showed that the patients whose depression remitted after 12 weeks of treatment had fewer cardiovascular events, both fatal and nonfatal, than those whose depression remained.[27] Although this was independent of treatment, it suggests that there may be cardiovascular benefit in

depression remission. Interpreted another way, it may suggest that the nonresponders reflected a subset of depressed patients that are vulnerable to cardiovascular adverse events. Reducing the depressive symptoms, if possible, may be protective.[28] Some potential reasons for this include placebo effect, the therapeutic effect of nurse-facilitated support, or the idea that depression that is comorbid with heart failure may be pathophysiologically unique.[28]

The Mortality and Mood in Depressed Heart Failure patients trial is in the process of evaluating the effects of escitalopram in heart failure patients at 12 to 24 months from randomization.[29]

The Heart Failure–A Controlled Trial Investigating Outcomes of Exercise Training study evaluated aerobic exercise as a therapy for depression in patients with heart failure. It was intended to evaluate whether exercise has an effect on depressive symptoms and if reduced depressive symptoms were associated with improved clinical outcomes. Heart Failure–A Controlled Trial Investigating Outcomes of Exercise Training was a multicenter, randomized clinical trial; it used the Beck Depression Inventory II (BDI-II) as a scale of depressive symptoms. The intervention was 3 supervised exercise sessions per week (total of 90 minutes) for 3 months. Modest reductions in all-cause mortality and all-cause hospitalization were found.[30]

Clinically significant depression was noted in 28% of the initial population, most of whom were white, married men with at least a high school education. Those who were more severely depressed were more likely to be taking an antidepressant (and also more likely to have worse heart failure). This population was equally distributed between the treatment and placebo group. The study showed that aerobic exercise resulted in a small, but significant, reduction in depressive symptoms in heart failure patients (1.75 point reduction in BDI-II scores compared with 0.98 point reduction in usual care). These differences were large in the subset with clinically significant depression or BDI-II scores of 14 or higher. Within this group, the aerobic exercise group showed a 2.2 point reduction versus 1.3 in the usual care group. Notably most patients were not clinically depressed and none was diagnosed with a new major depressive disorder during the study. Antidepressant use was allowed but equal between the 2 groups. It was difficult to determine if the observed differences imply that those who exercise had less depression or if depression resulted in less exercise. This study also confirmed that those with elevated depressive symptoms had a 20% increased risk of all-cause mortality and hospitalizations. The limitations were that the patients had to be willing and able to exercise; those who were more depressed may have been less able to engage in the exercise activities they were assigned. The BDI-II, although validated in detecting depressive symptoms, is not commonly used as a diagnostic tool of major depression, and only 28% of the patients had depressive symptoms based on the initial assessment, which is lower than that found in other evaluations of heart failure patients.[30]

Prior studies of exercise as a therapy for depression alone reported that 90 minutes per week was able to reduce depressive symptoms and 60 minutes per week could reduce the risk of relapse over a 1-year period.[31]

No specific studies have been done to evaluate the effects of psychotherapy in patients with heart failure, although it has been theorized that the frequent nursing contact in SADHART-CHF may have contributed to lessening of symptoms in both the treatment and the placebo groups.[27]

TREATMENT IMPLICATIONS

Although studies have had relatively disappointing outcomes with regard to reducing morbidity and mortality through treatment of depression, it is still recommended to screen the heart failure population for depression. As described above, those whose depression remits tend to have better cardiovascular outcomes. That the above studies did not establish a reliable way to improve cardiovascular function in this population may reflect more of a unique pathophysiology behind this depression and its treatment needs rather than futility in treatment. In addition, depression can influence patients' perception of their symptoms and potentially cause overreporting, which can lead to overuse of health services and possible iatrogenic harm. Screening may help distinguish symptoms of

depression from those of heart failure and may assist in patient perception of their disease.[32]

Furthermore, one study found that 70% of the study population with suspected major depression had not been diagnosed before, making this a quite underrecognized comorbid illness.[33] In addition, certain populations seem to be more responsive to treatment than others. For example, the SADHART-CHF study reported that men with heart failure and mild depression (Hamilton Depression Rating Scale ≤ 17) have almost a 2.5 times greater chance of achieving depression remission when compared with the rest of the study population.[28] However, in contrast, the patients with greater somatic presentations of their depression were less likely to remit.[28]

The American Heart Association has advocated routine screening for depression among cardiac patients with the Patient Health Questionnaire (PHQ-2) "at a minimum."[34] The PHQ-2 involves 2 questions whether they had: (1) little interest or pleasure in doing things and (2) feeling down, depressed, or hopeless over the past 2 weeks (**Table 1**). An assessment is positive if a patient endorses one or both of these questions and is negative if they deny both. This simple procedure has been found to have a 90% sensitivity and 69% specificity for the diagnosis of major depressive disorder among coronary heart disease patients.[35] In a study that evaluated hospitalized heart failure patients suspected of being depressed, increased 12-month all-cause mortality and mortality from cardiovascular causes were found to be significantly associated with a positive PHQ-2 screening. For the PHQ-2-positive population, all-cause mortality was 20%, whereas it was only 8% in the PHQ-2-negative group. Cardiovascular mortality was 14% of PHQ-2-positive and 6% of PHQ-2-negative group. This risk remained elevated even after adjusting for other markers of severity of disease. These results were also comparable to another study that evaluated heart

Table 1 PHQ-2				
Over the Past 2 weeks, How Often Have You Been Bothered by Any of the Following Problems	Not at All	Several Days	More than Half the Days	Nearly Every Day
1. Little interest or pleasure in doing things	0	1	2	3
2. Feeling down, depressed, or hopeless	0	1	2	3

This can be administered in a yes or no format. A cutoff of 3 has been identified as the optimal screening point.
From Kroenke K, Spitzer RL, Williams JB. The Patient Health Questionnaire-2: validity of a two-item depression screener. Med Care 2003;41(11):1290; with permission.

failure patients using the Beck Depression Index Inventory, a 21-item questionnaire.[36]

Many recommend using a PHQ-9 or more in-depth follow-up study if patients screen positive for a PHQ-2 because a diagnosis cannot be made from just this information (**Table 2**). The first 2 questions in PHQ-9 comprised the PHQ-2. Both can be self-administered.

The PHQ-9 scores the *Diagnostic and Statistical Manual of Mental Disorders* (Fourth Edition) (*DSM-IV*) criteria of major depression. This tool has been validated in primary care and obstetrics-gynecology clinics. A score ≥10 has a sensitivity of 88% and a specificity of 88% for major depression. Scores of 5, 10, 15, and 20 represent mild, moderate, moderately severe, and severe depression, respectively.[37]

The PHQ-9 addresses most of the *DSM-IV* criteria for a major depressive episode. To recapitulate these, 5 of the above symptoms must exist within the same 2-week period, with at least one of them being depressed mood or loss of interest/pleasure and this state must represent a change from previous functioning. The additional criteria are that these symptoms do not meet criteria for a mixed episode or the clinically significant distress or impairment in social, occupational, or other important areas of functioning,

are not due to direct physiologic effects of a substance or general medical condition, and are not better accounted for by bereavement or characterized by marked functional impairment, morbid preoccupation with worthlessness, active suicidal ideation, psychotic symptoms, or psychomotor retardation. A mixed episode exists when criteria for both a manic episode and a major depressive episode exist in conjunction nearly every day for at least a 1-week period. A mixed episode is not the only alternative in the differential, however. Other diagnoses include substance-induced or related depression, bipolar disorder, persistent depressive disorder (previously dysthymia), and schizoaffective disorder (**Table 3**).

It is frequently very helpful to get collateral information from family or close friends when evaluating for these disorders. In addition, although rating scales and diagnostic interviews are important in evaluating for depression, noticing affect, which may be constricted or flat, or generalized psychomotor retardation or restlessness can provide useful information.

There is admittedly overlap between certain symptoms of heart failure and somatic elements of depression. This overlap has raised concern that the somatic components of the PHQ-9 may enhance the relationship between depression

Table 2 PHQ-9				
Over the Last 2 weeks, How Often Have You Been Bothered by Any of the Following Problems?	**Not at All**	**Several Days**	**More than Half the Days**	**Nearly Every Day**
1. Little interest or pleasure in doing things	0	1	2	3
2. Feeling down, depressed, or hopeless	0	1	2	3
3. Trouble falling or staying asleep, or sleeping too much	0	1	2	3
4. Feeling tired or having little energy	0	1	2	3
5. Poor appetite or overeating	0	1	2	3
6. Feeling bad about yourself—or that you are a failure or have let yourself or your family down	0	1	2	3
7. Trouble concentrating on things, such as reading the newspaper or watching television	0	1	2	3
8. Moving or speaking so slowly that other people could have noticed? Or the opposite—being so fidgety or restless that you have been moving around a lot more than usual	0	1	2	3
9. Thoughts that you would be better off dead or of hurting yourself in some way	0	1	2	3

Table 3
Ways to screen for alternative psychiatric diagnoses

Substance-induced or -related depression	Careful history of alcohol and drug use
Bipolar disorder	Episodes (that last several days) of euphoria, sense of feeling on top of the world, excess accomplishment with increase in goal-directed activity, hyperenergized, lack of need for sleep, racing thoughts, pressured speech, increased risk-taking behavior (financially, sexually)
Schizoaffective disorder	Presence of paranoia, auditory or visual hallucinations, delusions

and cardiovascular outcomes when these are more a consequence of heart failure. To address this, multiple studies have divided the criteria of depression into affective and somatic components and looked at their association with cardiovascular outcome. They found that the affective depressive symptoms correlated with time to first cardiac event and all-cause mortality, while the physical symptoms did not; these were independent of health status, clinical, and sociodemographic characteristics,[38,39] which suggests that the PHQ-9 is an adequate way to measure depressive symptoms in patients with heart failure and make prognostic estimates.

TREATMENT CONSIDERATIONS

There are multiple things to consider when starting an antidepressant. Antidepressants are generally considered safe in cardiac populations but different classes have been associated with different risks. There has been a relative lack of randomized clinical trials evaluating individual antidepressants in heart failure patients; most have been done in patients with coronary artery disease. Therefore the existing data should be interpreted with caution. However, potential benefits lie not only in their effect on depressive symptoms but also in their cardiovascular effects.[40] For example, SSRIs may decrease thrombotic events by reducing platelet activation.[41] Treatment with tricyclic antidepressants and SNRIs has been associated with decreased pro-inflammatory markers, when compared with treatment with SSRIs, which may slow progression of heart failure.[14]

SSRIs are considered to be both efficacious and safe.[40] Some of the specific SSRIs studied in cardiovascular disease include sertraline, paroxetine, and fluoxetine.[42–44] Some SSRIs, such as citalopram, have a risk of QT prolongation at higher dosages.

Tricyclic antidepressants, such as amitriptyline and nortriptyline, have a theoretical increased

risk of arrhythmias. They have type 1A antiarrhythmic properties and therefore may cause atrioventricular block, bundle branch block, or QTc prolongation with subsequent increase in ventricular arrhythmias.[45] Monoamine oxidase inhibitors, such as selegiline, have known adverse effects on blood pressure as they can cause orthostatic hypotension and hypertensive crisis.[46]

To assess the effect accurately, a patient should be consistently taking a therapeutic dose for 4 to 6 weeks. Most side effects abate 10 to 14 days after initiation of the medication. This abatement does not apply to sexual dysfunction, however, so if this is a major concern, switching medications is appropriate (for example, from sertraline to bupropion). Other more general side effects can be particularly relevant in patients with heart failure, such as hypertension, hypotension, and hyponatremia. These side effects are outlined in **Box 1**. Serotonin syndrome, although rare, should be kept in mind when prescribing these medications. This syndrome consists of a constellation of symptoms including headache, agitation, confusion, hyperthermia, sweating, tachycardia, nausea, diarrhea, myoclonus, hyperreflexia, and tremor. Certain medications, listed below, have a higher risk of precipitating this (see **Box 1**). In general, a major depressive episode requires 6 months of continued intervention from the point of remission to the beginning of the taper. If patients have had 2 or more major depressive episodes in their lives, standard practice is to continue the effective care indefinitely.

QUALITY OF LIFE

It is common to assume a worse quality of life in patients with heart failure. It is notable that measures of heart failure severity, such as left ventricular ejection fraction, New York Heart Association functional class, and NT-proBNP levels, play only a small to negligible role in predicting quality of life. More specifically, multiple studies have shown the left ventricular ejection fraction does

---

Box 1
Depression care algorithm for CHF patients*

1. Screen all patients

   a. Start with PHQ-2 and follow-up with PHQ-9 or formal diagnostic interview

2. Psychoeducation

   a. Prevalence, prognostic implications

3. Offer treatment

   a. Omega-3 supplementation

   b. Aerobic exercise

   c. Psychosocial supportive intervention

   d. Medications—SSRIs found to be efficacious in reducing depressive symptoms in patients with coronary heart disease

      i. Common medications and their common side effects

         1. SSRIs (eg, Sertraline, Paroxetine, Fluoxetine), sexual dysfunction, gastrointestinal (GI; decreased appetite, nausea, diarrhea, constipation, dry mouth), central nervous system (insomnia, sedation, agitation, tremors, headache, dizziness)

         2. SNRIs (eg, Venlafaxine, Duloxetine), headache, nervousness, insomnia, sedation, GI, sexual dysfunction, Syndrome of inappropriate antidiuretic hormone secretion, hyponatremia, hypertension

         3. Norepinephrine-dopamine reuptake inhibitors (eg, Bupropion), dry mouth, constipation, nausea, weight gain, anorexia, myalgia, insomnia, dizziness, headache, agitation, anxiety, tremor, sweating, rash, hypertension

         4. Noradrenergic and specific serotonergic antidepressants (eg, Mirtazapine), GI, sedation, confusion, flulike symptoms, changes in urinary symptoms, hypotension, weight gain

      ii. Side effects

         1. Typically abate after 10 to 14 days of use, except sexual dysfunction

      iii. Consider drug-drug interactions

         1. Serotonin syndrome

            a. Antidepressants, opioids, stimulants, 5-HT1 agonists, herbs, mood stabilizers (lithium, valproate), antipsychotics (risperidone, olanzapine), antiemetics (ondansetron, metoclopramide), antibiotics (linezolid)

         2. QTc Prolongation

            a. SSRIs, antpsychotics, opioids, macrolides, fluoroquinolones, antiarrhythmics

4. When to refer to a psychiatrist

   a. Refractory mood symptoms

      i. Trials of 2 antidepressants

   b. Development of psychotic and/or manic symptoms

   c. Suicidal ideation

* Please note, this list is not meant to be all-inclusive but rather to serve as a general base for clinical decision making.

---

not correlate with perception of a patient's illness, and New York Heart Association class and NT-proBNP values have only a small correlation.[47] A large association was found between PHQ-9 score and quality of life in this patient population, which is particularly relevant because it can negatively affect therapy adherence, morbidity, mortality, and subsequent health care cost.[48–50]

FINANCIAL IMPLICATIONS

The economic burden of these diseases is immense. The annual cost in the United States for heart failure is over $33 billion.[4] Depression is among the several comorbid diseases associated with much higher cost when existing in conjunction with heart failure. The others are atrial fibrillation, coronary artery disease, chronic lung disease, diabetes, and hyperlipidemia. All of these lead to higher resource use. Depression has been found to account for 36% higher costs of care. To put this in perspective, diabetes was associated with 28%, chronic lung disease with 29%, hyperlipidemia with 21%, coronary artery disease with 14%, and atrial fibrillation with 15%.[51]

SUMMARY

The significance of depression as a comorbid illness in heart failure is large. As cited above, it is associated with increased morbidity and mortality, both all-cause and cardiovascular related. It has a large impact on quality of life with subsequent effects on effectiveness of care. In addition, it confers a large national economic cost. The exact pathophysiologic connection behind this depression and its most effective treatment has not yet been elucidated, but the potential for improved quality of life if treatment could be found is immense; the need for continued investigation is only growing.

REFERENCES

1. van den Broek KC, Defilippi CR, Christenson RH, et al. Predictive value of depressive symptoms and B-type natriuretic peptide for new-onset heart failure and mortality. Am J Cardiol 2011;107(5):723–9.
2. Rutledge T, Reis VA, Linke SE, et al. Depression in heart failure a meta-analytic review of prevalence, intervention effects, and associations with clinical outcomes. J Am Coll Cardiol 2006;48(8):1527–37.
3. Jiang W, Alexander J, Christopher E, et al. Relationship of depression to increased risk of mortality and rehospitalization in patients with congestive heart failure. Arch Intern Med 2001;161(15):1849–56.
4. Roger VL, Go AS, Lloyd-Jones DM, et al. Heart disease and stroke statistics–2012 update: a report from the American Heart Association. Circulation 2012;125(1):e2–220.
5. Prevention, C.f.D.C.a. An estimated 1 in 10 U.S. adults report depression. 2012, 2013. Available at: http://www.cdc.gov/features/dsdepression/. Accessed July 9, 2013.
6. Stewart S, MacIntyre K, Hole DJ, et al. More 'malignant' than cancer? Five-year survival following a first admission for heart failure. Eur J Heart Fail 2001;3(3):315–22.
7. Heidenreich PA, Trogdon JG, Khavjou OA, et al. Forecasting the future of cardiovascular disease in the United States: a policy statement from the American Heart Association. Circulation 2011;123(8):933–44.
8. Kato N, Kinugawa K, Shiga T, et al. Depressive symptoms are common and associated with adverse clinical outcomes in heart failure with reduced and preserved ejection fraction. J Cardiol 2012;60(1):23–30.
9. Munger MA, Johnson B, Amber IJ, et al. Circulating concentrations of proinflammatory cytokines in mild or moderate heart failure secondary to ischemic or idiopathic dilated cardiomyopathy. Am J Cardiol 1996;77(9):723–7.
10. Lanquillon S, Krieg JC, Bening-Abu-Shach U, et al. Cytokine production and treatment response in major depressive disorder. Neuropsychopharmacology 2000;22(4):370–9.
11. Nair N, Farmer C, Gongora E, et al. Commonality between depression and heart failure. Am J Cardiol 2012;109(5):768–72.
12. Blum A, Miller H. Pathophysiological role of cytokines in congestive heart failure. Annu Rev Med 2001;52:15–27.
13. Finkel MS, Oddis CV, Jacob TD, et al. Negative inotropic effects of cytokines on the heart mediated by nitric oxide. Science 1992;257(5068):387–9.
14. Tousoulis D, Drolias A, Antoniades C, et al. Antidepressive treatment as a modulator of inflammatory process in patients with heart failure: effects on proinflammatory cytokines and acute phase protein levels. Int J Cardiol 2009;134(2):238–43.
15. Holland DJ, Kumbhani DJ, Ahmed SH, et al. Effects of treatment on exercise tolerance, cardiac function, and mortality in heart failure with preserved ejection fraction. A meta-analysis. J Am Coll Cardiol 2011;57(16):1676–86.
16. Gorman JM, Sloan RP. Heart rate variability in depressive and anxiety disorders. Am Heart J 2000;140(Suppl 4):77–83.
17. Narang R, Cleland JG, Erhardt L, et al. Mode of death in chronic heart failure. A request and proposition for more accurate classification. Eur Heart J 1996;17(9):1390–403.
18. Kromhout D, Bosschieter EB, de Lezenne Coulander C. The inverse relation between fish consumption and 20-year mortality from coronary heart disease. N Engl J Med 1985;312(19):1205–9.
19. Frasure-Smith N, Lesperance F, Julien P. Major depression is associated with lower omega-3 fatty

acid levels in patients with recent acute coronary syndromes. Biol Psychiatry 2004;55(9):891–6.

20. Jiang W, Oken H, Fiuzat M, et al. Plasma omega-3 polyunsaturated fatty acids and survival in patients with chronic heart failure and major depressive disorder. J Cardiovasc Transl Res 2012;5(1):92–9.

21. Calder PC. Immunoregulatory and anti-inflammatory effects of n-3 polyunsaturated fatty acids. Braz J Med Biol Res 1998;31(4):467–90.

22. Simopoulos AP. The importance of the ratio of omega-6/omega-3 essential fatty acids. Biomed Pharmacother 2002;56(8):365–79.

23. Christensen JH, Christensen MS, Dyerberg J, et al. Heart rate variability and fatty acid content of blood cell membranes: a dose-response study with n-3 fatty acids. Am J Clin Nutr 1999;70(3):331–7.

24. Ghio S, Scelsi L, Latini R, et al. Effects of n-3 polyunsaturated fatty acids and of rosuvastatin on left ventricular function in chronic heart failure: a substudy of GISSI-HF trial. Eur J Heart Fail 2010; 12(12):1345–53.

25. Lin PY, Su KP. A meta-analytic review of double-blind, placebo-controlled trials of antidepressant efficacy of omega-3 fatty acids. J Clin Psychiatry 2007;68(7):1056–61.

26. Rivelli S, Jiang W. Depression and ischemic heart disease: what have we learned from clinical trials? Curr Opin Cardiol 2007;22(4):286–91.

27. O'Connor CM, Jiang W, Kuchibhatla M, et al. Safety and efficacy of sertraline for depression in patients with heart failure: results of the SADHART-CHF (Sertraline Against Depression and Heart Disease in Chronic Heart Failure) trial. J Am Coll Cardiol 2010;56(9):692–9.

28. Jiang W, Krishnan R, Kuchibhatla M, et al. Characteristics of depression remission and its relation with cardiovascular outcome among patients with chronic heart failure (from the SADHART-CHF Study). Am J Cardiol 2011;107(4):545–51.

29. Angermann CE, Gelbrich G, Störk S, et al. Rationale and design of a randomised, controlled, multicenter trial investigating the effects of selective serotonin re-uptake inhibition on morbidity, mortality and mood in depressed heart failure patients (MOOD-HF). Eur J Heart Fail 2007;9(12):1212–22.

30. Blumenthal JA, Babyak MA, O'Connor C, et al. Effects of exercise training on depressive symptoms in patients with chronic heart failure: the HF-ACTION randomized trial. JAMA 2012;308(5): 465–74.

31. Hoffman BM, Babyak MA, Craighead WE, et al. Exercise and pharmacotherapy in patients with major depression: one-year follow-up of the SMILE study. Psychosom Med 2011;73(2):127–33.

32. Rollman BL, Herbeck Belnap B, Mazumdar S, et al. A positive 2-item Patient Health Questionnaire depression screen among hospitalized heart failure patients is associated with elevated 12-month mortality. J Card Fail 2012;18(3):238–45.

33. Angermann CE, Gelbrich G, Störk S, et al. Somatic correlates of comorbid major depression in patients with systolic heart failure. Int J Cardiol 2011;147(1):66–73.

34. Lichtman JH, Bigger JT Jr, Blumenthal JA, et al. Depression and coronary heart disease: recommendations for screening, referral, and treatment: a science advisory from the American Heart Association Prevention Committee of the Council on Cardiovascular Nursing, Council on Clinical Cardiology, Council on Epidemiology and Prevention, and Interdisciplinary Council on Quality of Care and Outcomes Research: endorsed by the American Psychiatric Association. Circulation 2008; 118(17):1768–75.

35. McManus D, Pipkin SS, Whooley MA. Screening for depression in patients with coronary heart disease (data from the Heart and Soul Study). Am J Cardiol 2005;96(8):1076–81.

36. Jiang W, Kuchibhatla M, Clary GL, et al. Relationship between depressive symptoms and long-term mortality in patients with heart failure. Am Heart J 2007;154(1):102–8.

37. Kroenke K, Spitzer RL, Williams JB. The PHQ-9: validity of a brief depression severity measure. J Gen Intern Med 2001;16(9):606–13.

38. Lee KS, Lennie TA, Heo S, et al. Association of physical versus affective depressive symptoms with cardiac event-free survival in patients with heart failure. Psychosom Med 2012;74(5):452–8.

39. Schiffer AA, Pelle AJ, Smith OR, et al. Somatic versus cognitive symptoms of depression as predictors of all-cause mortality and health status in chronic heart failure. J Clin Psychiatry 2009; 70(12):1667–73.

40. Tousoulis D, Antonopoulos AS, Antoniades C, et al. Role of depression in heart failure–choosing the right antidepressive treatment. Int J Cardiol 2010;140(1): 12–8.

41. Alvarez W Jr, Pickworth KK. Safety of antidepressant drugs in the patient with cardiac disease: a review of the literature. Pharmacotherapy 2003;23(6): 754–71.

42. Glassman AH, O'Connor CM, Califf RM, et al. Sertraline treatment of major depression in patients with acute MI or unstable angina. JAMA 2002; 288(6):701–9.

43. Roose SP, Laghrissi-Thode F, Kennedy JS, et al. Comparison of paroxetine and nortriptyline in depressed patients with ischemic heart disease. JAMA 1998;279(4):287–91.

44. Lesperance F, Frasure-Smith N, Koszycki D, et al. Effects of citalopram and interpersonal psychotherapy on depression in patients with coronary artery disease: the Canadian Cardiac Randomized

Evaluation of Antidepressant and Psychotherapy Efficacy (CREATE) trial. JAMA 2007;297(4):367–79.

45. Deglin SM, Deglin JM, Chung EK. Drug-induced cardiovascular diseases. Drugs 1977;14(1):29–40.

46. Shapiro PA. Treatment of depression in patients with congestive heart failure. Heart Fail Rev 2009; 14(1):7–12.

47. Muller-Tasch T, Peters-Klimm F, Schellberg D, et al. Depression is a major determinant of quality of life in patients with chronic systolic heart failure in general practice. J Card Fail 2007;13(10):818–24.

48. Joynt KE, Whellan DJ, O'Connor CM. Why is depression bad for the failing heart? A review

of the mechanistic relationship between depression and heart failure. J Card Fail 2004;10(3): 258–71.

49. Junger J, Schellberg D, Möller-Tasch T, et al. Depression increasingly predicts mortality in the course of congestive heart failure. Eur J Heart Fail 2005;7(2):261–7.

50. Sullivan M, Simon G, Spertus J, et al. Depression-related costs in heart failure care. Arch Intern Med 2002;162(16):1860–6.

51. Smith DH, Johnson ES, Blough DK, et al. Predicting costs of care in heart failure patients. BMC Health Serv Res 2012;12:434.

Atrial Fibrillation and Congestive Heart Failure

Sudarone Thihalolipavan, MD[a],*,
Daniel P. Morin, MD, MPH, FHRS[a,b]

KEYWORDS

- Atrial fibrillation • Congestive heart failure • Atrial fibrillation ablation • Antiarrhythmics
- Atrio-ventricular node ablation

KEY POINTS

- Heart failure (HF) and atrial fibrillation (AF) commonly coexist and adversely affect mortality when found together.
- AF begets HF and HF begets AF.
- Rhythm restoration with antiarrhythmic drugs failed to show a mortality benefit but can be effective in improving symptoms.
- Nonpharmacologic treatment of AF may be of value in the HF population.

INTRODUCTION

Heart failure (HF) and atrial fibrillation (AF) frequently coexist, with an associated increase in morbidity and mortality. Together they impose a significant impact on the economy and strain health care resources. Each condition can promote the other, via complex structural, electrophysiological, and neurohormonal processes. Recent research has advanced the understanding of the underlying mechanisms responsible for these relationships, and further work may provide future insight into optimal management. This article reviews the epidemiology, pathophysiology, treatment options, and outcomes associated with these 2 conditions in combination.

EPIDEMIOLOGY OF HF AND AF

AF is the most common sustained arrhythmia among adults. It imposes a considerable public health burden, currently affecting greater than 2 million people in the United States. This statistic is increasing as the population ages.[1] HF is also a significant and growing epidemic, with nearly 5.7 million American adults affected currently and greater than 500,000 new patients diagnosed annually.[2] Furthermore, patients with HF are now living longer; this is in part due to improved survival from acute coronary syndrome and advances in the acute and chronic management of patients with HF. Thus, both AF and HF are common. They also carry significant morbidity and mortality.

Collectively, these disorders have a substantial impact on the economy and also on the utilization of health care resources. For example, HF hospital admissions account for greater than 6.5 million hospital days annually[3] and HF-related costs reach an estimated $34.4 billion each year. This total includes the cost of health care services, medications, and lost productivity.[4] AF accounts for 35% of all hospital admissions for arrhythmias.[3] The average estimated cost of medical care for

Dr Thihalolipavan has no disclosures.
Dr Morin has research grants from Boston Scientific and Medtronic and has received honoraria from Biotronik, Boston Scientific, CardioNet, Medtronic, St. Jude Medical, and Zoll.
[a] Department of Cardiology, Ochsner Medical Center, 1514 Jefferson Highway, New Orleans, LA 70121, USA;
[b] Department of Cardiology, Ochsner Clinical School, Queensland University School of Medicine, 1514 Jefferson Highway, New Orleans, LA 70121, USA
* Corresponding author.
E-mail address: sthihalolipavan@ochsner.org

Heart Failure Clin 10 (2014) 305–318
http://dx.doi.org/10.1016/j.hfc.2013.12.005
1551-7136/14/$ – see front matter © 2014 Elsevier Inc. All rights reserved.

each patient with AF is approximately $8700 per year higher than when AF is absent.[5] Overall, the national estimated annual cost of caring for AF is approximately $26 billion.[5]

PROGNOSTIC SIGNIFICANCE OF HF AND AF IN COMBINATION

AF and HF frequently coexist, in part because of common risk factors (eg, hypertension, coronary artery disease, diabetes mellitus, valvular disease) and also because of their common tendency to occur in patients with advanced age (**Figs. 1** and **2**).[6] The overall prevalence of AF among patients with HF has been reported to be 13% to 41%.[6–8] These figures include prevalence data from several HF trials, such as The Vasodilator in Heart Failure Trial, as well as the largest followed community cohort, the Framingham Heart Study. In the Framingham study, at the first diagnosis of HF among study participants, 24% had concurrent or prior AF and another 17% developed AF during follow-up. In addition, the proportion of patients with AF is increased in patients with advanced New York Heart Association (NYHA) functional classification, from less than 5% in class I to 49% in class IV (**Fig. 3**).[9]

Temporal analysis of Framingham Study participants showed that AF preceded HF just as frequently as HF preceded AF, and the development of the second condition led to a worse prognosis. There was some gender-based variability in these relationships, however. For example, when men with AF developed HF, their expected mortality increased (hazard ratio [HR] 2.7; 95% confidence interval [CI], 1.9–3.7), and these findings were similar among women. In contrast, women with HF demonstrated more severe compounding of mortality when they later developed AF (HR 2.7, 95% CI, 2.0–3.6) as compared with men (HR 1.6; 95% CI, 1.2–2.1).[6]

Subsequent trials have also reported consistently worse outcomes when HF and AF coexist. For example, data from a large population in the Studies of Left Ventricular Dysfunction (SOLVD) demonstrated that concomitant AF in HF patients led to increased hospitalization (21 compared with 13 events per 100 participant-years, $P<.001$) and increased overall mortality (34% vs 23% over an average of 33.4 ± 14.3 months, $P<.001$).[10] Recent retrospective data from patients enrolled in the *Get with the Guidelines—Heart Failure* program showed that among patients hospitalized for HF, the presence of AF on admission

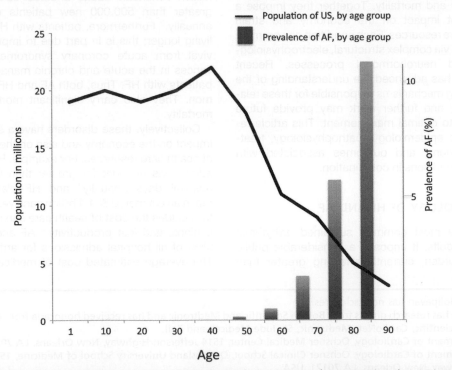

Fig. 1. Prevalence of AF according to age, and the US population by age, demonstrating that AF increases with age. (*Data from* Go AS, Hylek EM, Phillips KA, et al. Prevalence of diagnosed atrial fibrillation in adults: national implications for rhythm management and stroke prevention: the AnTicoagulation and Risk Factors in atrial fibrillation (ATRIA) study. JAMA 2001;285:2373; with permission.)

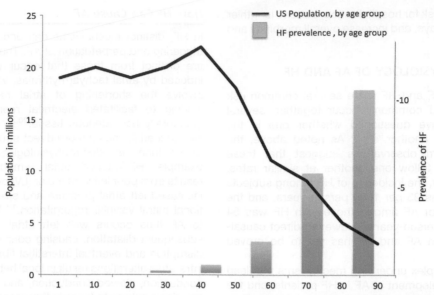

Fig. 2. Prevalence of HF according to age, and the US population by age, demonstrating the increase in HF with age. (*Adapted from* Roger VL, Go AS, Lloyd-Jones DM, et al. Heart disease and stroke statistics—2012 update: a report from the American Heart Association. Circulation 2012;125(1):e36; with permission.)

was independently associated with adverse outcomes, including hospital stays more frequently lasting for greater than 4 days (48.8% vs 41.5%, P<.001) and increased in-hospital mortality (4.0% vs 2.6%, P<.001).[11] In a meta-analysis by Mamas and colleagues[12] representing 20 studies including 9 randomized controlled trials (RCT) and totaling 32,946 patients, the coexistence of AF in HF was associated with increased mortality

(OR 1.33; 95% CI 1.2–2.1). Last, in a community-based cohort of 1664 patients with HF, with a median follow-up of 4 years, patients who developed AF after HF had a 2-fold increased risk of death when compared with HF patients without AF.[13] The poor prognosis found among patients with HF who developed AF is consistent in the findings of several prior HF trials.[14,15] In digest, AF and HF often coexist, and when they do, they confer

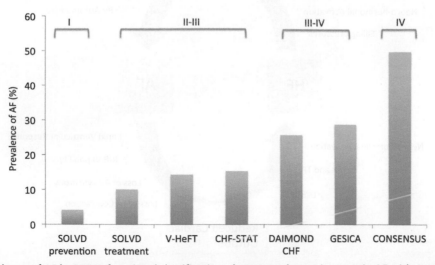

Fig. 3. Prevalence of AF by NYHA functional classification, demonstrating an increase in AF with worsening functional class. (*Adapted from* Maisel WH, Stevenson LW. Atrial fibrillation in heart failure: epidemiology, pathophysiology, and rationale for therapy. Am J Cardiol 2003;91:3; with permission.)

increased risk for hospitalization, portend lengthier inpatient stays, and increase overall morbidity and mortality.

PATHOPHYSIOLOGY OF AF AND HF

Because AF and HF share several common risk factors and commonly occur together, several authors have questioned whether one is the product of another.[9,16–18] As noted above, the Framingham observations suggest that these conditions follow one another at similar rates. Specifically, the incidence of HF among subjects with AF was 33 per 1000 person-years, and the incidence of AF among those with HF was 54 per 1000 person-years.[6] However, direct causality between AF and HF has yet to be proved definitively.

The complex underlying mechanisms that lead to the development of AF in HF patients, and the converse relationship, have been partially described. In patients with HF, there is evidence to support structural, neurohormonal, and electrical atrial remodeling—each of which may encourage the development of AF.[19–25] Likewise, AF can induce electrical and hemodynamic deterioration and can lead to tachycardia-mediated cardiomyopathy (**Fig. 4**).[26–28]

How HF Can Cause AF

In HF, distinct mechanisms can account for the triggering and perpetuation of AF. These changes are distinct from those that occur when AF is induced by atrial tachyarrhythmias, which mainly involve the shortening of atrial refractoriness leading to facilitated electrical reentry among structurally homogenous tissue.[20,21] In contrast, HF-induced AF has a more direct structural basis rather than an electrophysiological one. For example, HF-induced atrial remodeling often results from poor left ventricular (LV) performance, increased left atrial pressure and size, and functional mitral valvular regurgitation.[19] Vulnerability to AF thus occurs with left atrial stretch and subsequent dilatation, causing connective tissue disruption and eventual interstitial fibrosis. These intra-atrial alterations result in local heterogeneous conduction, slowed conduction, and local block, creating a substrate for arrhythmogenesis. In early observations supporting this mechanism, Boyden and colleagues[22,23] noted atrial fibrosis in canine and feline models of spontaneous HF. This observation was later confirmed in humans using electroanatomical mapping techniques.[21,24,25]

The hormonal milieu in HF patients can also lead to AF. For example, the renin-angiotensin system

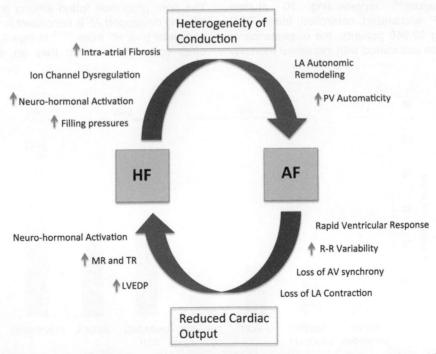

Fig. 4. The steps and interrelated pathways linking AF and HF. TR, tricuspid regurgitation. (*Adapted from* Anter E, Jessup M, Callans DJ. Atrial fibrillation and heart failure treatment considerations for a dual epidemic. Circulation 2009;119:2517; with permission.)

has an established role in remodeling in HF. Specifically, angiotensin II and aldosterone have proinflammatory properties (including via increased C-reactive protein activation) that can lead to the development of intra-atrial fibrosis in HF patients.[29–32] Attenuation of intra-atrial fibrosis in HF has been demonstrated in animal models with the use of angiotensin converting enzyme inhibitors (ACEi).[33] Similarly, ACEi use in patients with LV dysfunction has been associated with a decreased incidence of AF.[34,35] In further experimental models, aldosterone, a hormone implicated in HF, has been shown to be proarrhythmic when implanted subcutaneously in rats. Reil and colleagues[32] showed more inducible atrial arrhythmias in rats after aldosterone implantation than controls (100% vs 9%), and this effect occurred independently of LV hemodynamics.

Atrial arrhythmogenicity is also increased in HF. Increased automaticity occurs via changes in both ion channel expression and intracellular calcium dysregulation through decreased Na^{2+}/Ca^{2+} exchanger current.[20,36] Additional findings suggest that reduced L-type Ca^{2+} current as well as changes in potassium currents including the transient outward K^+ current (I_{to}) and slow delayed rectifier current (I_{Ks}) may adversely affect conduction velocity and refractoriness.

Recent in vivo findings suggest that left atrial autonomic remodeling, and its excitatory effects on pulmonary vein (PV) electrical activity, may also play a role in arrhythmogenesis. For example, Ng and colleagues[37] associated the initiation and maintenance of AF with autonomic remodeling in the posterior left atrium (LA) and PVs of HF-afflicted dogs. In rabbits with HF induced by rapid ventricular pacing, the PVs showed a higher frequency of irregular electrical activity, a higher incidence of early afterdepolarizations, and more delayed afterdepolarizations when compared with PVs in controls or the non-PV tissue of the LA.[38]

Endothelin-1 (ET1) is an autocrine and paracrine mediator with known mitogenic, inotropic, and arrhythmogenic activity in cardiac muscle.[39] Recently, increased levels of ET1 were found in patients with known AF when compared with those without AF. In addition, patients with HF also have elevated levels of ET1 that may facilitate the maintenance of AF. Among patients undergoing coronary artery bypass graft, valve repair, and/or Maze procedures, excised left atrial appendage tissue shows higher levels of ET1 varying directly with LA size, HF, AF persistence, and severity of mitral regurgitation.[40]

Thus, the development of AF in HF appears to be a multifactorial process, including early atrial enlargement, conduction heterogeneity from intra-atrial fibrosis, ion channel dysregulation, and autonomic remodeling. Future research elucidating these mechanisms may have therapeutic implications in the prevention and treatment of AF among HF patients.

How AF Can Cause HF

Several mechanisms are credited in the deterioration of cardiac transport function among patients with AF. Foremost, irregular R-R intervals evoked by variable atrioventricular (AV) conduction may themselves result in decreased ventricular filling, contractility, and output.[41] Irregular ventricular cycle lengths may culminate in increased left ventricular end diastolic pressure (LVEDP). This altered hemodynamic state may lead to an eventual reduction in cardiac output and function.[41] In addition, loss of organized contraction in atrial systole reduces the atrial contribution toward LV filling.

A rapid ventricular response in AF may cause a tachycardia-mediated cardiomyopathy, as first described by Gossage and Braxton Hicks[26] in 1913 and later verified when reproduced in an experimental pacing model in 1962.[28] As this is a known reversible form of cardiomyopathy, when HF and AF coexist, attempts at restoring normal rate often take precedence, whether this occurs via AV nodal blockade controlling the ventricular response in AF or via sinus rhythm restoration.

Few studies have investigated the development of HF in patients with AF. Byrne and colleagues[42] reported an ovine model of tachycardia-induced HF, in which the presence of AF in HF led to further LV deterioration. This model also showed increased plasma norepinephrine levels that were found to be independent of the heart rate. Interestingly and contrary to former studies, a decline in LVEDP was reported after the development of AF. This decline was attributed to decreased atrial contribution to LV end diastolic volume. Of note, Byrne demonstrated the change in LVEDP by echocardiographic assessment, whereas other investigators used left atrial pressure as a correlate for LVEDP.[41,43]

AF can lead to the development of LV dysfunction, whether by rapid ventricular response or by altered hemodynamics. These changes can also cause HF symptoms in patients with intact LV systolic function.

DIAGNOSIS OF AF AMONG PATIENTS WITH HF

The diagnosis of AF in HF patients can be made via an electrocardiogram, telemetry, or implanted device monitoring. Devices such as permanent pacemakers, implantable cardiac defibrillators, and cardiac resynchronization therapy defibrillators (CRT-Ds) continuously monitor AF occurrence and burden. Because AF can lead to more frequent HF hospitalization, routine monthly surveillance for AF using implantable devices has been suggested as a preventative measure.[44,45] Sarkar and colleagues[45] demonstrated in a pooled retrospective analysis of 1561 HF patients with CRT-D devices that the presence of AF (n = 519) implies a greater risk for HF hospitalization (HR 2.0, $P<.001$). In addition, 1 day of detected "high-burden" paroxysmal AF (defined as >6 hours of AF) with adequate rate control, defined as a heart rate less than 90 bpm, increases risk for HF hospitalization in the next 30 days (HR 3.4, $P<.001$).[45] High-burden AF with *poor* rate control further increased the risk of HF hospitalization (HR 5.9, $P<.001$).[45] Although prospective data are needed to determine if close surveillance may prevent HF hospitalizations, Sarkar and colleagues suggest that monthly monitoring can identify patients at higher near-term risk.

DIAGNOSIS OF HF AMONG PATIENTS WITH AF

The diagnosis of HF is most often made via clinical examination, but diagnostic tests such as brain natriuretic peptide (BNP) are often helpful.[46] However, AF patients have been shown to have elevated levels of BNP even in the absence of HF. In addition, a reduction in BNP level has been demonstrated after rhythm restoration by cardioversion, Maze operation, or pulmonary vein isolation (PVI), whether HF was present or absent.[47–51] Thus, the diagnostic utility of BNP may be limited in patients with AF.

TREATMENT OF AF AND HF
Medical Therapy: Anticoagulation

AF is a powerful risk factor for stroke and thromboembolism.[52] Among those with AF, comorbid conditions (HF, hypertension, age, diabetes, and prior stroke/transient ischemic attack [TIA]) are known to increase this risk. However, these other individual risk factors do not carry exact equivalent additional risk.[53–58] Notably, in the Framingham study, HF carried a 4-fold risk of thromboembolic events per year, whereas hypertension and coronary artery disease implied 3 times and twice the risk, respectively.[52] Other studies, including the Stroke Prevention in Atrial Fibrillation study (SPAF), have also demonstrated that LV dysfunction is a particularly significant independent risk factor for cerebrovascular accident (**Table 1**).[53–56,59–61] Despite this, commonly used risk stratification schemes, such as the $CHADS_2$ (congestive heart failure, hypertension, age, diabetes, stroke) and CHA_2DS_2-VASc (congestive heart failure, hypertension, age, diabetes, stroke, female gender, vascular disease) scores, assign similar risk to each "point." Both schemas divide patients into low-, intermediate-, and high-risk groups, with the incremental risk indicated by HF, hypertension, advanced age, and diabetes being the same (each amounting to one point of risk).

As evidence shows HF implies a truly higher relative risk than these other factors, the CHADS scoring system may underestimate the true risk of stroke and thromboembolism in patients with AF and HF. The concern is most relevant in the decision of whether to anticoagulate intermediate-risk patients ($CHADS_2$ or CHA_2DS_2-VASc score of 1) with isolated HF. Although AF patients at high stroke risk (score 2 or greater) clearly benefit from anticoagulation with oral anticoagulants (OACs, either vitamin K antagonists [VKAs] or the novel

Table 1
Summary of the results for structural heart disease (SHD) as a risk factor for stroke in patients with AF

Study, Year	N	SHD Definition	P Value
Cabin et al,[111] 1990	272	Structural heart disease (cardiomyopathy)	.037
SPAF III,[110] 1998	892	CHF	NS
Laupacis,[112] 1994	1593	CHF	NS
SPAF II,[54] 1995	854	LV dysfunction (LV FS <25%)	.2
Aronow et al,[59] 1998	312	LV dysfunction (LVEF <50)	.03
Ezekowitz et al,[60] 1998	1066	LV dysfunction (moderate to severe)	<.001
Pearce,[61] 1992	568	LV dysfunction	.03

Abbreviation: NS, nonsignificant.
Adapted from Hughes M, Lip GH. Stroke and thromboembolism in atrial fibrillation: a systematic review of stroke risk factors, risk stratification schema. Thromb Haemost 2008;99(2):298; and *Data from* Refs.[55,59–61,110,111]

oral anticoagulants [NOACs; see below in this section]), the data are less clear for patients with intermediate risk (score of 1) for whom either aspirin alone or oral anticoagulation are options.[62–64]

Recent data suggest that VKAs may be superior to antiplatelet agents alone among intermediate-risk patients with AF. Lee and colleagues[65] compared use of VKA versus antiplatelet agents in 422 patients over 2 years and reported an HR of 0.28 (95%, CI 0.10–0.79; $P = .016$) with the use of VKA, without a significant difference in major bleeding. Similarly, Gorin and colleagues[66] reported a lower rate of cerebrovascular accident and mortality with VKA of 8.4% versus non-VKA patients of 17.9%. Overall, VKAs appear to be superior to antiplatelet regimens in intermediate-risk patients, and the independent risk of stroke in patients with AF and HF is likely underestimated by commonly used risk stratification schemes. In addition, the OAC's risk of major bleeding may be less significant than previously estimated when compared with aspirin.[65]

With these findings in mind, the European Society of Cardiology AF management guidelines suggest treating CHA_2DS_2-VASc (score 1) with OAC and treating low-risk patients (score 0) with no anticoagulants or antiplatelets. In patients with CHADS scores of 1 or greater, the European Society of Cardiology recommends antiplatelet agents alone only if patients refuse OAC. Thus, it is reasonable to anticoagulate patients with HF as their only CHADS risk factor, using either VKA or an NOAC, as long as an obviously high adverse bleeding risk is not present. The HAS-BLED (hypertension, abnormal renal/liver function, stroke, bleeding history or predisposition, labile INR, elderly [age over 65], and drugs/alcohol) score can be used when assessing the risk of anticoagulation.[67]

The NOACs, dabigatran, rivaroxaban, and apixaban, have recently become US Food and Drug Administration approved for nonvalvular AF and are gaining widespread use. Although data from the RE-LY (Randomized Evaluation of Long-Term Anticoagulation Therapy) and ARISTOTLE (Apixaban for Reduction in Stroke and Other Thromboembolic Events in Atrial Fibrillation trial) trials (examining dabigatran and apixaban, respectively) showed antithrombotic superiority (while ROCKET AF (Rivaroxaban Once Daily Oral Direct Factor Xa Inhibition Compared with Vitamin K Antagonism for Prevention of Stroke and Embolism Trial in Atrial Fibrillation), examining rivaroxaban, demonstrated noninferiority) when compared with VKA, long-term data and experience are still needed.[68–70] Of note, HF patients often demonstrate variable renal function, which may influence

exposure to prescribed NOACs. In such patients, caution with the use of NOACs seems prudent.

Medical Therapy: Rate Control or Rhythm Control

Data from registry populations and study subsets suggest that AF is associated with adverse outcomes in patients with HF.[6,10–13,15] However, the theoretical benefit of rhythm control in patients with HF has never been established in RCT.

Early trials including SPAF demonstrated an increase in mortality associated with the use of antiarrhythmic medication.[57,71] The Atrial Fibrillation Follow-up Investigation of Rhythm Management trial (AFFIRM) was the largest randomized trial to compare the rate-control and rhythm-control strategies and demonstrated similar cumulative all-cause mortality at 5 years (24 vs 21%, $P = .08$).[72] Complementary analysis suggested that there was a gross mortality benefit to maintenance of sinus rhythm but that this effect was neutralized by an increase in mortality associated with antiarrhythmic use.[73] Other smaller randomized trials also showed similar mortality between rate and rhythm control. Specifically, these included the How to Treat Chronic Atrial Fibrillation study of 205 patients (1% vs 3%, $P = $ NS), Rate Control versus Electrical cardioversion for atrial fibrillation in 522 patients (7.0% vs 6.8%, $P = $ NS), and Strategies of Treatment of Atrial Fibrillation (8% vs 4%, $P = $ NS).[74–76] However, these populations had a relatively small number of patients with systolic dysfunction.

The AF in Congestive Heart Failure Trial, published in 2008, randomized 1376 patients with systolic dysfunction and AF to rhythm control versus rate control. Once again, there was no identified difference in overall survival, cardiovascular death, worsened HF, or stroke.[77] A related analysis reported in 2010 highlighted that there was no demonstrated benefit to sinus rhythm, and antiarrhythmic agents were associated with increased mortality,[78] in contrast with post-hoc analysis showing a mortality benefit from successful sinus rhythm maintenance in both AFFIRM and the Danish Investigations on Arrhythmia and Mortality on Dofetilide study (DIAMOND).[72,79] The authors stressed that the mortality benefit of maintaining sinus rhythm is likely outweighed by the incomplete efficacy of, and adverse effects related to, current antiarrhythmic drugs (AAD). Arguably, in older trials an increase in mortality could be accounted for by routine use of class 1 antiarrhythmics, which may themselves increase mortality in some populations. However, patients in the AF in congestive heart failure (CHF) trial instead received either amiodarone or dofetilide and still failed to demonstrate benefit.[74–77]

Medical Therapy: Symptomatology

Many patients with HF have significant symptoms while in AF than when they are in sinus rhythm (SR). Because patients with HF may be more dependent on the LA's contribution to LV filling, they may benefit more from restoration of SR than their counterparts without HF. However, although large randomized studies such as the AF-FRIM and AF in CHF trials examined the endpoint of mortality (and failed to show a benefit), symptom relief was not specifically studied.[72,77] In contrast, the Randomized Controlled Study of Rate versus Rhythm Control in Patients with Chronic Atrial Fibrillation and Heart Failure study demonstrated improved LV function ($P = .014$), lower NT-proBNP levels ($P = .05$), and improved quality of life ($P = .019$) at 1 year in patients assigned to rhythm control.[80] However, similar NYHA class ($P = .424$) and 6 minute walk test distance ($P = .342$) were reported between groups.[80] The management strategy of rhythm restoration with AADs is appropriate in HF patients with symptomatic AF, even given the rhythm control strategy's failure to show a clear mortality benefit compared with rate control.

Medical Therapy: Stroke Prevention

Although SPAF and AFFIRM showed similar stroke rates in patients with paroxysmal AF and permanent AF, a recent population-based observational study examined 16,325 patients receiving rhythm control therapy and 41,193 receiving rate control therapy, with a mean follow-up of 2.8 years. This study reported a lower rate of stroke/TIA with the rhythm control therapy (1.7 vs 2.5 per 100 person-years, $P<.001$). Although there were fewer patients with $CHADS_2$ scores greater than 2 in the rhythm control population, the lower rates of stroke/TIA were supported after propensity scoring.[81]

Overall, the use of AADs has yet to demonstrate any mortality benefit over rate control. Successful maintenance of sinus rhythm appears to be associated with improved outcome, but is balanced by the risks associated with AADs. Newer antiarrhythmics with improved safety profile and greater efficacy are sought, but recent progress has been disappointing.[82] Of note, the most recently approved agent, dronedarone, is contraindicated in the presence of a recent HF exacerbation requiring hospitalization, and also in permanent AF.[83] Newer antiarrhythmic therapies including vernakalant and ranolazine are being investigated

and may meet the promise of efficacy with improved safety.[84,85]

As noted above, studies of the electrophysiological changes associated with HF have concluded that atrial refractoriness is not shortened in HF. However, AAD in large part exert their benefit through prolonging myocardial refractoriness, thereby preventing reentry. This discrepancy could contribute to their reduced efficacy in HF.[21–25]

At present, it is reasonable to pursue rate control rather than rhythm restoration if symptoms are not different between SR and AF.

Medical Therapy: Non-antiarrhythmic Therapy

The potential impact of non-antiarrhythmic therapy for the primary prevention of AF in patients with known LV dysfunction should not be disregarded. These therapies treat the underlying condition while targeting substrates potentially responsible for the development of AF in HF. Retrospective analyses of large clinical trials have identified ACEi use among HF patients as an effective therapy in reducing the incidence of AF.[34,35] A substudy of the SOLVD trial demonstrated a lower AF incidence in patients treated with enalapril over 2.9 years (5.4 vs 24%; $P<.0001$).[35] Later, in the Valsartan Heart Failure Trial and the Candesartan in Heart failure: Assessment of Reduction in Mortality and Morbidity (CHARM) study, the use of angiotensin receptor blockers showed similar but more modest effects.[86,87] In CHARM, in which 6379 patients with symptomatic CHF were followed for the prespecified secondary endpoint of AF, incident AF was less frequent in the candesartan group (5.5 vs 6.7%; $P = .048$).

A meta-analysis of 7 large RCTs of β-blocker therapy found reduced risk (27% risk reduction) of AF among a total of 11,952 patients with HF.[88] More recently, the addition of eplerenone to an optimal HF regimen (including maximally tolerated ACEi or angiotensin receptor blockers therapy) demonstrated further risk reduction in new onset AF (HR 0.58, $P = .034$) in patients with left ventricular ejection fraction (LVEF) less than 35% and mild symptoms (NYHA II).[89] Although further randomized data are needed, the experience with these now conventional HF therapies has been positive in the primary prevention of AF in HF.

CATHETER-BASED ABLATION OF THE AV NODE AND BIVENTRICULAR PACING ("ABLATE AND PACE")

Implantation of a pacemaker (often, one with ventricular resynchronization therapy capacity) with subsequent radiofrequency ablation of the atrio-ventricular node (AVN) has been shown to be effective in AF patients with rapid ventricular response who are refractory to medical therapy.[90]

Patients with an implanted CRT device with persistent/permanent AF should be also undergo AV nodal ablation. Ineffective biventricular capture due to a high prevalence of fusion and pseudo-fusion beats was reported in CRT-treated patients with permanent AF, possibly limiting CRT's maximum benefit.[91] By eliminating rapid intrinsic ventricular activation, AVN ablation in these HF patients may optimize synchronized biventricular capture.[92] A recent meta-analysis, including mortality data from 450 patients in 3 nonrandomized trials, concluded that AVN ablation was associated with a reduction in all-cause (relative risk 0.42, $P<.001$) and cardiovascular mortality (relative risk 0.44, $P = .008$).[93] However, prospective randomized data are necessary to confirm these findings.

Surgical Therapy for AF

Surgical therapy for AF has existed since the 1980s with the development of the Cox Maze procedure. This operation has been reported to result in high rates of freedom from arrhythmia (93%) over an 8.5-year follow-up period.[94] However, the Maze procedures are complicated operations that involve cardiopulmonary bypass and carry an operative mortality of 3%.[95] More recent surgical PVI techniques using radiofrequency ablation and cryoablation have more than a decade of experience to report, despite few randomized trials. These techniques are less complicated than the Maze procedure and do not require an atriotomy nor additional time on cardiopulmonary bypass.[95] Procedural success with surgical PVI has been generally favorable but variable (50%–91%).[95]

A report of the Heart Rhythm Society Task Force on Catheter and Surgical Ablation of Atrial Fibrillation concluded that surgical ablation is indicated in symptomatic AF patients undergoing other cardiac surgical procedures, or in selected asymptomatic AF patients undergoing cardiac surgery (as is the case for many HF patients) in whom the ablation can be performed with minimal risk. In addition, the Task Force report states that stand-alone AF surgery should be considered for symptomatic AF patients who have failed medical management and prefer a surgical approach, or have failed one or more attempts at catheter ablation (CA), or are not candidates for CA.[96]

Catheter-Based PVI

In part due to the risks of medical antiarrhythmic therapy and its incomplete success in maintaining sinus rhythm, catheter-based ablation has emerged as a therapeutic option in the management of AF.[97] CA, most often with a goal of pulmonary vein electrical isolation (PVI), currently is accomplished using radiofrequency ablation and/or cyroablation-based techniques.[98,99] In cases refractory to at least one AAD, PVI has earned an American College of Cardiology/American Heart Association class I recommendation for therapy in patients with paroxysmal AF and normal or mildly reduced LV function.[97] Catheter-based ablation appears to be as good as, or better than, AAD therapy for the maintenance of sinus rhythm.[100,101]

In nonrandomized studies of HF patients with AF, catheter-based PVI has demonstrated benefit including improvements in cardiac function, exercise capacity, and quality of life.[102–105] Reports vary from 73% to 87% success in restoration of sinus rhythm at 1 year postprocedure in HF patients. In addition, improvements in LV function have been noted. For example, Hsu and colleagues[103] found an average increase in ejection fraction from 36% pre-CA to 57% post-CA, and Tondo and colleagues[104] found that LVEF increased from $33 \pm 2\%$ to $47 \pm 3\%$ ($P = .01$). In a recent open-label, blinded-endpoint trial, 52 symptomatic AF patients with LVEF less than 35% were followed for 12 months after randomization to PVI versus rate control. These investigators reported a success rate of 88% for maintaining sinus rhythm at 1 year in patients who underwent PVI. In addition, in the PVI arm, objective exercise performance improved, including peak oxygen consumption (+3.07 mL/kg/min, $P = .02$). Minnesota symptom scores were improved, BNP was lower, and trends toward improved 6-minute walk distance ($P = .10$) and LVEF ($P = .055$) were demonstrated.[106]

Long-term outcome data suggest that for several outcome measures, PVI outperforms AV node ablation and pacing.[105] Data from the Pulmonary-Vein Isolation for AF in Patients with Heart Failure trial show that those randomized to PVI had a significantly higher mean LVEF (35% vs 28%), a longer distance on the 6-minute walk test (340 vs 297 m), and a superior quality-of-life score.[107] In addition, in elderly patients there was a higher incidence of new HF at 5 years in the ablate-and-pace group when compared with those who underwent AF ablation (53% vs 24%).[108]

CA is rapidly evolving, and improvements in the efficacy and safety of this procedure occur frequently.[109] Although additional prospective data are needed, in patients with LV dysfunction, CA appears to be technically feasible without a higher procedural complication rate.[108] Catheter-based

PVI may also improve LV performance, reduce symptoms, and improve quality of life.

FINAL COMMENTS

AF and HF have a negative impact on one another and adversely affect mortality when found together. The poor prognosis of concomitant AF and HF is a consistent finding in several HF trials, leading to increased hospitalization and lengthier inpatient stays. Although comprehension of the combined AF/HF pathophysiology is progressing, further efforts are needed to elucidate the mechanisms involved. For patients with HF who are at risk for AF, frequent monitoring with the use of implantable devices may predict future events and may help to avoid hospitalization. Rhythm restoration with AAD, while often effective in terms of symptoms, continues to have limited efficacy in maintaining SR and has failed to show a mortality benefit. Thus, the existence of symptoms when the patient is in AF is the primary indication for rhythm restoration over rate control. Nonpharmacologic treatment of AF, including surgical techniques or CA, also may be of value in the HF population.

REFERENCES

1. Go AS, Hylek EM, Phillips KA, et al. Prevalence of diagnosed atrial fibrillation in adults; national implications for rhythm management and stroke prevention: the AnTicoagulation and Risk Factors in Atrial Fibrillation study (ATRIA). JAMA 2001;285:2370.

2. Roger VL, Go AS, Lloyd-Jones DM, et al. Heart disease and stroke statistics—2012 update: a report from the American Heart Association. Circulation 2012;125(1):e2–220.

3. Fuster V, Ryden LE, Asinger RW, et al. ACC/AHA/ESC Guidelines for the management of patients with atrial fibrillation: executive summary. Circulation 2001;104:2118–50.

4. Heidenriech PA, Trogdon JG, Khavjou OA, et al. Forecasting the future of cardiovascular disease in the United States: a policy statement from the American Heart Association. Circulation 2011;123(8):933–44.

5. Kim MH, Johnston SS, Chu BC, et al. Estimation of total incremental health care costs in patients with atrial fibrillation in the United States. Circ Cardiovasc Qual Outcomes 2011;4(3):313–20.

6. Wang TJ, Larson MG, Levy D, et al. Temporal relations of atrial fibrillation and congestive heart failure and their joint influence on mortality: the Framingham Heart Study. Circulation 2003;107:2920.

7. Stevenson WG, Stevenson LW, Middlekauff HR, et al. Improving survival for patients with atrial fibrillation and advanced heart failure. J Am Coll Cardiol 1996;28:1458.

8. Carson PE, Johnson GR, Dunkman WB, et al. The influence of atrial fibrillation on prognosis in mild to moderate heart failure. The V-HeFT Studies. The V-HeFT VA Cooperative Studies Group. Circulation 1993;87:V102–10.

9. Maisel WH, Stevenson LW. Atrial fibrillation in heart failure: epidemiology, pathophysiology, and rationale for therapy. Am J Cardiol 2003;91:2D–8D.

10. Dries DL, Exner DV, Gersh BJ, et al. Atrial fibrillation is associated with an increased risk for mortality and heart failure progression in patients with asymptomatic and symptomatic left ventricular systolic dysfunction a retrospective analysis of the SOLVD trials. J Am Coll Cardiol 1998;32:695–703.

11. Mountantonakis SE, Grau-Sepulveda MV, Bhatt DL, et al. Presence of atrial fibrillation is independently associated with adverse outcomes in patients hospitalized with heart failure: an analysis of get with the guidelines-heart failure. Circ Heart Fail 2012;5(2):191–201.

12. Mamas MA, Caldwell JC, Chako S, et al. A meta-analysis of the prognostic significance of atrial fibrillation in chronic heart failure. Eur J Heart Fail 2009;11:676–83.

13. Chamberlain AM, Redfield MM, Alonso A, et al. Atrial fibrillation and mortality in heart failure: a community study. Circ Heart Fail 2011;4:740–6.

14. Wasywich CA, Pope AJ, Somartne J, et al. Atrial fibrillation and the risk of death in patients with heart failure: a literature-based meta-analysis. Intern Med J 2010;40:347–56.

15. Mentz RJ, Chung MJ, Gheorghiade M, et al. Atrial fibrillation or flutter on initial electrocardiogram is associated with worse outcomes in patients admitted for worsening heart failure with reduced ejection fraction: findings from the EVEREST Trial. Am Heart J 2013;164(6):884–92.e2.

16. Lubitz SA, Benjamin EJ, Ellinor PT. Atrial fibrillation in congestive heart failure. Heart Fail Clin 2010;6(2):187–200.

17. Anter E, Jessup M, David J, et al. Atrial fibrillation and heart failure treatment considerations for a dual epidemic. Circulation 2009;119:2516–25.

18. Smit MD, Moes ML, Maass AH, et al. The importance of whether atrial fibrillation or heart failure develops first. Eur J Heart Fail 2012;14(9):1030–40.

19. Verheule S, Wilson E, Everett TT, et al. Alterations in atrial electrophysiology and tissue structure in a canine model of chronic atrial dilatation due to mitral regurgitation. Circulation 2003;107:2615–22.

20. Li D, Melnyk P, Feng J, et al. Effects of experimental heart failure on atrial cellular and ionic electrophysiology. Circulation 2000;101:2631–8.

21. Li D, Fareh S, Leung TK, et al. Promotion of atrial fibrillation by heart failure in dogs: atrial remodeling of a different sort. Circulation 1999;100:87–95.

22. Boyden PA, Tilley LP, Pham TD, et al. Effects of left atrial enlargement on atrial transmembrane potentials and structure in dogs with mitral valve fibrosis. Am J Cardiol 1982;49:1896–908.

23. Boyden PA, Tilley LP, Albala A, et al. Mechanisms for atrial arrhythmias associated with cardiomyopathy: a study of feline hearts with primary myocardial disease. Circulation 1984;69:1036–47.

24. Sanders P, Morton JB, Davidson NC, et al. Electrical remodeling of the atria in congestive heart failure: electrophysiological and electrophysiological and electroanatomic mapping in humans. Circulation 2003;108:1461–8.

25. Ohtani K, Yutani C, Nagata S, et al. High prevalence of atrial fibrosis in patients with dilated cardiomyopathy. J Am Coll Cardiol 1995;25:1162–9.

26. Gossage AM, Braxton Hicks JA. On auricular fibrillation. QJM 1913;6:435–40.

27. Philips E, Levine SA. Auricular fibrillation without other evidence of heart disease: a cause of reversible heart failure. Am J Med 1949;7:479.

28. Whipple GH, Sheffield LT, Woodman EG, et al. Reversible congestive heart failure due to chronic rapid stimulation of the normal heart. Proc N Engl Cardiovasc Soc 1962;20:39–40.

29. Everett TH, Olgin JE. Atrial fibrosis and the mechanisms of atrial fibrillation. Heart Rhythm 2007;4: S24–7.

30. Boos CJ, Anderson RA, Lip GY. Is atrial fibrillation an inflammatory disorder? Eur Heart J 2006;27: 136–49.

31. Boo CJ, Lip GY. Inflammation and atrial fibrillation: cause or effect? Heart 2008;94:133–4.

32. Reil JC, Hohl M, Selejan S, et al. Aldosterone promotes atrial fibrillation. Eur Heart J 2012;33: 2098–108.

33. Li D, Shinagawa K, Pang L, et al. Effects of angiotensin-converting enzyme inhibition on the development of the atrial fibrillation substrate in dogs with ventricular tachypacing-induced congestive heart failure. Circulation 2001;104:2608–14.

34. Vermes E, Tardif JC, Bourassa MG, et al. Enalapril decreases the incidence of atrial fibrillation in patients with left ventricular dysfunction: insight from the Studies Of Left Ventricular Dysfunction (SOLVD) trials. Circulation 2003;107:2926–31.

35. Pedersen OD, Bagger H, Kober L, et al. Trandolapril reduces the incidence of atrial fibrillation after acute myocardial infarction in patients with left ventricular dysfunction. Circulation 1999;100:376–80.

36. Ohkusa T, Ueyama T, Yamada J, et al. Alterations in cardiac sarcoplasmic reticulum Ca2+ regulatory proteins in the atrial tissue of patients with chronic atrial fibrillation. J Am Coll Cardiol 1999;34:255–63.

37. Ng J, Villuendas R, Cokic I, et al. Autonomic remodeling in the left atrium and pulmonary veins in heart failure: creation of a dynamic substrate for atrial fibrillation. Circ Arrhythm Electrophysiol 2011;4(3):388–96.

38. Chang SL, Chen YC, Yeh YH, et al. Heart failure enhances arrhythmogenesis in pulmonary veins. Clin Exp Pharmacol Physiol 2011;38(10):666–74.

39. Russell FD, Molenaar P. The human heart endothelin system: ET-1 synthesis, storage, release and effect. Trends Pharmacol Sci 2000;21:353–9.

40. Mayyas F, Niebauer M, Zurick A, et al. Association of left atrial endothelin-1 with atrial rhythm, size, and fibrosis in patients with structural heart disease. Circ Arrhythm Electrophysiol 2010;3(4): 369–79.

41. Clark DM, Plumb VJ, Epstein AE, et al. Hemodynamic effects of an irregular sequence of ventricular cycle lengths during atrial fibrillation. J Am Coll Cardiol 1997;30:1039–45.

42. Byrne M, Kaye DM, Power J. The synergism between atrial fibrillation and heart failure. J Card Fail 2008;14(4):320–6.

43. Lau CP, Leung WH, Wong CK, et al. Hemomodynamics of induced atrial fibrillation: a comparative assessment with sinus rhythm, atrial and ventricular pacing. Eur Heart J 1990;11:219–24.

44. Santini M, Gasparini M, Landolina M, et al. Device-detected atrial tachyarrhythmias predict adverse outcome in real-world patients with implantable biventricular defibrillators. J Am Coll Cardiol 2011;57: 167–72.

45. Sarkar S, Koehler J, Crossley GH, et al. Burden of atrial fibrillation and poor rate control detected by continuous monitoring and the risk for heart failure hospitalization. Am Heart J 2012;164: 616–24.

46. Maisel A, Mueller C, Adams K Jr, et al. State of the art: using natriuretic peptide levels in clinical practice. Eur J Heart Fail 2008;10(9):824–39.

47. Roy D, Paillard F, Cassidy D, et al. Atrial natriuretic factor during atrial fibrillation and supraventricular tachycardia. J Am Coll Cardiol 1987;9:509–14.

48. Rossi A, Enriquez-Sarano M, Burnett JC, et al. Natriuretic peptide levels in atrial fibrillation. J Am Coll Cardiol 2000;35:1256–62.

49. Inoue S, Murakami Y, Sano K, et al. Atrium as a source of brain natriuretic polypeptide in patients with atrial fibrillation. J Card Fail 2000;6:92–6.

50. Ohta Y, Shimada T, Yoshitomi H, et al. Drop in plasma brain natriuretic peptide levels after successful direct current cardioversion in chronic atrial fibrillation. Can J Cardiol 2001;17:415–20.

51. Wozakowska-Kaplon B. Effect of sinus rhythm restoration on plasma brain natriuretic peptide in patients with atrial fibrillation. Am J Cardiol 2004; 93:1555–8.

52. Wolf PA, Abbott RD, Kannel WB. Atrial fibrillation as an independent risk factor for stroke: the Framingham Study. Stroke 1991;22(8):983–8.

53. Risk factors for stroke and efficacy of antithrombotic therapy in atrial fibrillation. Analysis of pooled data from five randomized controlled trials. Arch Intern Med 1994;154:1449–57.

54. Stroke Prevention in Atrial Fibrillation Investigators. Risk factors for thromboembolism during aspirin therapy in patients with atrial fibrillation: the Stroke Prevention in Atrial Fibrillation Study. J Stroke Cerebrovasc Dis 1995;5:147–57.

55. Warfarin versus aspirin for prevention of thromboembolism in atrial fibrillation: Stroke Prevention in Atrial Fibrillation II Study. Lancet 1994;343:687–91.

56. Stroke prevention in Atrial Fibrillation Study. Final results. Circulation 1991;84:527–39.

57. Sato H, Ishikawa K, Kitabatake A, et al, Japan Atrial Fibrillation Stroke Trial Group. Low-dose aspirin for prevention of stroke in low-risk patients with atrial fibrillation: Japan atrial fibrillation stroke trial. Stroke 2006;37(2):447–51.

58. Lip GY. Anticoagulation therapy and the risk of stroke in patients with atrial fibrillation at 'moderate risk' [CHADS2 score=1]: simplifying stroke risk assessment and thromboprophylaxis in real-life clinical practice. Thromb Haemost 2010;103(4):683–5.

59. Aronow WS, Ahn C, Kronzon I, et al. Risk factors for new thromboembolic stroke in patient > or equal to 62 years of age with chronic atrial fibrillation. Am J Cardiol 1998;82:119–21.

60. Ezekowitz MD, Laupacis A, Boysen G, et al. Echocardiographic predictors of stroke in patients with atrial fibrillation: a prospective study of 1066 patients from 3 clinical trials. Arch Intern Med 1998; 158:1316–20.

61. Pearce LA. Predictors of thromboembolism in atrial fibrillation: II. Echocardiographic features of patients at risk. Ann Intern Med 1992;116:6–12.

62. Van Walraven C, Hart RG, Singer DE, et al. Oral anticoagulants vs aspirin in nonvalvular atrial fibrillation: an individual patient meta-analysis. JAMA 2002;288(19):2441–8.

63. Gage BF, Van Walraven C, Pearce L, et al. Selecting patients with atrial fibrillation for anticoagulation: stroke risk stratification in patients taking aspirin. Circulation 2004;110(16):2287–92.

64. Gage BF, Waterman AD, Shannon W, et al. Validation of clinical classification schemes for predicting stroke: results from the National Registry of Atrial Fibrillation. JAMA 2001;285(22):2864–70.

65. Lee BH, Park JS, Park JH, et al. The effect and safety of the anti-thrombotic therapies in patients with atrial fibrillation and CHADS2 score 1. J Cardiovasc Electrophysiol 2010;21(5):501–7.

66. Gorin L, Fauchier L, Nonin, et al. Antithrombotic treatment and the risk of death and stroke in patients with atrial fibrillation and a CHADS2 score=1. Thromb Haemost 2010;103:833–40.

67. Pisters R, Lane DA, Nieuwlaat R, et al. A novel user-friendly score (HAS-BLED) to assess 1-year risk of major bleeding in patients with atrial fibrillation: the Euro Heart Survey. Chest 2010;138(5): 1093–100.

68. Connolly SJ, Ezekowitz MD, Yusuf S, et al, RE-LY Steering Committee and Investigators. Dabigatran versus warfarin in patients with atrial fibrillation. N Engl J Med 2009;361:1139–51.

69. Patel MR, Mahaffey KW, Garg J, et al, ROCKET AF Investigators. Rivaroxaban versus warfarin in nonvalvular atrial fibrillation. N Engl J Med 2011;365: 883–91.

70. Granger CB, Alexander JH, McMurray JJ, et al, ARISTOTLE Committees and Investigators. Apixaban versus warfarin in patients with atrial fibrillation. N Engl J Med 2011;365:981–92.

71. Pratt CM, Moyé LA. The cardiac arrhythmia suppression trial casting suppression in a different light. Circulation 1995;91:245–7.

72. Van Gelder IC, Hagens VE, Bosker HA, et al, Rate Control Versus Electrical Cardioversion for Persistent Atrial Fibrillation Study Group. A comparison of rate control and rhythm control in patients with recurrent persistent atrial fibrillation. N Engl J Med 2002;347:1834–40.

73. Corley SD, Epstein AE, DiMarco JP, et al, AFFIRM Investigators. Relationships between sinus rhythm, treatment, and survival in the atrial fibrillation follow-up investigation of rhythm management (AFFIRM) study. Circulation 2004;109: 1509–13.

74. Opolski G, Torbicki A, Kosior DA, et al, Investigators of the Polish How to Treat Chronic Atrial Fibrillation Study. Rate control vs rhythm control in patients with nonvalvular persistent atrial fibrillation: the results of the polish how to treat chronic atrial fibrillation (HOT CAFE) study. Chest 2004; 126:476–86.

75. Carlsson J, Miketic S, Windeler J, et al, STAF Investigators. Randomized trial of rate-control versus rhythm-control in persistent atrial fibrillation: the strategies of treatment of atrial fibrillation (STAF) study. J Am Coll Cardiol 2003;41:1690–6.

76. Van Gelder IC, Hagens VE, Kingma JH, et al. Rate control versus electrical cardioversion for atrial fibrillation A randomised comparison of two treatment strategies concerning morbidity, mortality, quality of life and cost-benefit - the RACE study design. Neth Heart J 2002;10(3):118–22, 123–4.

77. Roy D, Talajic M, Nattel S, et al, Atrial Fibrillation and Congestive Heart Failure Investigators. Rhythm control versus rate control for atrial fibrillation and heart failure. N Engl J Med 2008;358: 2667–77.

78. Talajic M, Khairy P, Levesque S, et al, AF-CHF Investigators. Maintenance of sinus rhythm and survival in patients with heart failure and atrial fibrillation. J Am Coll Cardiol 2010;55(17):1796–802.

79. Pedersen OD, Bagger H, Keller N, et al. Efficacy of dofetilide in the treatment of atrial fibrillation–flutter in patients with reduced left ventricular function: a Danish investigations of arrhythmia and mortality on dofetilide (DIAMOND) sub-study. Circulation 2001;104:292–6.

80. Shelton RJ, Clark AL, Goode K, et al. A randomised, controlled study of rate versus rhythm control in patients with chronic atrial fibrillation and heart failure: (CAFÉ-II Study). Heart 2009; 95:924–30.

81. Tsadok MA, Jackevicius CA, Essebag V, et al. Rhythm versus rate control therapy and subsequent stroke or transient ischemic attack in patients with atrial fibrillation. Circulation 2012; 126(23):2680–7.

82. Hohnloser SH, Crijns HJ, van Eickels M, ATHENA Investigators. Effect of dronedarone on cardiovascular events in Atrial fibrillation. N Engl J Med 2009;360:668–78.

83. Køber L, Torp-Pedersen C, McMurray JJ, Dronedarone Study Group, et al. Increased mortality after dronedarone therapy for severe heart failure. N Engl J Med 2008;358:2678–87.

84. Tzeis S, Andrikopoulos G. Antiarrhythmic properties of ranolazine–from bench to bedside. Expert Opin Investig Drugs 2012;21(11):1733–41.

85. Blomström-Lundqvist C, Blomström P. Safety and efficacy of pharmacological cardioversion of atrial fibrillation using intravenous vernakalant, a new antiarrhythmic drug with atrial selectivity. Expert Opin Drug Saf 2012;11(4):671–9.

86. Ducharme A, Swedberg K, Pfeffer MA, et al. Prevention of atrial fibrillation in patients with symptomatic chronic heart failure by candesartan in Candesartan in Heart failure: Assessment of Reduction in Mortality and morbidity (CHARM) program. Am Heart J 2006;152(1):86–92.

87. Maggioni AP, Latini R, Carson PE, et al, Val-HeFT Investigators. Valsartan reduces the incidence of atrial fibrillation in patients with heart failure: results from the Valsartan Heart Failure Trial (Val-HeFT). Am Heart J 2005;149:548–57.

88. Nasr IA, Bouzamondo A, Hulot JS, et al. Prevention of atrial fibrillation onset by beta-blocker treatment in heart failure: a meta-analysis. Eur Heart J 2007; 28:457–62.

89. Swedberg K, Zannad F, McMurray JJ, et al. Eplerenone and atrial fibrillation in mild systolic: results from the EMPHAISIS-HF study. J Am Coll Cardiol 2012;59(18):1598–603.

90. Manolis AG, Katsivas AG, Lazaris EE, et al. Ventricular performance and quality of life in patients who underwent radiofrequency AV junction ablation and permanent pacemaker implantation due to medically refractory atrial tachyarrhythmias. J Interv Card Electrophysiol 1998;2:71–6.

91. Kamath GS, Cotiga D, Koneru JN, et al. The utility of 12-lead Holter monitoring in patients with permanent atrial fibrillation for the identification of nonresponders after cardiac resynchronization therapy. J Am Coll Cardiol 2009;53: 1050–5.

92. Gasparini M, Galimberti P. AV Junction ablation in heart failure patients with atrial fibrillation treated with cardiac resynchronization therapy: the picture is now clear! J Am Coll Cardiol 2012;59(8): 727–9.

93. Ganesan AN, Brooks AG, Roberts-Thomson KC, et al. Role of AV nodal ablation in cardiac resynchronization in patients with coexistent atrial fibrillation and heart failure a systematic review. J Am Coll Cardiol 2012;59(8):719–26.

94. Cox JL, Schuessler RB, Lappas DG, et al. An 8 1/2-year clinical experience with surgery for atrial fibrillation. Ann Surg 1996;224:267–73.

95. Lee A. The surgical treatment of atrial fibrillation. Surg Clin North Am 2009;89(4):1001–20, x–xi.

96. Calkins H, Brugada J, Packer DL, et al. HRS/EHRA/ECAS expert Consensus Statement on catheter and surgical ablation of atrial fibrillation: recommendations for personnel, policy, procedures and follow-up. A report of the Heart Rhythm Society (HRS) Task Force on catheter and surgical ablation of atrial fibrillation. Heart Rhythm 2007;4(6):816–61.

97. Anderson JL, Halperin JL, Albert NM, et al. Management of patients with atrial fibrillation (Compilation of 2006 ACCF/AHA/ESC and 2011 ACCF/AHA/HRS Recommendations): a report of the American College of Cardiology/American Heart Association Task Force on Practice Guidelines. Circulation 2013;127:1916–26.

98. Haissaguerre M, Jais P, Shah DC, et al. Spontaneous initiation of atrial fibrillation by ectopic beats originating in the pulmonary veins. N Engl J Med 1998;339:659–66.

99. Nademanee K, McKenzie J, Kosar E, et al. A new approach for catheter ablation of atrial fibrillation: mapping of the electrophysiologic substrate. J Am Coll Cardiol 2004;43:2044–53.

100. Cosedis Nielsen J, Johannessen A, Raatikainen P, et al. Radiofrequency ablation as initial therapy in paroxysmal atrial fibrillation. N Engl J Med 2012; 367(17):1587–95.

101. Pappone C, Vicedomini G, Augello G, et al. Radiofrequency catheter ablation and antiarrhythmic drug therapy: a prospective, randomized, 4-year follow-up trial: the APAF study. Circ Arrhythm Electrophysiol 2011;4(6):808–14.

102. Chen MS, Marrouche NF, Khaykin Y, et al. Pulmonary vein isolation for the treatment of atrial fibrillation in patients with impaired systolic function. J Am Coll Cardiol 2004;43:1004–9.

103. Hsu LF, Jais P, Sanders P, et al. Catheter ablation for atrial fibrillation in congestive heart failure. N Engl J Med 2004;351:2373–83.

104. Tondo C, Mantica M, Russo G, et al. Pulmonary vein vestibule ablation for the control of atrial fibrillation in patients with impaired left ventricular function. Pacing Clin Electrophysiol 2006;29:962–70.

105. Gentlesk PJ, Sauer WH, Gerstenfeld EP, et al. Reversal of left ventricular dysfunction following ablation of atrial fibrillation. J Cardiovasc Electrophysiol 2007;18:9–14.

106. Jones DG, Haldar SK, Hussain W, et al. A randomized trial to assess catheter ablation versus rate control in the management of persistent atrial fibrillation in heart failure. J Am Coll Cardiol 2013;61(18):1894–903.

107. Khan MN, Jaïs P, Cummings J, PABA-CHF Investigators, et al. Pulmonary-vein isolation for atrial fibrillation in patients with heart failure. N Engl J Med 2008;359:1778–85.

108. Hsieh MH, Tai CT, Lee SH, et al. Catheter ablation of atrial fibrillation versus atrioventricular junction ablation plus pacing therapy for elderly patients with medically refractory paroxysmal atrial fibrillation. J Cardiovasc Electrophysiol 2005;16:457–61.

109. Wilton SB, Fundytus A, Ghali WA, et al. Meta-analysis of the effectiveness and safety of catheter ablation of atrial fibrillation in patients with versus without left ventricular systolic dysfunction. Am J Cardiol 2010;106(9):1284–91.

110. Patients with nonvalvular atrial fibrillation at low risk of stroke during treatment with aspirin: stroke prevention in atrial fibrillation III study. The SPAF III Writing Committee for the Stroke Prevention in Atrial Fibrillation Investigators. JAMA 1998; 279(16):1273–7.

111. Cabin HS, Clubb KS, Hall C, et al. Risk for systemic embolization of atrial fibrillation without mitral stenosis. Am J Cardiol 1990;65(16):1112–6.

112. Laupacis A, Boysen G, Connolly S, et al. Risk factors for stroke and efficacy of antithrombotic therapy in atrial fibrillation: Analysis of pooled data from five randomized controlled trials. Arch Int Med 1994;154:1449–57.

Obesity Paradox, Cachexia, Frailty, and Heart Failure

Carl J. Lavie, MD[a,b,c,*], Alban De Schutter, MD[a],
Martin A. Alpert, MD[d], Mandeep R. Mehra, MD[e],
Richard V. Milani, MD[a], Hector O. Ventura, MD[a]

KEYWORDS

- Obesity • Heart failure • Cachexia • Frailty

KEY POINTS

- Overweight and obesity adversely affect hemodynamics and ventricular structure and function, and greatly increase the prevalence of heart failure (HF).
- An obesity paradox exists, because overweight and obese patients with HF, by body mass index, body fat, and waist circumference, seem to have a better prognosis than do their leaner counterparts with HF.
- Frailty and cardiac cachexia are associated with poor clinical prognosis in many conditions, including HF.
- Low levels of cardiorespiratory fitness (CRF) are associated with a poor prognosis in HF and, in this group, as opposed to patients with HF with better CRF, a strong obesity paradox exists, with the leaner patients with low CRF having a particularly poor prognosis.
- Purposeful weight loss in HF remains controversial, although this therapy seems warranted, especially with severe obesity.

Overweight and obesity, which are typically defined by body mass index (BMI) criteria, have numerous adverse effects on general, and particularly, cardiovascular (CV), health.[1,2] Obesity is a major risk factor for both coronary heart disease (CHD) and hypertension (HTN), which are the two strongest risk factors for development of heart failure (HF). In addition, obesity adversely affects CV structure and function, causing systolic, and especially diastolic, left ventricular (LV) dysfunction. Therefore, overweight and obesity are potent risk factors for the development of HF.[2]

Despite the adverse affects of obesity on CV risk factors and the development of CV disease, including HF, numerous studies have shown an obesity paradox, meaning that overweight and obese patients with HF have a better prognosis than do their leaner counterparts, with the leanest patients with HF, including the frail and cachectic,[2–4] having a particularly poor prognosis.

This article describes the hemodynamic effects of weight on CV structure and function, and addresses the impact of overweight/obesity on the incidence and prevalence of HF. It also describes

[a] Department of Cardiovascular Diseases, John Ochsner Heart and Vascular Institute, Ochsner Clinical School, University of Queensland School of Medicine, 1514 Jefferson Highway, New Orleans, LA 70121-2483, USA; [b] Cardiac Rehabilitation, Exercise Laboratories, John Ochsner Heart and Vascular Institute, Ochsner Clinical School, University of Queensland School of Medicine, 1514 Jefferson Highway, New Orleans, LA 70121-2483, USA; [c] Department of Preventive Medicine, Pennington Biomedical Research Center, Louisiana State University System, 6400 Perkins Road, Baton Rouge, LA 70808, USA; [d] Division of Cardiovascular Medicine, University of Missouri School of Medicine, Room CE-338, 5 Hospital Drive, Columbia, MO 65202, USA; [e] BWH Heart and Vascular Center and Harvard Medical School, Brigham and Women's Hospital, 75 Francis Street, A Building, 3rd Floor, Room AB324, Boston, MA 02115, USA
* Corresponding author. Cardiac Rehabilitation, Exercise Laboratories, John Ochsner Heart and Vascular Institute, Ochsner Clinical School, University of Queensland School of Medicine, 1514 Jefferson Highway, New Orleans, LA 70121-2483.
E-mail address: clavie@ochsner.org

Heart Failure Clin 10 (2014) 319–326
http://dx.doi.org/10.1016/j.hfc.2013.12.002
1551-7136/14/$ – see front matter © 2014 Elsevier Inc. All rights reserved.

the obesity paradox, and especially the adverse effects of cachexia and frailty on HF prognosis. In addition, potential implications of weight loss and exercise training (ET; aerobic/dynamic, as well as isometric/resistance) for the treatment of HF are discussed, particularly in frail and/or cachectic patients.

IMPACT OF OBESITY ON HEMODYNAMICS AND VENTRICULAR STRUCTURE AND FUNCTION

We recently reviewed the detailed evidence showing the adverse affects of overweight/obesity on central and peripheral hemodynamics, as well as on cardiac structure and function (**Box 1**, **Fig. 1**).[2] Although the impact of obesity on LV structure and function are well recognized, the right ventricle is also adversely affected by obesity, especially morbid obesity. Cardiac cachexia in chronic HF with systolic dysfunction was recently associated with right ventricular (RV) dysfunction independent of LV systolic dysfunction, which correlates with cachexia and prognosis.[4,5] Fat mass loss rather than lean body mass loss was noted in this study, a finding that is counter to conventional understanding. It may be that fat loss represents an earlier event as cachexia becomes manifest, a finding that may be used to assess prognosis at a time when the syndrome may be influenced therapeutically, although this contention remains speculative.

OBESITY AND HF PREVALENCE

Substantial data suggest an increase in HF incidence and prevalence in overweight and obesity.[2] In 5881 Framingham Heart Study participants, Kenchaiah and colleagues[6] showed a 5% increase in HF in men and 7% increase in HF in women for every 1 kg/m^2 increase in BMI during a 14-year follow-up; the increase in HF risk was noted across all BMI categories. In a study of 74 morbidly obese patients, nearly one-third had clinical evidence of HF, with the probability of HF increasing greatly with the duration of morbid obesity; prevalence rates exceeded 70% at 20 years and 90% at 30 years.[7]

OBESITY PARADOX AND HF

Horwich and colleagues[8] were among the first to show an obesity paradox in HF, in that the best prognosis occurred in the overweight patients with HF, followed closely by obese patients with HF based on BMI classification. In contrast, the worst prognosis occurred in the underweight or cachectic patients with HF (who typically have a

Box 1
Effects of obesity on cardiac performance

1. Hemodynamics
   i. Increased blood volume
   ii. Increased stroke volume
   iii. Increased arterial pressure
   iv. Increased LV wall stress
   v. Pulmonary artery hypertension
2. Cardiac structure
   i. LV concentric remodeling
   ii. LV hypertrophy (eccentric and concentric)
   iii. Left atrial enlargement
   iv. RV hypertrophy
3. Cardiac function
   i. LV diastolic dysfunction
   ii. LV systolic dysfunction
   iii. RV failure
4. Inflammation
   i. Increased C-reactive protein
   ii. Overexpression of tumor necrosis factor
5. Neurohumoral
   i. Insulin resistance and hyperinsulinemia
   ii. Leptin insensitivity and hyperleptinemia
   iii. Reduced adiponectin
   iv. Sympathetic nervous system activation
   v. Activation of renin-angiotensin-aldosterone system
   vi. Overexpression of peroxisome proliferator-activator receptor
6. Cellular
   i. Hypertrophy
   ii. Apoptosis
   iii. Fibrosis

Abbreviation: RV, right ventricular.
From Lavie CJ, Alpert MA, Arena R, et al. Impact of obesity and the obesity paradox on prevalence and prognosis in heart failure. JACC Heart Fail 2013;1(2):93–102; with permission.

poor prognosis in most general health and CV situations) and followed closely by the patients with normal BMI and HF (**Fig. 2**).[8] We previously showed that this obesity paradox was noted with percent body fat (BF) as well as with BMI (**Fig. 3**),[9] because for every 1% increase in percent BF there was a 13% independent reduction in

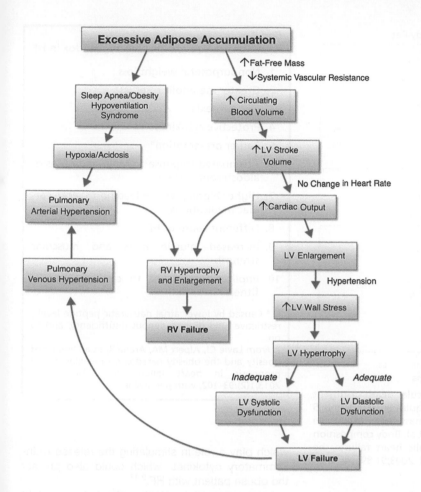

Excessive Adipose Accumulation

↑Fat-Free Mass
↓Systemic Vascular Resistance

Sleep Apnea/Obesity Hypoventilation Syndrome

↑ Circulating Blood Volume

Hypoxia/Acidosis

↑LV Stroke Volume

No Change in Heart Rate

Pulmonary Arterial Hypertension

↑Cardiac Output

Pulmonary Venous Hypertension

RV Hypertrophy and Enlargement

LV Enlargement

Hypertension

RV Failure

↑LV Wall Stress

LV Hypertrophy

Inadequate   Adequate

LV Systolic Dysfunction   LV Diastolic Dysfunction

LV Failure

Fig. 1. The central hemodynamic, cardiac structural abnormalities and alterations in ventricular function that may occur in severely obese patients and predispose them to HF. LV hypertrophy in severe obesity may be eccentric or concentric. In uncomplicated (normotensive) severe obesity, eccentric LV hypertrophy predominates. In severely obese patients with long-standing systemic hypertension, concentric LV hypertrophy is frequently observed and may occur more commonly than eccentric LV hypertrophy. Whether and to what extent metabolic disturbances such as lipotoxicity, insulin resistance, leptin resistance, and alterations of the renin-angiotensin-aldosterone system contribute to obesity cardiomyopathy in humans is uncertain. RV, right ventricular. (*From* Lavie CJ, Alpert MA, Arena R, et al. Impact of obesity and the obesity paradox on prevalence and prognosis in heart failure. JACC Heart Fail 2013;1(2):93–102; with permission.)

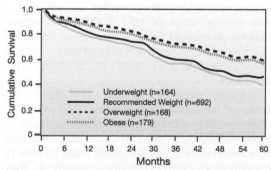

Fig. 2. Risk-adjusted survival curves for the 4 BMI categories at 5 years in a study of 1203 patients with moderate to severe HF. Survival was significantly better in the overweight and obese categories. (*From* Horwich TB, Fonarow GC, Hamilton MA, et al. The relationship between obesity and mortality in patients with heart failure. J Am Coll Cardiol 2001;38:789–95; with permission.)

major CV events. A recent study by Clark and colleagues[10] showed that both higher BMI and higher waist circumference (WC) were associated with better HF event–free survival. In an analysis of in-hospital mortality in more than 100,000 patients with decompensated HF, Fonarow and colleagues[11] showed that higher BMI was associated with lower in-hospital mortality. In this large study, for every 5-unit increase in BMI, in-hospital mortality was reduced by approximately 10%. In a study of 7599 symptomatic patients with HF with either reduced or preserved systolic function, Kenchaiah and colleagues[12] showed that underweight patients and patients with normal BMI have a higher mortality than did overweight and obese patients with HF, but this increased mortality was prominently noted in those without volume overload and peripheral edema.

Several years ago, in a large meta-analysis of 9 observational studies of nearly 30,000 patients with HF, Oreopoulos and colleagues[13] showed that, compared with patients with HF with normal

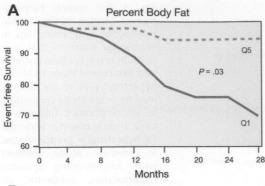

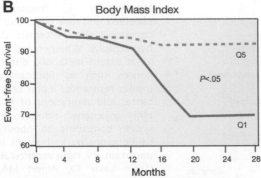

Fig. 3. Freedom from cardiovascular death or urgent transplantation in patients in quintiles (Q) 1 and 5 for percent BF (*A*) and body mass index (*B*). (*From* Lavie CJ, Osman AF, Milani RV, et al. Body composition and prognosis in chronic systolic heart failure: the obesity paradox. Am J Cardiol 2003;91:891–4; with permission.)

BMI, those overweight and obese patients with HF had significant reductions in all-cause (−16% and −33%, respectively) and CV mortality (−19% and −40%, respectively).

MECHANISMS FOR OBESITY PARADOX IN HF

Although there are several potential mechanisms for the obesity paradox in patients with CV diseases and in HF (**Box 2**),[2] the exact reason for this relationship remains difficult to reconcile. HF is a catabolic state, and obese patients may have more metabolic reserve.[2] Frail and cachectic patients (discussed later) experience greater morbidity and higher mortality in many disease states, including HF.[2,4] Adipose tissue is also known to produce soluble tumor necrosis factor-alpha receptors, and this could have a protective effect in overweight and obese patients with greater adipose tissue.[14] Other cytokines and neuroendocrine profiles in overweight/obese patients with HF may be protective. Higher levels of circulating lipoproteins in obese patients with HF may bind and then detoxify lipopolysaccharides,

---

Box 2
Potential reasons for the obesity paradox in HF

1. Nonpurposeful weight loss
2. Greater metabolic reserves
3. Less cachexia
4. Protective cytokines
5. Earlier presentation[a]
6. Attenuated response to renin-angiotensin-aldosterone system
7. Higher blood pressure leading to more cardiac medications
8. Different cause of HF
9. Increased muscle mass and muscular strength
10. Implications related to cardiorespiratory fitness

[a] Caused by lower atrial natriuretic peptide levels, restrictive lung disease, venous insufficiency, and so on.

From Lavie CJ, Alpert MA, Arena R, et al. Impact of obesity and the obesity paradox on prevalence and prognosis in heart failure. JACC Heart Fail 2013;1(2):93–102; with permission.

---

which play a role in stimulating the release of inflammatory cytokines, which could also protect the obese patient with HF.[2,15]

Another potential protective effect of overweight and obesity in HF is caused by the reduced expression of circulating natriuretic peptides.[2] We showed that obese patients with HF have suppressed B-type natriuretic peptide levels, which could lead to obese patients with HF presenting earlier with volume accumulation occurring at a less severe stage of HF.[2,16] Moreover, obese patients in general have an attenuated response to the renin-angiotensin-aldosterone system (RAAS), which may lead to a better HF prognosis.[1,2]

In theory, because overweight and obesity are known to increase levels of arterial blood pressure, obese patients with HF typically have high levels of blood pressure and more HTN than do their leaner counterparts. Not only are obese patients able to tolerate more cardioprotective medications, they may also be able to do so at higher, more therapeutic doses, including β-blockers, RAAS inhibitors, and aldosterone antagonists.[1,2]

In addition, as assessed later, various aspects of body composition, including BF and lean or muscle mass, and physical fitness (PF), including both cardiorespiratory fitness (CRF) and muscle fitness (MF), may affect prognosis in many patients with CV diseases, including HF.[17,18]

IMPACT OF SEVERE OR CLASS III OBESITY

Although an obesity paradox exists for most CV diseases, being noted in HTN, atrial fibrillation, and CHD,[1] in addition to HF,[2] there is also substantial evidence that the degree of obesity significantly influences prognosis.[18–22] For example, even in the general population, Flegal and colleagues[23] recently analyzed 97 studies of nearly 2.9 million subjects and noted that obese subjects, including all grades, had worse survival than subjects with normal BMI. However optimal survival in this meta-analysis seemed to occur in the overweight BMI group (BMI, 25–30 kg/m^2) who had a significantly (6%) lower mortality than did the subjects with normal BMI. In addition, the mildly obese (class I obese with BMI 30–35 kg/m^2) also had a 5% lower mortality than did the normal BMI group, which was nearly statistically significant.

In patients with CHD, several recent studies suggest that the relationship between adiposity and prognosis may represent more of an overweight paradox or a lean paradox, as opposed to a true obesity paradox.[24–26] As shown in the population-based data, overweight patients with CHD also seem to do particularly well. We suggested that a lean paradox may be present, because patients with both a low BF (<25% in men and <35% in women) and low BMI (<25 kg/m^2)[25] and, most recently, both a low BF and a low lean mass (or nonfat mass)[27] seem to do particularly poorly. In CHD, the obesity paradox may not apply to the more extreme, morbid, or class III ($\geq$40 kg/m^2) obese.

The impact of morbid or class III obesity on HF prevalence and prognosis is the most concerning, because recent statistics suggest that morbid obesity has been increasing more than obesity per se.[1,20] This level of extreme obesity has deleterious affects on CV structure and function, and, as discussed previously, greatly increases the prevalence of HF.[2,6,7] Unlike less severe degrees of obesity, in which an obesity paradox seems to exist, studies suggest that class III obesity is associated with a poor HF prognosis.[19–22]

IMPACT OF FRAILTY/CACHEXIA ON HF

Frailty is defined as a biological syndrome characterized by declining overall function and loss of resistance to stresses, and this is known to be associated with increased morbidity, mortality, and health care use, especially in the elderly population, who have a high prevalence of HF.[3] Few studies have investigated the prognostic role of frailty in HF populations, but this has typically predicted death in HF, and a recent study indicated that frailty was highly prevalent among community patients with HF, and this predicted a marked increased risk for emergency department visits and hospitalizations, independently of other comorbidities.[3]

Cachexia is an especially serious accompaniment of advanced HF syndrome.[4] Unintentional weight loss carries a greater burden of morbidity and mortality for most medical conditions, and the same is true for HF.[1,2,4] A limitation of most studies examining the obesity paradox is failure to control the nonpurposeful weight loss before study entry, which could be expected to be associated with a poor prognosis. In advanced HF, cachexia and wasting seem to be independent predictors of increased mortality.[4] To an extent, overweight and obesity may represent the reverse of cachexia, or reverse epidemiology.[28]

To a large extent, cardiac cachexia is likely a multifactorial and poorly understood syndrome in advanced HF.[4] Melenovsky and colleagues[5] recently provided observational correlations that made the connection between cardiac cachexia and the prognostic implications to fat mass (more than muscle mass) loss and provided an insight into the association and implications of unintentional weight loss with echocardiographic evidence of varying degrees of RV dysfunction.[4,5,29] Fat loss may precede lean muscle mass loss as cardiac cachexia becomes manifest, and fat loss may signal the onset of a declining prognosis in HF. Although the data made the link between cardiac cachexia and RV dysfunction,[29] these two disorders likely represent an epiphenomenon in advanced stages of HF rather than a true cause-and-effect relationship.[4] Nevertheless, targeting cardiac cachexia therapeutically may require identifying and tracking early signals, such as the combined role of anorexia and RV dysfunction in HF.

In cachexia, therapy could be intended to prevent and treat anorexia by using ghrelin analogues to stimulate appetite[30] or by hypothalamic inhibition of signals via the type IV melanocortin receptor.[31] Lean mass catabolic pathways could be targeted by replenishing reduced testosterone levels[32] or by using molecules such as soluble myostatin decoy receptors.[33] We have previously addressed the potential use of omega-3 polyunsaturated fatty acids in HF; low doses have been associated with reductions in mortality and HF hospitalizations and higher doses may provide antiinflammatory and anabolic effects that may particularly benefit cardiac cachexia.[34,35]

IMPACT OF PF IN HF

Associated with frailty/cachexia in HF is the potentially important role of PF, including both CRF and MF, in HF prognosis.[27,36] High levels of CRF are associated with a good prognosis, and high levels of CRF remain protective and largely negate the adverse effects of traditional CV risk factors and diseases on subsequent prognosis.[36] Although the ideal situation is to be free from chronic diseases and to have a high level of CRF, in most circumstances, patients with CV risk factors and diseases and high CRF have lower mortality than do patients without these conditions but with low CRF. Considering this, low levels of CRF may be the strongest risk factor for CV diseases and total mortality.[36,37]

High levels of CRF, including high levels of peak oxygen consumption (peak Vo_2), are associated with better prognosis in most CV diseases, including CHD and HF.[36,37] In addition, we have shown that CRF strongly mitigates the impact of adiposity on subsequent prognosis.[38,39] In both CHD and HF, some studies have suggested that the obesity paradox is only present in those with low levels of CRF.[38–40] In a recent study of 2066 patients with HF from a cardiopulmonary stress testing database, those patients with a preserved peak Vo_2 (>14 mL/kg/min) have a favorable prognosis and no obesity paradox was present (Fig. 4).[39] In contrast, a strong obesity paradox was apparent in those with poor CRF (<14 mL/kg/min), with the leaner patients with HF (even excluding underweight patients with HF) having a particularly high mortality during follow-up.

IMPACT OF ET IN HF

Concerning the importance of CRF and MF, the potential for aerobic ET to improve CRF and resistance training (RT) to improve MF seems obvious.[27,41] ET has numerous potential benefits, including improvement in peak Vo_2, central hemodynamics, peripheral vascular and skeletal muscle function, autonomic nervous system function, and overall functional capacity.[41,42] Most ET studies in HF have shown 15% to 17% improvements in peak Vo_2, with 25% to 35% reductions in major CV events, hospitalizations, and mortality.[41,43] However, the most well-known study of ET and HF is the recent HF-ACTION (Heart Failure: A Controlled Trial Investigating Outcomes of Exercise Training),[44] which only produced a modest improvement in peak Vo_2 of 4%, reflecting a lower adherence to ET intervention in this trial. Therefore, after a median follow-up of 30 months in 2333 class II to IV patients with systolic HF, a nonsignificant 7% reduction in the combined end point of all-cause mortality or hospitalizations was noted, but, after adjustment for prespecified predictors of mortality, the primary end point was significantly reduced (by 11%). In addition, this trial found a close relationship between volume of ET and clinical prognosis, with 30% reduction in mortality and hospitalizations noted in the subgroup of subjects who achieved their ET prescription guidelines.[45] Based on the considerable body of data, ET was recognized by the American College of Cardiology Foundation (ACCF)/American Heart Association (AHA) as a class I level in 2005, which was confirmed in the latest guidelines.[21] Moving patients with HF out of the lowest

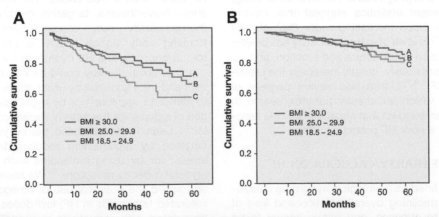

Fig. 4. Kaplan-Meier analyses according to BMI with (A) the low-cardiorespiratory-fitness (CRF) group (O_2 consumption, <14 mL O_2 kg^{-1} min^{-1}; log rank, 11.7; P = .003) and (B) high CRF group (O_2 consumption, ≥14 mL O_2 kg^{-1} min^{-1}; log rank, 1.72; P = .42). (From Lavie CJ, De Schutter A, Patel DA, et al. Does fitness completely explain the obesity paradox? Am Heart J 2013;166(1):1–3; with permission.)

levels of CRF seems to be associated with potentially marked improvements in clinical outcomes. Considering the importance of MF for overall CV prognosis, it is reasonable to also include RT with the aerobic ET for patients with HF.[27,41,42]

INTENTIONAL WEIGHT REDUCTION IN HF

One of the most effective long-term therapies for the hemodynamics and cardiac structural changes associated with obesity, most of which adversely affect HF, is intentional weight loss via structured dietary and ET programs or bariatric surgery.[2,7] Despite this evidence, and considering the previously shown obesity paradox and the adverse impact of cardiac cachexia and frailty on HF prognosis, the major HF societies have various recommendations regarding intentional weight loss intervention in HF. The AHA previously recommended weight loss in HF only with BMI greater than 40 kg/m², the Heart Failure Society of America for BMI greater than 35 kg/m², and both the European Society of Cardiology and the Canadian Cardiovascular Society recommended weight loss for BMI greater than 30 kg/m².[2] Because of the lack of definitive large-scale clinical trials on the role of weight loss in HF to make firm recommendations, the most recent HF guidelines from ACCF/AHA do not provide any firm recommendations for purposeful weight loss in HF.[21] Nevertheless, they recognize the poor prognosis in morbid obesity and more severely obese patients.[21,22] Therefore, based on the constellation of data, recommendations for purposeful weight loss for HF in the setting of BMI greater than or equal to 40 kg/m² seem sound, and this seems particularly reasonable with BMI greater than or equal to 35 kg/m².[19–21] In less severe obesity and overweight in patients with HF, weight reduction seems to be beneficial to improve symptoms and functional classification, but data on major clinical prognosis are lacking.[2,20]

SUMMARY

Although obesity adversely affects hemodynamics and LV structure and function, leading to systolic and, especially, diastolic HF, an obesity paradox exists, in that at least the overweight and mildly obese have a better prognosis than do normal-weight patients with HF. In contrast, frailty and cardiac cachexia, particularly, are associated with a poor prognosis. Efforts to improve CRF and lean muscle mass/muscular strength or MF in HF are needed to improve overall prognosis, with weight loss reserved for severe degrees of obesity.

REFERENCES

1. Lavie CJ, Milani RV, Ventura HO. Obesity and cardiovascular disease: risk factor, paradox, and impact of weight loss. J Am Coll Cardiol 2009;53:1925–32.
2. Lavie CJ, Alpert MA, Arena R, et al. Impact of obesity and the and the obesity paradox on prevalence and prognosis in heart failure. JACC Heart Fail 2013;1(2):93–102.
3. McNallan SM, Singh M, Chamberlain AM, et al. Frailty and healthcare utilization among patients with heart failure in the community. J Am Coll Cardiol 2013;1(2):135–41.
4. Mehra MR. Fat, cachexia and the right ventricle in heart failure. J Am Coll Cardiol 2013;62(18):1671–3.
5. Melenovsky V, Kotrc M, Borlaug BA, et al. Relationships between right ventricular function, body composition and prognosis in advanced heart failure. J Am Coll Cardiol 2013;62(18):1660–70.
6. Kenchaiah S, Evans JC, Levy D, et al. Obesity and the risk of heart failure. N Engl J Med 2002;347:305–13.
7. Alpert MS, Terry BE, Mulekar M, et al. Cardiac morphology and left ventricular function in morbidly obese patients with and without congestive heart failure and effect of weight loss. Am J Cardiol 1997;80:736–40.
8. Horwich TB, Fonarow GC, Hamilton MA, et al. The relationship between obesity and mortality in patients with heart failure. J Am Coll Cardiol 2001;38:789–95.
9. Lavie CJ, Osman AF, Milani RV, et al. Body composition and prognosis in chronic systolic heart failure: the obesity paradox. Am J Cardiol 2003;91:891–4.
10. Clark AL, Chyu J, Horwich TB. The obesity paradox in men versus women with systolic heart failure. Am J Cardiol 2012;110:77–82.
11. Fonarow GC, Srikanthan P, Costanzo MR, et al. An obesity paradox in acute heart failure: analysis of body mass index and in hospital mortality for 108,927 patients in the Acute Decompensated Heart Failure National Registry. Am Heart J 2007;153:74–81.
12. Kenchaiah S, Pocock SJ, Wang D, et al. Body mass index and prognosis in patients with chronic heart failure: insights from the Candesartan in Heart Failure: Assessment of Reduction in Mortality and Morbidity (CHARM) program. Circulation 2007;116:627–36.
13. Oreopoulos A, Padwal R, Kalantar-Zadeh K, et al. Body mass index and mortality in heart failure: a meta-analysis. Am Heart J 2008;156:13–22.
14. Mohamed-Ali V, Goodrick S, Bulmer K, et al. Production of soluble tumor necrosis factor receptors by human subcutaneous adipose tissue in vivo. Am J Physiol 1999;277:E971–5.
15. Rauchhaus M, Coats AJ, Anker SD. The endotoxin-lipoprotein hypothesis. Lancet 2000;356:930–3.

16. Mehra MR, Uber PA, Parh MH, et al. Obesity and suppressed B-type natriuretic peptide levels in heart failure. J Am Coll Cardiol 2004;43:1590–5.

17. Kaminsky LA, Arena R, Beckie TM, et al. The importance of cardiorespiratory fitness in the United States: the need for a national registry: a policy statement from the American Heart Association. Circulation 2013;127(5):652–62.

18. Artero EG, Lee DC, Lavie CJ, et al. Effects of muscular strength on cardiovascular risk factors and prognosis. J Cardiopulm Rehabil Prev 2012; 32:351–8.

19. Nagarajan V, Cauthern CA, Starling RC, et al. Prognosis of morbid obesity patients with advanced heart failure. Congest Heart Fail 2013;19:160–4.

20. Lavie CJ, Vetura HO. Analyzing the weight of evidence on the obesity paradox and heart failure – Is there a limit to the madness? Congest Heart Fail 2013;19:158–9.

21. Writing Committee Members, Yancy CW, Jessup M, Bozkurt B, et al. 2013 ACCF/AHA guideline for the management of heart failure: a report of the American College of Cardiology Foundation/American Heart Association Task Force on Practice Guidelines. Circulation 2013;128(16):e240–319.

22. Habbu A, Lakkis NM, Dokainish H. The obesity paradox: fact or fiction? Am J Cardiol 2006;98:944–8.

23. Flegal KM, Kit BK, Orpana H, et al. Association of all-cause mortality with overweight and obesity using standard body mass index categories: a systematic review and meta-analysis. JAMA 2013;309:71–82.

24. Azimi A, Charlot MG, Torp-Pedersen C, et al. Moderate overweight is beneficial and severe obesity detrimental for patients with documented atherosclerotic heart disease. Heart 2013;99(9):655–60. http://dx.doi.org/10.1136/heartjnl-2012-303066.

25. Lavie CK, De Schutter A, Patel D, et al. Body composition and coronary heart disease mortality: an obesity or a lean paradox? Mayo Clin Proc 2011;86:857–64.

26. Lavie CJ, De Schutter A, Milani RV. Is there an obesity, overweight, or lean paradox in coronary disease? Getting to the 'fat' of the matter. Heart 2013; 99(9):596–8.

27. Lavie CJ, De Schutter A, Patel DA, et al. Body composition and survival in stable coronary heart disease: impact of lean mass index and body fat in the "obesity paradox". J Am Coll Cardiol 2012;60:1374–80.

28. Lavie CJ, Mehra MR, Milani RV. Obesity and heart failure prognosis: paradox or reverse epidemiology? Eur Heart J 2005;26(1):5–7.

29. Anker SD, Sharma R. The syndrome of cardiac cachexia. Int J Cardiol 2002;85(1):51–66.

30. Palus S, Schur R, Akashi YJ, et al. Ghrelin and its analogues, BIM-28131 and BIM-28125, improve body weight and regulate the expression of MuRF-1 in a rat heart failure model. PLoS One 2011;6(11):e26865. http://dx.doi.org/10.1371/journal.pone.0026865.

31. Suzuki M, Narita M, Ashikawa M, et al. Changes in the melanocortin receptors in the hypothalamus of a rat model of cancer cachexia. Synapse 2012; 66(8):747–51.

32. Stout M, Tew GA, Doll H, et al. Testosterone therapy during exercise rehabilitation in male patients with chronic heart failure who have low testosterone status: a double-blind randomized controlled feasibility study. Am Heart J 2012;164(6):893–901.

33. Han HQ, Zhou X, Mitch WE, et al. Myostatin/activin pathway antagonism: molecular basis and therapeutic potential. Int J Biochem Cell Biol 2013; 45(10):2333–47. http://dx.doi.org/10.1016/j.biocel.2013.05.019. pii:S1357–2725(13)00163-5.

34. Mehra MR, Lavie CJ, Ventura HO, et al. Fish oils produce anti-inflammatory effects and improve body weight in severe heart failure. J Heart Lung Transplant 2006;25(7):834–8.

35. Lavie CJ, Milani RV, Mehra MR, et al. Omega-3 polyunsaturated fatty acids and cardiovascular diseases. J Am Coll Cardiol 2009;54(7):585–94.

36. Lavie CJ, De Schutter A, Patel DA, et al. New insights into the "obesity paradox" and cardiovascular outcomes. J Glycomics Lipidomics 2012;2:2.

37. Lavie CJ, Swift DL, Johannsen NM, et al. Physical fitness–an often forgotten cardiovascular risk factor. J Glycomics Lipidomics 2012;2:2.

38. McAuley PA, Artero EG, Sui X, et al. The obesity paradox, cardiorespiratory fitness, and coronary heart disease. Mayo Clin Proc 2012;87:443–51.

39. Lavie CJ, Cahalin LP, Chase P, et al. Impact of cardiorespiratory fitness on the obesity paradox in patients with heart failure. Mayo Clin Proc 2013;88: 251–8.

40. Lavie CJ, De Schutter A, Patel DA, et al. Does fitness completely explain the obesity paradox? Am Heart J 2013;166(1):1–3.

41. Lavie CJ, Berra K, Arena R. Formal cardiac rehabilitation and exercise training programs in heart failure. J Cardiopulm Rehabil Prev 2013;33:209–11.

42. Lavie CJ, Arena R, Earnest CP. High-intensity interval training in patients with cardiovascular diseases and heart transplantation. J Heart Lung Transplant 2013;32(11):1056–8.

43. Piepoli MF, Davos C, Francis DP, et al, ExTraMATCH Collaborative. Exercise Training Meta-analysis of Trials in Patients with Chronic Heart Failure (ExTraMATCH). BMJ 2004;328(7433):189.

44. O'Connor CM, Whellan DJ, Lee KL, et al, HF-ACTION Investigators. Efficacy and safety of exercise training in patients with chronic heart failure: HF-ACTION randomized controlled trial. JAMA 2009;301:1439–50.

45. Keteyian SJ, Leifer ES, Houston-Miller N, et al, HF-ACTION Investigators. Relation between volume of exercise and clinical outcomes in patients with heart failure. J Am Coll Cardiol 2012;60(19):601899–905.

The Impact of Peripheral Arterial Disease on Patients with Congestive Heart Failure

Amit N. Keswani, MD, Christopher J. White, MD*

KEYWORDS

- Congestive heart failure • Peripheral arterial disease • Peripheral angioplasty

KEY POINTS

- Peripheral arterial disease (PAD) is quite prevalent in patients with congestive heart failure (CHF).
- PAD and CHF share several similar risk factors.
- Patients with PAD and concomitant CHF have increased hospitalizations as well as worse overall prognosis.
- Risk factor modification and supervised exercise training are effective treatments of patients with PAD.
- A comprehensive, multidisciplinary approach to patients with PAD and CHF is needed to potentially improve patient outcomes.

INTRODUCTION AND BACKGROUND

Peripheral arterial disease (PAD) includes a large group of arterial disorders in which atherosclerosis is the predominant etiology. Atherosclerotic PAD leads to progressive stenosis/occlusion, or aneurysmal dilation of noncoronary arteries that supply the brain, visceral organs, and limbs. Lower extremity PAD is the preferred clinical term that should be used to denote stenotic, occlusive, and/or aneurysmal diseases of the abdominal aorta and lower extremities.[1] Atherosclerosis remains the most common cause of PAD, although many other additional pathologic processes can contribute to stenosis or aneurysms of the noncoronary arterial circulation.

Congestive heart failure (CHF) also has been implicated in increased patient morbidity and mortality, and has been shown that, along with other comorbid illnesses commonly occurring within this disease, often comprise synergistic negative

outcomes. As an independent risk factor, PAD has been shown to cause worse patient outcomes.[2–6] CHF and PAD share risk factors, pathophysiology, treatment strategies, and prognostic features, with a worse overall prognosis in patients who have concurrent CHF and PAD.[7–11]

The presence of PAD is associated with a twofold increase in the prevalence of CHF.[12] Shared risk factors for CHF and PAD include increased age, diabetes, tobacco use, atherosclerosis, and poor renal function.[2,13] The self-reported prevalence of cardiovascular disease (CVD) in the United States (coronary heart disease, CHF, or stroke) was 12.9%.[14] The prevalence of PAD in patients with CHF across 3 racial/ethnic groups was 17.1%.[14] PAD is most commonly asymptomatic, so it is underdiagnosed in the general population.[6] In matched patients with PAD and CHF, all-cause mortality occurred in 43% of the patients with CHF with PAD and 33% of the patients with CHF without PAD, and the patients with CHF without

Department of Cardiology, Ochsner Clinic Foundation, Ochsner Clinical School, University of Queensland, New Orleans, LA, USA
* Corresponding author. Department of Cardiology, Ochsner Clinic Foundation, Ochsner Clinical School, University of Queensland, 1514 Jefferson Highway, Jefferson, LA 70121.
E-mail address: cwhite@ochsner.org

Heart Failure Clin 10 (2014) 327–338
http://dx.doi.org/10.1016/j.hfc.2013.10.006
1551-7136/14/$ – see front matter © 2014 Elsevier Inc. All rights reserved.

PAD had significantly greater survival than patients with PAD.[8]

The health care utilization of patients with concomitant PAD and CHF is significantly increased when compared with utilization of patients with CHF without PAD.[8] The Controlled Rosuvastatin Multinational Trial in Heart Failure Trial (CORONA) found that 12.7% of patients with CHF had PAD (**Figs. 1** and **2, Table 1**).[7]

Patients with PAD were more likely to be hospitalized for cardiovascular reasons and were at greater risk of cardiovascular death as well as all-cause mortality. In the Upon further analysis of the Heart Failure–A Controlled Trial Investigating Outcomes in Exercise Training (HF-ACTION) trial, patients with PAD and CHF had decreased baseline functional capacity compared with patients with CHF without PAD, and those with PAD had substantially worse clinical outcomes (**Fig. 3, Table 2**).[11]

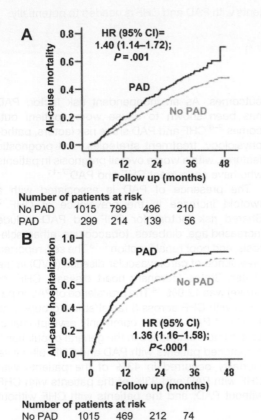

Fig. 1. Kaplan Meier plots for all-cause mortality (*A*) and all-cause hospitalization (*B*) by a history of PAD. (*From* Ahmed MI, Aronow WS, Criqui MH, et al. Effects of peripheral arterial disease on outcomes in advanced chronic systolic heart failure: a propensity-matched study. Circ Heart Fail 2010;3(1):121; with permission.)

More recent studies show that more than 50% of patients with clinically evident CHF have normal left ventricular ejection fraction[15,16] and are now referred to as "heart failure with preserved ejection fraction" (HFpEF) as compared with "heart failure with reduced ejection fraction" (HFrEF). The overall prognosis of patients with HFpEF is similar to the prognosis of patients with HFrEF.[15,16] PAD had a more deleterious effect in patients with HFpEF compared with those with HFrEF, which points to a role for ventriculo-vascular coupling in the development of HFpEF.[10]

In this article, we review lower extremity PAD, those without symptoms but an abnormal ankle brachial index, intermittent claudication, and critical limb ischemia, and their impact for patients with CHF.

EPIDEMIOLOGIC INSIGHTS BETWEEN PAD AND CHF

The documented worldwide prevalence of lower extremity PAD ranges from 3% to 12%.[1,17–21] The PAD Awareness, Risk, and Treatment: New Resources for Survival (PARTNERS) program included 6979 subjects, and found the prevalence of PAD almost 30% in individuals at high risk for PAD (50–69 years of age and diabetes mellitus or >10 pack-year history of smoking, or >70 years of age). This study also demonstrated a significant overlap of disease and showed 16% of patients had concomitant PAD and CVD, which included patients with CHF.[22]

PAD disproportionately affects individuals who are older, African American, and current smokers, and those who have diabetes or abnormal renal function. PAD in those who are Caucasian has a prevalence of 13.2%, 22.8% in African American individuals, and 13.7% among Hispanic individuals.[23] The prevalence of concomitant CHF and PAD in those who are Caucasian is 25.9%, African American is 13.7%, and Hispanic is 13.4%.[14] Additional studies demonstrate an increased prevalence of CHF in patients with PAD ranging from 5.3% to 13.9%.[12,22,24]

PATHOPHYSIOLOGY AND RISK FACTORS

Although no single targeted study addresses actual treatment of concomitant PAD and CHF, current guidelines recommend treatment to reduce several similarly associated risk factors in CHF and PAD.[25,26] Atherosclerosis is the most common cause of lower extremity PAD and risk factors for development of atherosclerosis include hypertension, diabetes, and cigarette smoking.[20] Patients with known atherosclerotic disease are

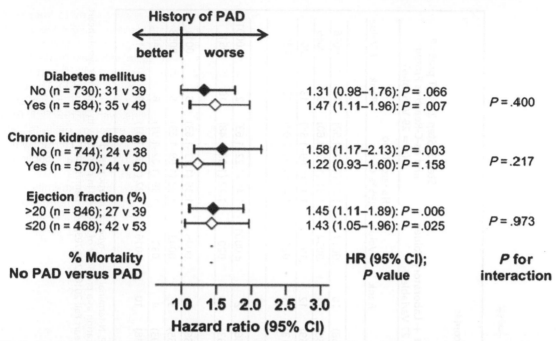

Fig. 2. Association between PAD and all-cause mortality in subgroups of propensity score-matched patients in the BEST trial. (*From* Ahmed MI, Aronow WS, Criqui MH, et al. Effects of peripheral arterial disease on outcomes in advanced chronic systolic heart failure: a propensity-matched study. Circ Heart Fail 2010;3(1):121; with permission.)

also more likely to develop CHF as well as PAD, and current guidelines recommend modifying these risk factors associated with the development of atherosclerosis.[19,27,28]

Hypertension (HTN) is a known risk factor for atherosclerosis and development of both PAD and CHF.[29–34] Additionally, hypertension is identified as a recognized risk of development of both HFpEF and HFrEF.[25,35,36] Long-term treatment of both systolic and diastolic hypertension has been shown to reduce the risk of incident CHF by 50%.[37–40]

Cigarette smoking and diabetes are additional risk factors for development of lower extremity PAD and CHF. Cigarette smoking is 2 to 3 times more likely to cause lower extremity PAD than coronary artery disease.[41] Tobacco use is also strongly associated as an independent risk factor for CHF.[36,42] The presence of diabetes mellitus increases the risk of lower extremity PAD by twofold to fourfold.[43–45] Additionally, insulin resistance has been shown to be an important risk factor in development of CHF.[42,46–48]

The prevalence of smoking and diabetes in patients with concomitant PAD and CVD when compared with the reference group in the PARTNERS study is increased. In patients with concomitant PAD and CVD, the prevalence of

smokers was 64% and significantly higher when compared with the study reference group, which was 50%. The prevalence of diabetes mellitus in patients with concomitant PAD and CVD was significantly higher (44%) when compared with the reference group (34%) in the PARTNERS study.[22]

DIAGNOSTIC ISSUES

A careful and detailed history and physical examination is essential in the assessment of patients with CHF as well as distinguishing PAD from nonvascular causes of lower extremity pain. When assessing patients for PAD, fewer than 20% report typical symptoms of intermittent claudication (leg-muscle discomfort on exertion that is relieved with rest), making this assessment a clinical challenge.[49]

In the assessment of PAD, it is important to delineate chronic stable PAD (intermittent claudication) from chronic critical PAD (critical limb ischemia [CLI]), as this will help drive treatment and therapy. Chronic stable PAD classically presents as intermittent claudication, and physical examination findings include changes in skin color, decreased pulses, cool extremities, and decreased hair distribution. However many patients with PAD are

Table 1
Multivariable analysis: intermittent claudication as an independent predictor of clinical outcomes

Type of End Point	Step 1: Adjusted for Demographic/Clinical Variables (n = 20 Variables)			Step 2: Step 1 + Laboratory Values (n = 27 Variables)			Step 3: Step 2 + NT proBNP and hs-C-Reactive Protein (n = 29 Variables)		
	Hazard Ratio (95% CI)	Rank	P Value	Hazard Ratio (95% CI)	Rank	P Value	Hazard Ratio (95% CI)	Rank	P Value
Mortality									
All-cause (n = 934)	1.40 (1.18–1.67)	7	.0002	1.33 (1.11–1.58)	10	.0017	1.27 (1.07–1.52)	12	.0076
Cardiovascular death (n = 725)	1.43 (1.17–1.75)	7	.0005	1.35 (1.11–1.65)	11	.0034	1.31 (1.07–1.60)	9	.0089
Sudden death (n = 407)	1.28 (0.97–1.69)	9	.0835	1.21 (0.91–1.59)	12	.19	1.17 (0.89–1.55)	13	.26
Death due to worsening heart failure (n = 230)	1.61 (1.14–2.27)	8	.0064	1.50 (1.06–2.13)	11	.021	1.46 (1.03–2.07)	10	.035
Hospitalizations									
Cardiovascular cause (n = 1452)	1.45 (1.25–1.67)	3	<.0001	1.44 (1.24–1.66)	2	<.0001	1.41 (1.22–1.63)	2	<.0001
Worsening heart failure (n = 823)	1.30 (1.07–1.58)	8	.0075	1.26 (1.04–1.53)	10	.020	1.22 (1.00–1.48)	10	.051
Combined end points									
Primary (n = 883)	1.43 (1.19–1.72)	6	.0001	1.38 (1.15–1.66)	9	.0005	1.36 (1.13–1.63)	5	.0011
Coronary (n = 741)	1.37 (1.12–1.68)	3	.0021	1.34 (1.10–1.65)	5	.0042	1.33 (1.09–1.63)	5	.0058
Athero-thrombotic (n = 284)	1.41 (1.03–1.93)	4	.0034	1.41 (1.03–1.93)	4	.033	1.39 (1.02–1.91)	6	.040
Death or heart failure hospitalization (n = 1376)	1.32 (1.14–1.53)	7	.0003	1.27 (1.10–1.48)	10	.0016	1.22 (1.05–1.41)	9	.011

Abbreviations: CI, confidence interval; hs-C-Reactive Protein, high-sensitivity C-reactive protein; NT proBNP, N-terminal pro-B-type natriuretic peptide.
From Inglis SC, McMurray JJ, Böhm M, et al, on behalf of the CORONA Study Group. Intermittent claudication as a predictor of outcome in patients with ischaemic systolic heart failure: analysis of the Controlled Rosuvastatin Multinational Trial in Heart Failure trial (CORONA). Eur J Heart Fail 2010;12(7):703; with permission.

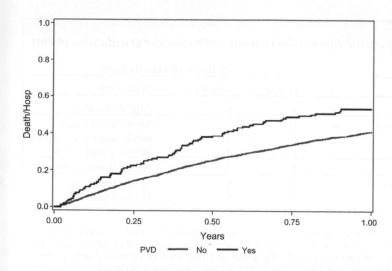

Fig. 3. Unadjusted Kaplan-Meier curve demonstrating time to all-cause death or all-cause hospitalization by presence or absence of PAD. (*From* Jones WS, Clare R, Ellis SJ, et al. Effect of peripheral arterial disease on functional and clinical outcomes in patients with heart failure (from HF-ACTION). Am J Cardiol 2011;108(3):383; with permission.)

either asymptomatic or present with atypical symptoms, such as leg fatigue, difficulty walking, and leg pain that is not typical of claudication.[17,18,22,50–52] Chronic critical PAD includes more severe symptoms, such as ischemic rest pain, nonhealing ulcers, or gangrene attributed to proven PAD (abnormal Ankle Brachial Index [ABI] <0.5), and has a higher risk of tissue loss, which will require

a more urgent revascularization strategy. There currently exist 2 classification systems for severity of lower extremity PAD: the Fontaine system and the Rutherford system (**Table 3**).[20]

Screening and diagnosis of PAD can be performed using noninvasive techniques, such as the Edinburgh Claudication Questionnaire[53] and the ABI,[54] which are both simple and noninvasive

Table 2
Unadjusted Kaplan–Meier event rates, unadjusted and adjusted effects of peripheral arterial disease for primary and secondary end points

End Point	Kaplan–Meier 1-Year Rate Estimates		PAD Effect in Unadjusted Cox Proportional Hazards Model			PAD Effect in Adjusted Cox Proportional Hazards Model		
	No PAD	PAD	Wald Chi-Square	HR (95% CI)	P Value	Wald Chi-Square	HR (95% CI)	P Value
All-cause death or all-cause hospitalization	0.410	0.535	17.9	1.49 (1.24–1.79)	<.001	6.4	1.31 (1.06–1.62)	.011
All-cause death	0.045	0.110	21.9	2.07 (1.53–2.81)	<.001	3.3	1.36 (0.98–1.91)	.070
Cardiovascular death or cardiovascular hospitalization	0.318	0.414	14.4	1.47 (1.20–1.79)	<.001	8.8	1.41 (1.12–1.76)	.003
Cardiovascular death or heart failure hospitalization	0.149	0.210	21.5	1.76 (1.39–2.24)	<.001	15.2	1.72 (1.31–2.26)	<.001

Abbreviations: CI, confidence interval; HR, hazard ratio; PAD, peripheral arterial disease.
From Jones WS, Clare R, Ellis SJ, et al. Effect of peripheral arterial disease on functional and clinical outcomes in patients with heart failure (from HF-ACTION). Am J Cardiol 2011;108(3):383; with permission.

Table 3
Clinical staging of lower extremity arterial disease with Fontaine and Rutherford Classification of PAD

Fontaine Classification			↔	Rutherford Classification		
Stage	Symptoms		↔	Grade	Category	Symptoms
I	Asymptomatic		↔	0	0	Asymptomatic
II	Intermittent claudication		↔	I	1	Mild claudication
				I	2	Moderate claudication
				I	3	Severe claudication
III	Ischemic rest pain		↔	II	4	Ischemic rest pain
IV	Ulceration or gangrene		↔	III	5	Minor tissue loss
				III	6	Major tissue loss

↔, signifies equivalency in classification systems.
From European Stroke Organization, Tendera M, Aboyans V, et al. ESC Guidelines on the diagnosis and treatment of peripheral artery diseases: document covering atherosclerotic disease of extracranial carotid and vertebral, mesenteric, renal, upper and lower extremity arteries: the Task Force on the Diagnosis and Treatment of Peripheral Artery Diseases of the European Society of Cardiology (ESC). Eur Heart J 2011;32(22):2851–90; with permission of Oxford University Press (UK) (c).

tools that have been validated as reliable and reproducible tests for the detection of lower extremity PAD (**Fig. 4**).

The Edinburgh Claudication Questionnaire identifies intermittent claudication and the location of the pain and severity (grade 1 or 2). It has been validated to have a sensitivity of 91% and specificity of 99%[53]; however, because many cases of PAD are not symptomatic or have atypical symptoms, it will underestimate cases of PAD if used alone.

The single best screening test in a patient suspected of PAD is the ABI. The ABI is the ratio of the highest systolic arm blood pressure to the highest systolic ankle blood pressure, obtained with a handheld continuous-wave Doppler and blood pressure cuff. A ratio lower than 0.9 is considered abnormal, and lower than 0.4 is often associated with limb-threatening ischemia.[54] Falsely elevated ABI readings in noncompressible heavily calcified vessels commonly seen in diabetic individuals or patients with renal failure can be assessed with a

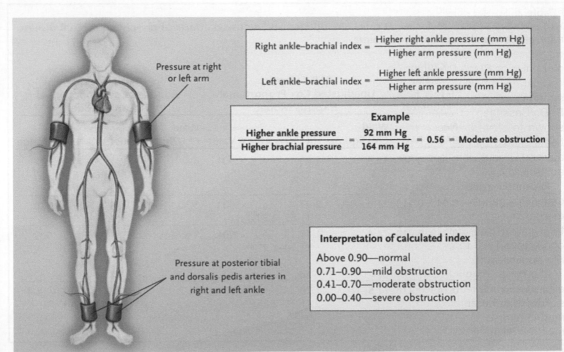

$$\text{Right ankle–brachial index} = \frac{\text{Higher right ankle pressure (mm Hg)}}{\text{Higher arm pressure (mm Hg)}}$$

$$\text{Left ankle–brachial index} = \frac{\text{Higher left ankle pressure (mm Hg)}}{\text{Higher arm pressure (mm Hg)}}$$

Pressure at right or left arm

Example

$$\frac{\text{Higher ankle pressure}}{\text{Higher brachial pressure}} = \frac{92 \text{ mm Hg}}{164 \text{ mm Hg}} = 0.56 = \text{Moderate obstruction}$$

Pressure at posterior tibial and dorsalis pedis arteries in right and left ankle

Interpretation of calculated index

Above 0.90—normal
0.71–0.90—mild obstruction
0.41–0.70—moderate obstruction
0.00–0.40—severe obstruction

Fig. 4. Ankle-brachial index. (*From* White C. Intermittent claudication. N Engl J Med 2007;356(12):1243; with permission. Copyright © 2007 Massachusetts Medical Society.)

toe-brachial index performed with a small plethysmographic cuff on the great or second toe. Exercise testing is useful to determine the presence of PAD when the resting ABI is normal and/or to document the severity of symptom limitation and degree of improvement after treatment in patients with claudication. Although computed tomography and magnetic resonance angiography (MRA) are helpful, the gold standard for the diagnosis and evaluation of lower extremity PAD is invasive digital subtraction angiography and is necessary if endovascular intervention is planned.[52]

THERAPEUTIC ISSUES
Chronic Stable PAD

Treatment of chronic stable lower extremity PAD and CHF includes risk factor modification, a supervised exercise program, pharmacologic therapy, and revascularization.

Risk Factor Modification

Risk factor targets for patients with concomitant PAD and CHF include hypertension, smoking cessation, lipid management, and optimal glycemic control. Hypertension is a major risk factor for development of PAD and CHF. However, there are no data evaluating whether antihypertensive therapy alters the progression of claudication, but has been shown to prevent the development of CHF.[17] Health care providers should lower both systolic and diastolic blood pressure in accordance with current published guidelines, including the most recent report of the Joint National Committee on Prevention, Detection, Evaluation and Treatment of High Blood Pressure.[25,55,56]

Cigarette smoking has been shown to have a strong association with development of CHF and PAD. Cessation of cigarette smoking has been shown to slow the progression of PAD.[57,58] Patients should be evaluated at each visit, strongly advised about the hazards of smoking, and advised to quit.[25,27,56]

The third report of the National Cholesterol Education Program (NCEP) Expert Panel on detection, evaluation, and treatment of high blood cholesterol in adults (Adult Treatment Panel [ATP] III) considered PAD to be a coronary heart disease risk equivalent.[59]

A number of cholesterol-lowering trials have evaluated the effects on PAD and CHF. Regression of femoral atherosclerosis,[60] a lower rate of new or worsening claudication,[61] and improvements in walking distance and pain-free walking time[62–64] have been described. Aggressive treatment of dyslipidemia with statins reduces the likelihood of development of CHF and PAD in patients

at risk.[65,66] In the case of concomitant CHF and PAD, because patients with known atherosclerotic disease are likely to develop heart failure, current guidelines recommend clinicians control these vascular risk factors appropriately. Patients with lower extremity PAD are classified as "high risk" and recommend a low-density lipoprotein (LDL) target of less than 100 mg/dL. Additionally, patients classified as "very high risk" (defined as the presence of PAD and multiple risk factors, such as diabetes, cigarette smoking, and metabolic syndrome) recommend an LDL goal of less than 70 mg/dL.[59,67]

Although no randomized controlled trial has directly evaluated the effects of antidiabetic therapy on lower extremity PAD, the Diabetes Control and Complications Trial of patients with type 1 diabetes mellitus found that intensive insulin therapy had a tendency to lower PAD events, such as claudication, peripheral revascularization, or amputation, but was not statistically significant, but did decrease the risk of microvascular events, such as nephropathy and retinopathy.[68] Insulin resistance, with or without diabetes mellitus, has been shown to be a risk factor in the development of CHF.[42,46–48] Currently, guidelines for both CHF and PAD endorse aggressive reduction in glycosylated hemoglobin with a goal of less than 7.0%, although there are insufficient data to show that this strategy reduces the risk of CHF and concomitant PAD.[19,25]

Exercise

Exercise training (or regular physical activity) has been shown to be safe and effective for patients with CHF who are able to participate to improve their functional status.[69–71] Additionally, supervised exercise (cardiac rehabilitation) has been shown to improve functional capacity, exercise duration, and mortality in patients with CHF.[72,73] With regard to lower extremity PAD and intermittent claudication, multiple clinical trials and meta-analyses have demonstrated the feasibility and benefit for supervised exercise therapy (not unsupervised exercise).[74–78] One systematic review demonstrated that combination of percutaneous transluminal angioplasty (PTA) and exercise (supervised exercise therapy or exercise advice) may produce greater changes in walking distance compared with exercise or PTA alone in patients with lower extremity PAD.[74] Per current evidence, patients with PAD and CHF should be encouraged to enroll in a supervised exercise program if they are able to participate to improve functional capacity, exercise duration, lower hospitalization, and decrease morbidity and mortality.[19,25,73]

Pharmacologic

Current guidelines for patients with PAD and concurrent CHF include antiplatelet or antithrombotic therapy, which is currently recommended to reduce the risk of myocardial infarction (MI), stroke, or vascular death in individuals with atherosclerotic lower extremity PAD.[79] Current guidelines recommend use of Aspirin (75–325 mg) as safe and effective antiplatelet therapy to reduce the risk of MI, stroke, or vascular death in individuals with atherosclerotic PAD, and clopidogrel is a recommended alternative therapy.

Cilostazol is a phosphodiesterase inhibitor that suppresses platelet aggregation and is a direct arterial vasodilator and is currently recommended in patients with PAD.[80] However, because other oral phosphodiesterase inhibitors used for inotropic therapy have caused increased mortality in patients with advanced heart failure, cilostazol is contraindicated in patients with heart failure of any severity.[81] Pentoxyfilline is not recommended, as its clinical effectiveness is not established. Cilostazol should be avoided in patients with CHF and reduced systolic left ventricular function per current guidelines; however, this warning does not specify the heart failure classification or degree of severity that should be avoided. Although none of the current trials to date have found a significant increase in mortality or major cardiovascular events in patients with cilostazol, this recommendation is based on prior studies with oral milrinone therapy (another phosphodiesterase 3 inhibitor) in patients with heart failure.[25,82]

Revascularization

Patients with intermittent claudication should be selected for revascularization based on the severity of their symptoms causing significant functional disability, following failure of medical and exercise therapies with appropriate vascular anatomy for revascularization and a favorable risk/benefit ratio.[3] In a study of patients with life-style–limiting chronic stable PAD (intermittent claudication) who have aorto-iliac disease, improvement in peak walk time (PWT) over 6 months and quality of life (QOL) were noted in groups who received supervised exercise and stent revascularization. The benefits of PWT were greater among those with supervised exercise; however, the greatest improvement in QOL was shown in the stent revascularization group.[78] This study suggested that both treatment strategies are superior to optimal medical therapy in patients with aorto-iliac PAD. Supervised exercise should be an initial strategy in these patients, but if patients do not respond, then revascularization

would be appropriate. In general, patients with claudication progress to limb loss at a rate of less than 5% per year, and therefore, revascularization is reserved for those patients with favorable anatomy who (1) fail conservative therapy and have life-style–limiting symptoms or (2) have vocational-limiting symptoms.[52]

Patients with chronic critical PAD (critical limb ischemia) typically have more extensive disease than patients with intermittent claudication and require a more urgent revascularization approach to prevent tissue loss.[1] The clinical outcomes for patients with CLI overall is poor and within 3 months of presentation, 12% will require amputation and 9% will die.[83] Therapy is centered around restoring pulsatile flow to the distal limb as quickly as possible with as low a procedural morbidity as possible with the emphasis more on amputation-free survival than long-term vessel patency. Before intervention, patients should undergo noninvasive imaging studies, such as duplex ultrasound, MRA, computed tomography angiography, and/or catheter angiography to determine a suitable revascularization approach. Percutaneous procedures are generally preferred to open surgical approaches initially, an "endovascular first approach" due to the lower comorbidity, mortality rates, shorter hospital stay, and patient preference.

TREATING COMORBIDITIES

Caring for patients with CHF and PAD requires a strong focus on the treatment of serious comorbidities to improve the overall prognosis. PAD in patients with CHF has been associated with increased mortality, increased health care utilization, and worse health outcomes.[7,8,10,11,14] Current evidence supports a multidisciplinary approach for the care of patients with CHF by using risk factor modification, and revascularization for atherosclerotic ischemia producing lesions when necessary.[84,85] Patients with CHF and PAD have been shown to benefit from supervised exercise training, and the authors strongly support enrolling patients in such programs.

SUMMARY

Currently, PAD remains a largely underdiagnosed disease because of the lack of clinical symptoms, atypical symptoms (ie, leg fatigue), and the lack of appropriate screening by primary care providers. The relationship between CHF and PAD is commonly overlooked and requires an increased focus on PAD as an important comorbidity in patients with CHF. This requires a comprehensive, team-based approach to the prevention and treatment of these patients with PVD and CHF. Based on our evidence and current guidelines, patients who are smokers, and have known coronary artery disease and/or diabetes mellitus should have an ABI performed to screen for PAD.

Obtaining ABI measurements in these patients at risk also with concomitant CHF will enhance PAD detection in this specific population. Increased screening for comorbidities, such as PAD in patients with CHF, will ultimately yield a greater recognition of PAD, which will enable clinicians to begin treatment sooner (such as risk factor modification, exercise programs, and revascularization) and potentially mitigate the adverse consequences of PAD and atherosclerosis in patients with CHF.

REFERENCES

1. Hirsch AT, Haskal ZJ, Hertzer NR, et al. ACC/AHA 2005 Practice Guidelines for the management of patients with peripheral arterial disease (lower extremity, renal, mesenteric, and abdominal aortic): a collaborative report from the American Association for Vascular Surgery/Society for Vascular Surgery, Society for Cardiovascular Angiography and Interventions, Society for Vascular Medicine and Biology, Society of Interventional Radiology, and the ACC/AHA Task Force on Practice Guidelines (Writing Committee to Develop Guidelines for the Management of Patients With Peripheral Arterial Disease): endorsed by the American Association of Cardiovascular and Pulmonary Rehabilitation; National Heart, Lung, and Blood Institute; Society for Vascular Nursing; TransAtlantic Inter-Society Consensus; and Vascular Disease Foundation. Circulation 2006;113(11):e463–654.

2. Nakata S, Yokoi Y, Matsumoto R, et al. Long-term cardiovascular outcomes following ischemic heart disease in patients with and without peripheral vascular disease. Osaka City Med J 2008;54(1):21–30.

3. Bertomeu V, Morillas P, Gonzalez-Juanatey JR, et al. Prevalence and prognostic influence of peripheral arterial disease in patients >or=40 years old admitted into hospital following an acute coronary event. Eur J Vasc Endovasc Surg 2008;36(2):189–96.

4. Cotter G, Cannon CP, McCabe CH, et al. Prior peripheral arterial disease and cerebrovascular disease are independent predictors of adverse outcome in patients with acute coronary syndromes: are we doing enough? Results from the Orbofiban in Patients with Unstable Coronary Syndromes-Thrombolysis In Myocardial Infarction (OPUS-TIMI) 16 study. Am Heart J 2003;145(4):622–7.

5. Makowsky MJ, McAlister FA, Galbraith PD, et al. Lower extremity peripheral arterial disease in individuals with coronary artery disease: prognostic importance, care gaps, and impact of therapy. Am Heart J 2008;155(2):348–55.

6. McDermott MM, Guralnik JM, Ferrucci L, et al. Asymptomatic peripheral arterial disease is associated with more adverse lower extremity characteristics than intermittent claudication. Circulation 2008;117(19):2484–91.

7. Inglis SC, McMurray JJ, Bohm M, et al. Intermittent claudication as a predictor of outcome in patients with ischaemic systolic heart failure: analysis of the Controlled Rosuvastatin Multinational Trial in Heart Failure trial (CORONA). Eur J Heart Fail 2010;12(7):698–705.

8. Ahmed MI, Aronow WS, Criqui MH, et al. Effects of peripheral arterial disease on outcomes in advanced chronic systolic heart failure: a propensity-matched study. Circ Heart Fail 2010;3(1):118–24.

9. Hebert K, Beltran J, Tamariz L, et al. Evidence-based medication adherence in Hispanic patients with systolic heart failure in a disease management program. Congest Heart Fail 2010;16(4):175–80.

10. Edelmann F, Stahrenberg R, Gelbrich G, et al. Contribution of comorbidities to functional impairment is higher in heart failure with preserved than with reduced ejection fraction. Clin Res Cardiol 2011;100(9):755–64.

11. Jones WS, Clare R, Ellis SJ, et al. Effect of peripheral arterial disease on functional and clinical outcomes in patients with heart failure (from HF-ACTION). Am J Cardiol 2011;108(3):380–4.

12. Anand RG, Ventura HO, Mehra MR. Is heart failure more prevalent in patients with peripheral arterial disease? A meta-analysis. Congest Heart Fail 2007;13(6):319–22.

13. Selvin E, Erlinger TP. Prevalence of and risk factors for peripheral arterial disease in the United States: results from the National Health and Nutrition Examination Survey, 1999–2000. Circulation 2004;110(6):738–43.

14. Hebert K, Lopez B, Michael C, et al. The prevalence of peripheral arterial disease in patients with heart failure by race and ethnicity. Congest Heart Fail 2010;16(3):118–21.

15. Owan TE, Hodge DO, Herges RM, et al. Trends in prevalence and outcome of heart failure with preserved ejection fraction. N Engl J Med 2006;355(3):251–9.

16. Lee DS, Gona P, Vasan RS, et al. Relation of disease pathogenesis and risk factors to heart failure with preserved or reduced ejection fraction: insights from the Framingham Heart Study of the National Heart, Lung, and Blood Institute. Circulation 2009;119(24):3070–7.

17. Norgren L, Hiatt WR, Dormandy JA, et al. Inter-Society Consensus for the Management of

Peripheral Arterial Disease (TASC II). J Vasc Surg 2007;45(Suppl S):S5–67.

18. Olin JW, Sealove BA. Peripheral artery disease: current insight into the disease and its diagnosis and management. Mayo Clin Proc 2010;85(7):678–92.

19. Rooke TW, Hirsch AT, Misra S, et al. Management of patients with peripheral artery disease (compilation of 2005 and 2011 ACCF/AHA Guideline Recommendations): a report of the American College of Cardiology Foundation/American Heart Association Task Force on Practice Guidelines. J Am Coll Cardiol 2013;61(14):1555–70.

20. Dormandy JA, Rutherford RB. Management of peripheral arterial disease (PAD). TASC Working Group. TransAtlantic Inter-Society Consensus (TASC). J Vasc Surg 2000;31(1 Pt 2):S1–296.

21. Novo S. Classification, epidemiology, risk factors, and natural history of peripheral arterial disease. Diabetes Obes Metab 2002;4(Suppl 2):S1–6.

22. Hirsch AT, Criqui MH, Treat-Jacobson D, et al. Peripheral arterial disease detection, awareness, and treatment in primary care. JAMA 2001; 286(11):1317–24.

23. Collins TC, Petersen NJ, Suarez-Almazor M, et al. The prevalence of peripheral arterial disease in a racially diverse population. Arch Intern Med 2003; 163(12):1469–74.

24. Newman AB, Shemanski L, Manolio TA, et al. Ankle-arm index as a predictor of cardiovascular disease and mortality in the Cardiovascular Health Study. The Cardiovascular Health Study Group. Arterioscler Thromb Vasc Biol 1999;19(3):538–45.

25. Yancy CW, Jessup M, Bozkurt B, et al. 2013 ACCF/AHA Guideline for the Management of Heart Failure: a Report of the American College of Cardiology Foundation/American Heart Association Task Force on Practice Guidelines. Circulation 2013; 128:1810–52.

26. Hirsch AT, Haskal ZJ, Hertzer NR, et al. ACC/AHA 2005 guidelines for the management of patients with peripheral arterial disease (lower extremity, renal, mesenteric, and abdominal aortic): executive summary a collaborative report from the American Association for Vascular Surgery/Society for Vascular Surgery, Society for Cardiovascular Angiography and Interventions, Society for Vascular Medicine and Biology, Society of Interventional Radiology, and the ACC/AHA Task Force on Practice Guidelines (Writing Committee to Develop Guidelines for the Management of Patients With Peripheral Arterial Disease) endorsed by the American Association of Cardiovascular and Pulmonary Rehabilitation; National Heart, Lung, and Blood Institute; Society for Vascular Nursing; TransAtlantic Inter-Society Consensus; and Vascular Disease Foundation. J Am Coll Cardiol 2006;47(6): 1239–312.

27. Smith SC Jr, Benjamin EJ, Bonow RO, et al. AHA/ACCF Secondary Prevention and Risk Reduction Therapy for Patients with Coronary and other Atherosclerotic Vascular Disease: 2011 update: a guideline from the American Heart Association and American College of Cardiology Foundation. Circulation 2011;124(22):2458–73.

28. Yancy CW, Jessup M, Bozkurt B, et al. 2013 ACCF/AHA Guideline for the Management of Heart Failure: a Report of the American College of Cardiology Foundation/American Heart Association Task Force on Practice Guidelines. J Am Coll Cardiol 2013;62:e147–239.

29. Wilhelmsen L, Rosengren A, Lappas G. Hospitalizations for atrial fibrillation in the general male population: morbidity and risk factors. J Intern Med 2001;250(5):382–9.

30. Levy D, Larson MG, Vasan RS, et al. The progression from hypertension to congestive heart failure. JAMA 1996;275(20):1557–62.

31. Kostis JB, Davis BR, Cutler J, et al. Prevention of heart failure by antihypertensive drug treatment in older persons with isolated systolic hypertension. SHEP Cooperative Research Group. JAMA 1997; 278(3):212–6.

32. Effects of treatment on morbidity in hypertension. II. Results in patients with diastolic blood pressure averaging 90 through 114 mm Hg. JAMA 1970; 213(7):1143–52.

33. Izzo JL Jr, Gradman AH. Mechanisms and management of hypertensive heart disease: from left ventricular hypertrophy to heart failure. Med Clin North Am 2004;88(5):1257–71.

34. Baker DW. Prevention of heart failure. J Card Fail 2002;8(5):333–46.

35. Jong P, Yusuf S, Rousseau MF, et al. Effect of enalapril on 12-year survival and life expectancy in patients with left ventricular systolic dysfunction: a follow-up study. Lancet 2003;361(9372):1843–8.

36. Scirica BM, Morrow DA, Cannon CP, et al. Intensive statin therapy and the risk of hospitalization for heart failure after an acute coronary syndrome in the PROVE IT-TIMI 22 study. J Am Coll Cardiol 2006;47(11):2326–31.

37. Goda A, Lund LH, Mancini D. The heart failure survival score outperforms the peak oxygen consumption for heart transplantation selection in the era of device therapy. J Heart Lung Transplant 2011;30(3):315–25.

38. Grady KL, Jalowiec A, White-Williams C. Predictors of quality of life in patients at one year after heart transplantation. J Heart Lung Transplant 1999; 18(3):202–10.

39. Kobashigawa JA, Leaf DA, Lee N, et al. A controlled trial of exercise rehabilitation after heart transplantation. N Engl J Med 1999;340(4): 272–7.

40. Grady KL, Jalowiec A, White-Williams C. Improvement in quality of life in patients with heart failure who undergo transplantation. J Heart Lung Transplant 1996;15(8):749–57.

41. Price JF, Mowbray PI, Lee AJ, et al. Relationship between smoking and cardiovascular risk factors in the development of peripheral arterial disease and coronary artery disease: Edinburgh Artery Study. Eur Heart J 1999;20(5):344–53.

42. Klotz S, Deng MC, Hanafy D, et al. Reversible pulmonary hypertension in heart transplant candidates—pretransplant evaluation and outcome after orthotopic heart transplantation. Eur J Heart Fail 2003;5(5):645–53.

43. Newman AB, Siscovick DS, Manolio TA, et al. Ankle-arm index as a marker of atherosclerosis in the Cardiovascular Health Study. Cardiovascular Heart Study (CHS) Collaborative Research Group. Circulation 1993;88(3):837–45.

44. Hiatt WR, Hoag S, Hamman RF. Effect of diagnostic criteria on the prevalence of peripheral arterial disease. The San Luis Valley Diabetes Study. Circulation 1995;91(5):1472–9.

45. Beks PJ, Mackaay AJ, de Neeling JN, et al. Peripheral arterial disease in relation to glycaemic level in an elderly Caucasian population: the Hoorn study. Diabetologia 1995;38(1):86–96.

46. Kirklin JK, Naftel DC, Bourge RC, et al. Evolving trends in risk profiles and causes of death after heart transplantation: a ten-year multi-institutional study. J Thorac Cardiovasc Surg 2003;125(4):881–90.

47. Kuppahally SS, Valantine HA, Weisshaar D, et al. Outcome in cardiac recipients of donor hearts with increased left ventricular wall thickness. Am J Transplant 2007;7(10):2388–95.

48. Radovancevic B, McGiffin DC, Kobashigawa JA, et al. Retransplantation in 7,290 primary transplant patients: a 10-year multi-institutional study. J Heart Lung Transplant 2003;22(8):862–8.

49. McDermott MM, Liu K, Greenland P, et al. Functional decline in peripheral arterial disease: associations with the ankle brachial index and leg symptoms. JAMA 2004;292(4):453–61.

50. European Stroke Organisation, Tendera M, Aboyans V, et al. ESC Guidelines on the diagnosis and treatment of peripheral artery diseases: document covering atherosclerotic disease of extracranial carotid and vertebral, mesenteric, renal, upper and lower extremity arteries: the Task Force on the Diagnosis and Treatment of Peripheral Artery Diseases of the European Society of Cardiology (ESC). Eur Heart J 2011;32(22):2851–906.

51. McDermott MM, Greenland P, Liu K, et al. Leg symptoms in peripheral arterial disease: associated clinical characteristics and functional impairment. JAMA 2001;286(13):1599–606.

52. White CJ, Gray WA. Endovascular therapies for peripheral arterial disease: an evidence-based review. Circulation 2007;116(19):2203–15.

53. Leng GC, Fowkes FG. The Edinburgh Claudication Questionnaire: an improved version of the WHO/Rose Questionnaire for use in epidemiological surveys. J Clin Epidemiol 1992;45(10):1101–9.

54. Grenon SM, Gagnon J, Hsiang Y. Video in clinical medicine. Ankle-brachial index for assessment of peripheral arterial disease. N Engl J Med 2009;361(19):e40.

55. Chobanian AV, Bakris GL, Black HR, et al. Seventh report of the Joint National Committee on Prevention, Detection, Evaluation, and Treatment of High Blood Pressure. Hypertension 2003;42(6):1206–52.

56. Rooke TW, Hirsch AT, Misra S, et al. 2011 ACCF/AHA Focused Update of the Guideline for the Management of Patients With Peripheral Artery Disease (updating the 2005 guideline): a report of the American College of Cardiology Foundation/American Heart Association Task Force on Practice Guidelines. J Am Coll Cardiol 2011;58(19):2020–45.

57. Ameli FM, Stein M, Provan JL, et al. The effect of postoperative smoking on femoropopliteal bypass grafts. Ann Vasc Surg 1989;3(1):20–5.

58. Quick CR, Cotton LT. The measured effect of stopping smoking on intermittent claudication. Br J Surg 1982;69(Suppl):S24–6.

59. National Cholesterol Education Program (NCEP) Expert Panel on Detection, Evaluation, and Treatment of High Blood Cholesterol in Adults (Adult Treatment Panel III). Third Report of the National Cholesterol Education Program (NCEP) Expert Panel on Detection, Evaluation, and Treatment of High Blood Cholesterol in Adults (Adult Treatment Panel III) final report. Circulation 2002;106(25):3143–421.

60. de Groot E, Jukema JW, Montauban van Swijndregt AD, et al. B-mode ultrasound assessment of pravastatin treatment effect on carotid and femoral artery walls and its correlations with coronary arteriographic findings: a report of the Regression Growth Evaluation Statin Study (REGRESS). J Am Coll Cardiol 1998;31(7):1561–7.

61. Pedersen TR, Kjekshus J, Pyorala K, et al. Effect of simvastatin on ischemic signs and symptoms in the Scandinavian simvastatin survival study (4S). Am J Cardiol 1998;81(3):333–5.

62. Aronow WS, Nayak D, Woodworth S, et al. Effect of simvastatin versus placebo on treadmill exercise time until the onset of intermittent claudication in older patients with peripheral arterial disease at six months and at one year after treatment. Am J Cardiol 2003;92(6):711–2.

63. Mohler ER 3rd, Hiatt WR, Creager MA. Cholesterol reduction with atorvastatin improves walking

distance in patients with peripheral arterial disease. Circulation 2003;108(12):1481–6.

64. Mondillo S, Ballo P, Barbati R, et al. Effects of simvastatin on walking performance and symptoms of intermittent claudication in hypercholesterolemic patients with peripheral vascular disease. Am J Med 2003;114(5):359–64.

65. Mills EJ, Rachlis B, Wu P, et al. Primary prevention of cardiovascular mortality and events with statin treatments: a network meta-analysis involving more than 65,000 patients. J Am Coll Cardiol 2008;52(22):1769–81.

66. Taylor F, Ward K, Moore TH, et al. Statins for the primary prevention of cardiovascular disease. Cochrane Database Syst Rev 2011;(1):CD004816.

67. Grundy SM, Cleeman JI, Merz CN, et al. Implications of recent clinical trials for the National Cholesterol Education Program Adult Treatment Panel III guidelines. Circulation 2004;110(2):227–39.

68. Effect of intensive diabetes management on macrovascular events and risk factors in the Diabetes Control and Complications Trial. Am J Cardiol 1995;75(14):894–903.

69. Davies EJ, Moxham T, Rees K, et al. Exercise training for systolic heart failure: Cochrane systematic review and meta-analysis. Eur J Heart Fail 2010;12(7):706–15.

70. McKelvie RS. Exercise training in patients with heart failure: clinical outcomes, safety, and indications. Heart Fail Rev 2008;13(1):3–11.

71. O'Connor CM, Whellan DJ, Lee KL, et al. Efficacy and safety of exercise training in patients with chronic heart failure: HF-ACTION randomized controlled trial. JAMA 2009;301(14):1439–50.

72. Smart N, Marwick TH. Exercise training for patients with heart failure: a systematic review of factors that improve mortality and morbidity. Am J Med 2004; 116(10):693–706.

73. Piepoli MF, Davos C, Francis DP, et al. Exercise training meta-analysis of trials in patients with chronic heart failure (ExTraMATCH). BMJ 2004; 328(7433):189.

74. Frans FA, Bipat S, Reekers JA, et al. Systematic review of exercise training or percutaneous transluminal angioplasty for intermittent claudication. Br J Surg 2012;99(1):16–28.

75. Gardner AW, Skinner JS, Bryant CX, et al. Stair climbing elicits a lower cardiovascular demand than walking in claudication patients. J Cardiopulm Rehabil 1995;15(2):134–42.

76. Hiatt WR, Regensteiner JG, Hargarten ME, et al. Benefit of exercise conditioning for patients with peripheral arterial disease. Circulation 1990;81(2): 602–9.

77. Leng GC, Fowler B, Ernst E. Exercise for intermittent claudication. Cochrane Database Syst Rev 2000;(2):CD000990.

78. Murphy TP, Cutlip DE, Regensteiner JG, et al. Supervised exercise versus primary stenting for claudication resulting from aortoiliac peripheral artery disease: six-month outcomes from the claudication: exercise versus endoluminal revascularization (CLEVER) study. Circulation 2012;125(1):130–9.

79. Hirsch AT, Haskal ZJ, Hertzer NR, et al. ACC/AHA Guidelines for the Management of Patients with Peripheral Arterial Disease (lower extremity, renal, mesenteric, and abdominal aortic): a collaborative report from the American Associations for Vascular Surgery/Society for Vascular Surgery, Society for Cardiovascular Angiography and Interventions, Society for Vascular Medicine and Biology, Society of Interventional Radiology, and the ACC/AHA Task Force on Practice Guidelines (writing committee to develop guidelines for the management of patients with peripheral arterial disease)—summary of recommendations. J Vasc Interv Radiol 2006;17(9): 1383–97 [quiz: 1398].

80. Reilly MP, Mohler ER 3rd. Cilostazol: treatment of intermittent claudication. Ann Pharmacother 2001; 35(1):48–56.

81. Drugs for intermittent claudication. Med Lett Drugs Ther 2004;46(1176):13–5.

82. Packer M, Carver JR, Rodeheffer RJ, et al. Effect of oral milrinone on mortality in severe chronic heart failure. The PROMISE Study Research Group. N Engl J Med 1991;325(21):1468–75.

83. Jamsen T, Manninen H, Tulla H, et al. The final outcome of primary infrainguinal percutaneous transluminal angioplasty in 100 consecutive patients with chronic critical limb ischemia. J Vasc Interv Radiol 2002;13(5):455–63.

84. McAlister FA, Stewart S, Ferrua S, et al. Multidisciplinary strategies for the management of heart failure patients at high risk for admission: a systematic review of randomized trials. J Am Coll Cardiol 2004;44(4):810–9.

85. Inglis SC, Clark RA, McAlister FA, et al. Which components of heart failure programmes are effective? A systematic review and meta-analysis of the outcomes of structured telephone support or telemonitoring as the primary component of chronic heart failure management in 8323 patients: Abridged Cochrane Review. Eur J Heart Fail 2011; 13(9):1028–40.

Cardiovascular Comorbidity in Rheumatic Diseases
A Focus on Heart Failure

Kerry Wright, MBBS[a], Cynthia S. Crowson, MS[a,b],*,
Sherine E. Gabriel, MD, MSc[a,b]

KEYWORDS

- Rheumatoid arthritis • Cardiovascular disease • Systemic lupus erythematosus • Heart failure

KEY POINTS

- There is an increased risk of cardiovascular disease–related mortality associated with systemic rheumatic diseases, which is not explained entirely by traditional cardiovascular risk factors and is likely related to both inflammation and immune-mediated mechanisms.
- The risk of heart failure in rheumatic arthritis (RA) is almost twice that of the general population; although it has been associated with worse outcomes, the treatment of heart failure in RA remains less aggressive.
- Aggressive control of rheumatic disease activity in conjunction with traditional cardiovascular risk factor modification is important in the management of patients with RA, although the impact on long-term outcomes remains incompletely understood.

INTRODUCTION

The increased risk of cardiovascular disease (CVD) associated with rheumatologic conditions is well recognized and has been described extensively in systemic lupus erythematosus (SLE), rheumatoid arthritis (RA), and, more recently, ankylosing spondylitis (AS) and psoriatic arthritis.

There is evidence to support the role of inflammation in the pathogenesis of CVD in this population, but the exact mechanism remains incompletely understood. Given the mortality gap that exists between patients with rheumatic diseases and the general population, early recognition, modification of risk factors, and control of disease activity will likely be pivotal in improving outcomes in this population.[1]

RA
Epidemiologic Insights

RA is a common rheumatic disease, estimated to have a prevalence of approximately 1%, and is seen 2 to 3 times more frequently among women.[2] The lifetime risk of RA has been estimated as 3.6% in women and 1.7% in men.[3]

Cardiovascular-Related Mortality and Ischemic Heart Disease in RA

Patients with RA have a higher risk of mortality when compared with the general population, which is largely a result of increased cardiovascular (CV) death (**Fig. 1**).[4,5] There is a 50% increased risk of CV mortality among patients with RA

Funding Source: This work was supported by the National Institute of Arthritis and Musculoskeletal and Skin Diseases, part of the National Institutes of Health, under award number R01AR46849 and the National Institute on Aging of the National Institutes of Health under award number R01AG034676. The content is solely the responsibility of the authors and does not necessarily represent the official views of the National Institutes of Health.

Financial Disclosures: The authors have nothing to disclose.

a Division of Rheumatology, Department of Medicine, Mayo Clinic, 200 First Street Southwest, Rochester, MN 55905, USA; b Department of Health Sciences Research, Mayo Clinic, 200 First Street Southwest, Rochester, MN 55905, USA

* Corresponding author.

E-mail address: crowson@mayo.edu

Heart Failure Clin 10 (2014) 339–352

http://dx.doi.org/10.1016/j.hfc.2013.10.003

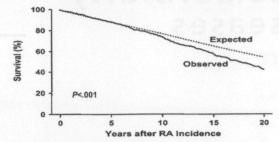

Fig. 1. Survival in RA compared with expected survival in the general population. (*From* Gabriel SE, Crowson CS, Kremers HM, et al. Survival in rheumatoid arthritis: a population-based analysis of trends over 40 years. Arthritis Rheum 2003;48(1):56; with permission.)

compared with the general population, with heart failure (HF) being a significant contributor to the observed excess mortality.[6,7]

The risk of ischemic heart disease (IHD) is significantly higher among patients with RA when compared with the general population.[8–10] In a large prospective cohort study of 114,342 women with RA and no prior CVD, the relative risk of myocardial infarction (MI) (after adjusting for CV risk factors) was 2.0 (95% confidence interval [CI] 1.23–3.29) compared with the general population.[11] Population-based studies have also shown that patients with RA are more likely to have unrecognized coronary heart disease (CHD) and are almost twice as likely to experience sudden death when compared with the general population (hazard ratio [HR] 1.94, 95% CI 1.06–3.55).[10]

The increased risk of coronary artery disease among patients with RA has been attributed to accelerated atherosclerosis in the presence of systemic inflammation.[12,13] Although coronary artery disease is the major cause of HF in the general population, accounting for 62% of all cases, its contribution to the development of HF in RA is not as compelling.[14] The excess risk of HF is not

explained by clinical IHD.[15] Patients with RA presenting with incident HF are less likely to have a preceding history of IHD compared with non-RA patients (24% compared with 35% among non-RA patients, $P = .02$).[16] This fact may be explained, in part, by the increased risk of unrecognized CHD described earlier.

HF in RA

The increased risk of developing HF among patients with RA is well described.[9,17,18] A population-based incidence cohort of patients with RA over a 40-year period demonstrated a higher incidence of HF among patients with RA compared with a cohort of non-RA patients. After adjusting for age, sex, IHD, and traditional CV risk factors, the risk of developing HF (defined according to the Framingham Heart Study Criteria) among patients with RA was almost twice that of non-RA patients (HR 1.87, 95% CI 1.47–2.39), with an increase in cumulative incidence observed over time (**Fig. 2**). The higher incidence of HF was seen among all age groups, but it tended to be increased in women compared with men (relative risk [RR] 1.9, 95% CI 1.4–2.5 vs RR 1.3 95% CI 0.9–2.0).[15]

Compared with the general population, HF in patients with RA seems to be more frequently associated with diastolic dysfunction.[19,20] After adjusting for age, sex, and history of IHD, patients with RA have been shown to be twice as likely to have preserved ejection fraction (odds ratio [OR] 1.90, 95% CI 0.98–3.67) (**Fig. 3**).[16] When HF with reduced ejection fraction does occur in patients with RA, it is seen much more frequently in men (HR 3.7, 95% CI 1.8–7.7).[21] Diastolic dysfunction is a predictor for incident HF independent of the traditional CV risk factors, including age, hypertension, diabetes, and coronary artery disease (HR 1.81, 95% CI 1.01–3.48).[22,23] Echocardiographic

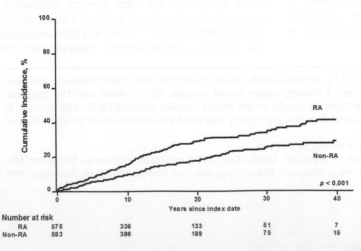

Number at risk				
RA	575	336	133	51	7
Non-RA	583	386	189	75	15

Fig. 2. Comparison of the cumulative incidence of congestive HF in the RA cohort and the non-RA cohort, according to the number of years since the index date, adjusting for the competing risk of death. (*From* Nicola PJ, Maradit-Kremers H, Roger VL, et al. The risk of congestive heart failure in rheumatoid arthritis: a population based study over 46 years. Arthritis Rheum 2005;52(2):416; with permission.)

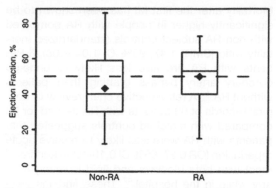

Fig. 3. Distribution of ejection fraction (EF) between patients with RA and non-RA patients at the onset of HF. Data are presented as box plots: The boxes represent the 25th to 75th percentiles, the vertical lines represent the 10th and 90th percentiles, the diamonds represent the means, the lines within the boxes represent the medians, and the broken line represents the 50% EF reference. (*From* Davis JM 3rd, Roger VL, Crowson CS. The presentation and outcome of heart failure in patients with rheumatoid arthritis differs from that in the general population. Arthritis Rheum 2008;58(9):2606; with permission.)

findings of diastolic dysfunction have also been shown to be associated with an increase in all-cause and cardiac mortality.[24–26]

Role of Traditional CV Risk Factors

The increased risk of CHD and HF among patients with RA is not explained by an increased incidence of the traditional CV risk factors; in fact, some traditional risk factors may play a paradoxic role in RA.[10,18,27]

Age is a major determinant for CVD risk in the general population. Indeed, the impact of aging on the CV risk in patients with RA may be even

greater than for the general population. Recently, a population-based inception cohort of patients with RA with no prior CVD history demonstrated that the effect of age on CVD risk was almost twice that in the general population in men and more than twice that in women. The impact of age on CVD risk in seronegative patients and among patients younger than 50 years was similar to that seen in the general population.[28]

Diabetes mellitus, hypertension, dyslipidemia, and alcohol use/abuse have not been described more frequently in patients with RA when compared with patients without RA.[15,16,18,29] The prevalence of smoking is higher among patients with RA, but this risk factor alone is unlikely to account for the increased CVD risk.[27,29,30]

Obesity seems to play a paradoxic role in its contribution to CVD risk in patients with RA, with a lower body mass index (BMI) associated with increased CV risk in one study.[29] Davis and colleagues[16] also described a lower prevalence of obesity at baseline among subjects with RA with incident HF compared with non-RA subjects (60% vs 71%, *P* = .03). Patients with RA with a higher BMI have lower mortality rates than that seen in thinner patients independent of RA onset, age, duration, and smoking status.[31]

Lipids also seem to play a paradoxic role with respect to CV risk among patients with RA, with lower total cholesterol being significantly associated with a higher CV risk (**Fig. 4**).[32] High-density lipoprotein, low-density lipoprotein (LDL), and total cholesterol levels may be reduced in patients with untreated RA and later increase with suppression of inflammation through treatment, although the increase in LDL cholesterol associated with RA treatment does not seem to confer a higher CV risk.[33–35] Patients with RA tended to have a lower likelihood of achieving therapeutic LDL goals

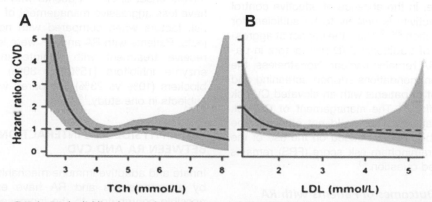

Fig. 4. HRs for CVD in RA (*solid lines*) according to (*A*) total cholesterol (TCh) and (*B*) LDL. Shaded areas represent 95% CIs. (*From* Myasoedova E, Crowson CS, Kremers HM. Lipid paradox in rheumatoid arthritis: the impact of serum lipid measures and systemic inflammation on the risk of cardiovascular disease. Ann Rheum Dis 2011;70(3):484; with permission.)

following statin use. Increased erythrocyte sedimentation rate (ESR) is associated with a lower likelihood of achieving LDL targets, which underscores the importance of control of disease activity in risk-factor modification.[36]

Screening for Traditional CV Risk Factors in RA

Despite the increased awareness of the higher risk of CVD among patients with RA, screening and management of traditional CV risk factors in this population remains inadequate.[37] In one study, a significant proportion of patients with RA and hyperlipidemia with sufficiently high risk to warrant statin use were not receiving treatment with statins.[38] Similarly, hypertension among patients with RA remains underdiagnosed and undertreated.[39]

The association between CV risk factors and CV events seems to be weaker among patients with RA compared with the general population. Male gender, smoking, and personal cardiac history have a weaker relative association with CV events in patients with RA compared with non-RA patients.[29] Overall, the proportion of risk attributable to traditional CV risk factors was 23% lower in subjects with RA than in non-RA subjects in one study.[18]

Taken together, these data suggest that the higher risk of CVD in RA is not explained by a higher prevalence of CV risk factors or an increased impact of CV risk factors. Instead, recent data have suggested that RA may be an independent CV risk factor. Notably, the magnitude of risk conferred by RA as an independent CV risk factor is comparable with the magnitude of risk associated with diabetes mellitus.[40,41]

Because RA disease activity has repeatedly been shown to be significantly associated with higher CVD risk, modification of traditional risk factors alone, in the absence of effective control of disease activity is unlikely to be sufficient for CV risk reduction.[29,42] Thus, the impact of aggressive control of traditional CVD risk factors in patients with RA remains unclear. Nonetheless, the current recommendations support screening and management of patients with an elevated CV risk when identified.[38] The management of CV risk factors in patients who would not otherwise be deemed to be high risk based on the use of the traditional Framingham risk score (FRS) remains an unresolved question.[43]

Prognosis/Outcomes of Patients with RA

Studies have suggested that patients with RA have worse short- and long-term outcomes following MI compared with the general population.[44,45]

Mortality after the first MI has been shown to be significantly higher in people with RA compared with non-RA subject controls (standardized mortality ratio [SMR] 1.47, 95% CI 1.04–2.08).[46] Patients with RA are also less likely to undergo coronary artery bypass grafting than patients without RA.[10] A retrospective chart review of hospital records of 90 patients with RA treated for MI compared with matched controls suggested that patients with RA were less likely to receive acute reperfusion (OR 0.27, 95% CI 0.10–0.64) and treatment with beta-blockers and lipid-lowering therapy while in the hospital.[47] These findings were not reproduced in a recent larger cross-sectional study of 13,029 patients with RA conducted between 2003 and 2005, which, in contrast, demonstrated a higher rate of percutaneous intervention (OR 1.27, 95% CI, 1.17–1.39) and a greater likelihood of thrombolytic use (OR 1.38, 95% CI 1.10–1.71) compared with the general population. This study also suggested improved in-hospital mortality when compared with the general population.[48] It is unclear if the observed disparities are a reflection of different practice patterns based on the different populations in which these studies were conducted, and further investigation is warranted.

The prognosis of patients with HF and RA is also worse compared with non-RA patients based on population-based data derived from Olmsted County, Minnesota, which demonstrated a higher 30-day (15.5% vs 6.6%, $P = .001$) and 1-year mortality (35% vs 19.3%, $P = .01$) after the onset of HF among patients with RA compared with non-RA subjects. The risk of death at 30 days was 2.39 fold higher (95% CI 1.36–4.18) and 2.02 fold (95% CI 1.40–2.90) higher at 1 year. Among those subjects who survived the first year, there was no difference in overall survival after the onset of HF.[16] Patients with RA seem to have less aggressive management of HF and CV risk factors when compared with non-RA subjects. Patients with RA and HF were less likely to receive treatment with angiotensin-converting enzyme inhibitors (15% vs 30%) and beta-blockers (10% vs 23%) compared with non-RA subjects in one study.[16]

PATHOPHYSIOLOGIC INTERACTIONS BETWEEN RA AND CVD

Innate and adaptive immune mechanisms shared by atherosclerosis and RA have emerged as possible contributors to the increased CVD risk seen in this population. There is evidence from both human and animal studies that toll-like receptor signaling plays a role in driving the production of cytokines in synovium and in the activation of atherosclerotic lesions.[49] HLA–DRB1 is a major gene that has been shown to be associated with RA susceptibility and has also been shown to potentially confer an increased risk of CHD, suggesting a role for adaptive immunity in the pathogenesis of both diseases.[50–52] The loss of expression of CD28, which is a costimulatory molecule present on CD4 T cells (CD28 null cells), has been associated with RA and, in particular, with more aggressive disease manifestations.[53] Higher levels of CD28 null cells have been seen in patients with RA with evidence of preclinical atherosclerosis compared with controls.[54] CD28 null cells identified in atherosclerotic plaque has been shown to play a role in the mediation of the inflammatory process.[55]

Chronic inflammation plays an important role in development of HF, but the mechanism by which this increases the risk of myocardial dysfunction and HF remains incompletely understood. Elevated inflammatory markers (C-reactive protein [CRP], interleukin 6 [IL-6], and tumor necrosis factor [TNF] alpha) are associated with an increased risk for left ventricular (LV) hypertrophy, diastolic dysfunction, and development of HF in the general population, with higher levels conferring greater risk.[56–58] Among patients with advanced HF, higher levels of TNF alpha and IL-6 have also been associated with increased mortality.[59]

In patients with RA, elevated levels of IL-6 have also been demonstrated to confer a higher risk of diastolic dysfunction (OR 1.2 per 2.8 pg/mL, 95% CI 1.02–1.4) and have been associated with premature coronary atherosclerosis, even after adjustment for CV risk factors.[13,60]

Systemic inflammation as evidenced by persistently elevated ESR levels among patients with RA has been shown to confer a 2-fold increased risk (HR 2.03, 95% CI 1.45–2.83) for CV death among patients with RA even after adjustment for traditional CV risk factors. There also seems to be an increasing risk with higher ESR levels.[21,61] Among patients with RA, higher ESR levels were seen in the 6-month period before the development of HF than any other time during the follow-up period, which also supports the potential for inflammatory mechanisms to be involved in the pathogenesis of HF (Fig. 5).[62]

Abnormal Myocardial Structure and Function in RA

Patients with RA are more likely to have abnormal LV geometry (higher LV mass and LV hypertrophy) than healthy people without RA. These abnormalities are associated with an increased risk of CVD. For example, there is a strong association between increased LV mass (seen in patients with RA) and incident HF (HR 1.4 per 10% increment, P<.0001).[63,64] Patients with RA with abnormal LV geometry are also significantly more likely to have LV concentric remodeling (OR 4.73, 95% CI 2.85–7.83), which is associated with a higher risk of incident CHD.[64,65]

Speckle tracking echocardiography is an advanced echocardiographic modality for detection of myocardial changes during contraction and relaxation (ie, myocardial strain).[66,67] A recent population-based study of 87 patients with RA using this imaging modality showed a reduction in LV and right ventricular strain among patients with RA when compared with the general population, which correlated with markers of disease severity.[68] Although larger studies are needed to confirm these findings, this modality may be useful in detecting early myocardial changes in RA.[66,67]

Impact of Disease Characteristics of RA

The disease characteristics of RA seem to influence the risk of development of CVD and CV mortality, with rheumatoid factor (RF) positivity

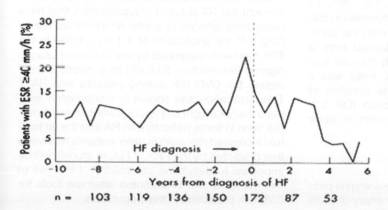

Fig. 5. Erythrocyte sedimentation rate (ESR) levels before and after development of HF. (*From* Maradit-Kremers H, Nicola PJ, Crowson CS, et al. Raised erythrocyte sedimentation rate signals heart failure in patients with rheumatoid arthritis. Ann Rheum Dis 2007;66(1):76–80; with permission.)

and disease severity conferring the greatest risk.[61,69]

RF positivity is a significant predictor of CV events including HF all-cause and CV mortality among the general population, suggesting a role for antibodies in the pathogenesis of CVD.[69,70] Among RF-negative subjects, after adjusting for age, sex, IHD, and CV risk factors, the increased risk of HF was no longer significant in a population-based cohort study but remained significant with a 2.5-fold increased risk among RF-positive subjects (adjusted HR 2.59, 95% CI 1.95–3.43).[15] Severe extra-articular manifestations of disease are associated with a higher likelihood of developing HF (HR 3.1, 95% CI 1.9–5.1) even after adjustment for CV risk factors.[21] The presence of rheumatoid lung disease and RA vasculitis, which are markers of disease severity, has also been associated with a greater likelihood of CV death.[61]

Impact of Disease Duration

There is evidence to suggest that the increased CVD risk in RA may predate the clinical manifestations of the disease, with evidence of atherosclerosis and coronary artery disease predating the diagnosis.[71] Following the diagnosis of RA, the relationship between the disease duration and CVD outcomes is less clear. A recent meta-analysis suggested that the SMR was higher among noninception cohorts. A population-based inception cohort study of patients with RA did not identify an association with risk of coronary artery disease and disease duration, but there was an increased risk of events in the 2-year period before meeting the American College of Rheumatology's (ACR) criteria for RA.[61] Another population-based study found no increased risk of IHD in the 5-year period before the RA diagnosis (adjusted OR 1.2, 95% CI 0.6–2.4).[72] However, this population noted a significantly increased risk of IHD in years 1 to 4 after the RA diagnosis (RR 1.5, 95% CI 1.2–1.7).[73] The risk of diastolic dysfunction in patients with RA may be associated with the duration of disease based on data derived from a population-based cohort study that showed that after adjusting for CV risk factors, there was a significant association between the duration of the disease and diastolic dysfunction (OR 3.2, 95% CI 1.8–5.4), similar to that seen in other studies.[74,75]

DIAGNOSTIC ISSUES

Patients with RA are less likely to have angina pectoris as a manifestation of coronary artery disease

(OR 0.58, 95% CI 0.34–0.99), more likely to have silent MI (OR 5.86, 95% CI 1.29–26.64) compared with the general population, and less likely to have typical electrocardiogram findings at presentation.[10,45] The difference in clinical presentation may contribute to delays in the recognition and treatment of patients with RA and emphasizes the importance of a high index of suspicion in these patients.

Clinical features of HF typically seen in the general population are less likely to be evident at presentation in patients with RA. Population studies of incident HF in patients with RA showed that they are less likely to have dyspnea on exertion, orthopnea, or paroxysmal nocturnal dyspnea at presentation. Patients with RA in this study were also more likely to have rales compared with non-RA subjects and less likely to have elevated blood pressures at presentation.[16]

B-Type Natriuretic Peptide

Elevated levels of B-type natriuretic peptide (BNP) are predictive of LV diastolic dysfunction (LVDD) on echocardiography in the general population and are useful in the evaluation of suspected HF.[76] Among patients without clinical CVD, those with RA were more likely to have elevated BNP than non-RA subjects (16% vs 9%, P<.001). Patients with RA with abnormal BNP are more likely to have LVDD compared with those with normal BNP, but the specificity compared with non-RA patients (89% vs 94%, P = .02) and the positive predictive value (25%) of elevated BNP in patients with RA is low (25%) and is, therefore, not a good screening tool.[77] The duration of RA and CRP levels is independently associated with N-terminal proBNP.[78]

CV Risk Scores in RA

There is a need for risk scores that accurately estimate the risk of CVD among patients with RA.

Given that the current risk scores do not take into account the RA disease characteristics that have been demonstrated to confer an increased risk of CVD,[37,67] the application of a 1.5 multiplier to the FRS has been suggested by the European League Against Rheumatism (EULAR) as a means of estimating the CVD risk among patients with RA.[42] This application was shown to inadequately estimate the risk in light of a re-equivalent or even lower risk seen in some patients with RA and the up to 3-fold increased risk seen in older patients relative to that predicted by the FRS.[79] Future studies will be important to determine the validity of the use of this multiplier and to establish alternate tools for CVD risk prediction in this population.

IMPACT OF MEDICATIONS USED IN TREATMENT OF RA ON HF

Medications used for the treatment of RA may have opposing effects on CV risk; although a reduction in disease activity is associated with a lower risk of CV outcomes, the potential for increased CV risk remains with the use of certain drugs.

Glucocorticoids

Glucocorticoids are frequently used in the treatment of RA primarily for short-term control of disease activity but may also have disease-modifying benefits. The use of glucocorticoids has been associated with an increased risk of CVD based on observational studies in the general population.[80,81] Among patients with RA, population-based studies have shown a higher risk of CV events (MI, HF, and CV death) associated with glucocorticoid exposure, with higher exposure associated with a 3-fold increased risk of CV events in one study (HR 3.06, 95% CI 1.81–5.18). The increased risk was not seen in patients who were RF negative and in those taking lower doses of glucocorticoids (average daily dose of ≤7.5 mg).[82] Current use of glucocorticoids has been associated with a 2-fold increased risk of HF (HR 2.0, 95% CI 1.3–3.2) and increased risk of hospitalization for HF (HR 1.4, 95% CI 1.03–1.8).[21,83] Glucocorticoid use in patients with RA, when indicated, should be limited in dose and duration given the dose-dependent increase in the risk observed.

Nonsteroidal Antiinflammatory Medications

The use of Cox-2 inhibitors and nonsteroidal antiinflammatory drugs (NSAIDs) is associated with an increased risk of MI, relapse of HF, and hypertension, which are greatest in patients with a prior history of CVD.[84,85] The use of nonselective NSAIDs, however, has not been shown to be associated with an increased risk of incident HF in patients with RA without a prior history. Use of NSAIDs and Cox-2 inhibitors should, therefore, be avoided in patients with RA with a history of CVD.

Disease-Modifying Antirheumatic Drugs

There is evidence to suggest that control of disease activity is associated with a reduction in CV risk. A case-control study of patients with RA with no history of HF showed that patients treated with disease-modifying antirheumatic drugs (DMARDs) had a 30% lower rate of hospitalization for HF when compared with no DMARD use.[86]

Data from population-based cohort studies showed that patients treated with methotrexate were half as likely to develop HF compared with nonusers (HR 0.5, 95% CI 0.3–0.9).[21] The use of methotrexate in patients with RA was associated with a 60% reduction in all-cause mortality and a 70% reduction in CV mortality in one study.[87] A reduction in CV events in patients treated with methotrexate was also suggested by 2 recent systematic reviews.[88,89]

Methotrexate has been the most widely studied of the disease-modifying agents with regard to the impact on CV risk, but there is a suggestion that the use of other traditional DMARDs (hydroxychloroquine, sulfasalazine, and leflunomide) may also be associated with a lower CV risk.[90,91]

Biologic Response Modifiers

Of the biologic response modifiers used for the treatment of RA, anti-TNF agents have garnered the most attention for their impact on HF given the initial investigations into their role as a potential therapeutic agent. Trials of etanercept and infliximab failed to demonstrate any treatment benefit and, in the case of infliximab, suggested a potential harm with a higher rate of HF and hospitalization.[92–95]

Among patients with RA, the risk associated with the use of anti-TNF agents remains less clear. Data from observational cohort studies and long-term extension studies of patients with RA treated with anti-TNF agents have failed to show an increased risk of new or worsening HF. The possibility of a decreased risk associated with anti-TNF therapy has also been suggested.[86,96] In a large observational cohort of 13,171 patients with RA, HF was significantly less common in anti-TNF–treated patients (3.1% [180/5832] vs 3.8% [281/7339], P<.05). Patients in this study who received infliximab were less likely to have a history of CVD than those who did not (47.8% vs 54.4% [4820/8864]), which may be reflective of the awareness of the treating clinician of the Food and Drug Administration's warnings that arose out of the trials of anti-TNF agents in HF.[17] The applicability of these results to all patients with RA remains unclear In the absence of randomized controlled clinical trial data.[97] Nevertheless, the ACR's current recommendations for patients with HF recommend against the use of anti-TNF agents in patients with NYHA class III/IV HF with an ejection fraction of 50% or less.[98]

SLE

Coronary artery disease is a well-recognized cause of morbidity and mortality among patients with SLE, with autopsy evidence of atherosclerosis in up to 50% of patients.[99,100]

The risk of MI in patients with SLE (after adjusting for CV risk factors) has been estimated to be between 2 and 9 times greater than the general population depending on the study setting.[101,102] The increased relative risk is especially striking in young women, with a prospective cohort study estimating that women in the 35- to 44-year-old age group were more than 50 times more likely to have an MI compared with women of a similar age.[102]

Premature atherosclerosis is a recognized complication of SLE, which is associated with significant morbidity and mortality, with subclinical evidence detected more frequently among patients with SLE than the general population. Coronary calcification (a known marker of atherosclerosis) was seen more commonly among patients with SLE with no prior history of coronary artery disease when compared with control subjects (20 out of 65 vs 6 out of 69, $P = .002$).[103] Evidence of carotid plaque on ultrasound was more common in 197 patients with SLE compared with matched controls (37.1% vs 15.2%, $P<.001$).[104] Age, male gender, longer disease duration, higher damage scores, and longer duration of steroid therapy have been associated with a higher risk for subclinical atherosclerosis.[103–106]

The role of the innate immune system in the pathogenesis of SLE and associated CVD is an area of ongoing research. Type 1 interferon has been implicated in animal studies through its impact on recruitment of T cells and macrophages into atherosclerotic lesions and endothelial dysfunction.[107,108]

HF

The risk of HF is higher among patients with SLE. Women with SLE were 3.8 times more likely to be admitted to hospital for HF than age-matched patients without SLE in one study.[109] Tissue Doppler and strain imaging in patients with SLE with no signs of HF were more likely to show evidence of systolic and diastolic dysfunction when compared with a matched healthy control group.[110]

A total of 173 patients with SLE (with no evidence of coronary artery disease or valvular disease) compared with an age- and gender-matched reference group without SLE were more likely to have increased LV mass (38.3 vs 32.8 g/m^2, $P<.001$) on echocardiogram, suggesting that this may be a possible mechanism behind the increased risk seen in this population.[111]

Traditional CV Risk Factors

Studies of CV risk factors suggest that patients with SLE are more likely to be hypertensive than the general population, with an RR of 2.59 (95% CI 1.79–3.75) in one study.[103,104,112] In a case control study of 250 women with SLE examining risk factors for CHD, hyperlipidemia and smoking were not seen more frequently compared with controls.[112] The prevalence of traditional CV risk factors is higher among patients with SLE, but the increased risk is not explained by traditional risk factors.[113–115] Among 263 patients with SLE attending a lupus clinic, after adjusting for baseline CV risk using the FRS, the increase in the RR for nonfatal MI was 10.1 and 17.0 for death caused by CHD, suggesting that the increased risk is unlikely to be explained by traditional CV risk factors and is likely contributed, in part, by the chronic inflammation and the resulting increase in risk of atherosclerosis.[116,117]

AS

AS represents the prototype of the spondyloarthropathies and is characterized by axial disease, enthesitis, and oligoarthritis. Although the risk of CVD in patients with AS has not been as well defined as in RA, there has been heightened awareness of the risk of CVD in this population.[118–121] A recent retrospective cohort study using population-based administrative data from 8616 patients with AS reported, the sex standardized prevalence ratio for IHD was 1.37 (95% CI 1.31–1.44) and for HF was 1.34 (95% CI 1.26–1.42).[119]

PSORIASIS AND PSORIATIC ARTHRITIS

Both psoriasis and psoriatic arthritis have been shown to be associated with an increased risk of CV disease relative to the general population. The prevalence of traditional CV risk factors has been demonstrated to be higher among patients with psoriasis; but even after adjusting for these variables, the risk of IHD remains high (OR 1.78, 95% CI 1.51–2.11), with recent studies suggesting that psoriasis may be an independent risk factor for MI.[122–124] Patients with psoriatic arthritis are more likely to have evidence of preclinical atherosclerosis and are at an increased risk of CVD relative to the general population.[121,125–127] Among 648 patients with psoriatic arthritis enrolled in the University of Toronto database, the risk of MI (standardized prevalence ratio 2.57, 95% CI 1.73–3.80) and angina (1.97, 95% CI 1.24–3.12) was significantly higher than that of the general population, with increased risk seen in patients with more severe psoriasis.[128]

Although data on the increased risk of CVD among patients with psoriatic arthritis and AS are emerging, they have been recognized to be important factors contributing to increased mortality and morbidity in this patient population and represent an area of ongoing research; the EULAR's current recommendations for CV risk management recognize these as risk factors.[42]

SUMMARY

CVD remains a significant comorbidity associated with rheumatic diseases contributing to the higher mortality rate relative to the general population.

The risk of HF has been best described in RA, which is more frequently associated with diastolic dysfunction. Patients with RA are less likely to present with typical features of HF or IHD, which underscores the importance of awareness on the part of treating clinicians for a high index of suspicion for CVD in the absence of the clinical features that are typically seen in the general population. The mortality rate after an MI is higher among patients with RA, which is potentially related to less aggressive treatment approaches in this population. Patients with RA and HF are treated less aggressively and have worse outcomes compared with the general population. Increased awareness of a higher CVD risk may ultimately translate into better treatment outcomes in the future.

The pathogenesis of the increased CVD risk seen in this population remains incompletely understood; but the role of systemic inflammation in the pathogenesis of premature atherosclerosis, IHD, and HF has been illustrated. Innate and adaptive immune mechanisms shared by CV diseases and systemic rheumatic diseases have been identified and are promising areas for expanding understanding of the pathogenesis of the increased risk as well as the identification of potential novel treatment targets.

It has been recognized that the increased risk of CVD in rheumatic diseases is not explained in entirety by the traditional CV risk factors. Isolated treatment of CV risk factors in the absence of adequate control of disease activity is unlikely to effectively reduce the CV risk; therefore, the current treatment strategies are focused on targeting both of these areas. Traditional CV risk factor identification and treatment is suboptimal among patients with RA; it remains unclear if the treatment targets used for the general population are applicable, especially in light of the paradoxic role of some risk factors.

Treatment strategies for the rheumatic diseases frequently involve the use of glucocorticoids and NSAIDs, both of which have been associated with a higher risk of CVD. Among patients with known CVD and rheumatic diseases, the use of glucocorticoids and NSAIDs should be avoided or minimized. There has been no increased risk associated with the use of traditional DMARDs; in fact, methotrexate use has been associated with improved CV outcomes, likely reflecting the impact of better control of disease activity. The safety of anti-TNF agents in patients with RA and HF remains less well defined and will warrant further study.

REFERENCES

1. Gonzalez A, Maradit Kremers H, Crowson CS, et al. The widening mortality gap between rheumatoid arthritis patients and the general population. Arthritis Rheum 2007;56(11):3583–7.
2. Spector TD. Rheumatoid arthritis. Rheum Dis Clin North Am 1990;16(3):513–37.
3. Crowson CS, Matteson EL, Myasoedova E, et al. The lifetime risk of adult-onset rheumatoid arthritis and other inflammatory autoimmune rheumatic diseases. Arthritis Rheum 2011;63(3):633–9.
4. Gabriel SE, Crowson CS, Kremers HM, et al. Survival in rheumatoid arthritis: a population-based analysis of trends over 40 years. Arthritis Rheum 2003;48(1):54–8.
5. Gabriel SE. Cardiovascular morbidity and mortality in rheumatoid arthritis. Am J Med 2008;121(10 Suppl 1):S9–14.
6. Avina-Zubieta JA, Choi HK, Sadatsafavi M, et al. Risk of cardiovascular mortality in patients with rheumatoid arthritis: a meta-analysis of observational studies. Arthritis Rheum 2008;59(12):1690–7.
7. Nicola PJ, Crowson CS, Maradit-Kremers H, et al. Contribution of congestive heart failure and ischemic heart disease to excess mortality in rheumatoid arthritis. Arthritis Rheum 2006;54(1):60–7.
8. Watson DJ, Rhodes T, Guess HA. All-cause mortality and vascular events among patients with rheumatoid arthritis, osteoarthritis, or no arthritis in the UK General Practice Research Database. J Rheumatol 2003;30(6):1196–202.
9. Wolfe F, Freundlich B, Straus WL. Increase in cardiovascular and cerebrovascular disease prevalence in rheumatoid arthritis. J Rheumatol 2003; 30(1):36–40.
10. Maradit-Kremers H, Crowson CS, Nicola PJ, et al. Increased unrecognized coronary heart disease and sudden deaths in rheumatoid arthritis: a population-based cohort study. Arthritis Rheum 2005;52(2):402–11.
11. Solomon DH, Karlson EW, Rimm EB, et al. Cardiovascular morbidity and mortality in women diagnosed with rheumatoid arthritis. Circulation 2003; 107(9):1303–7.

12. Van Doornum S, McColl G, Wicks IP. Accelerated atherosclerosis: an extra-articular feature of rheumatoid arthritis? Arthritis Rheum 2002;46(4):862–73.

13. Rho YH, Chung CP, Oeser A, et al. Inflammatory mediators and premature coronary atherosclerosis in rheumatoid arthritis. Arthritis Rheum 2009; 61(11):1580–5.

14. He J, Ogden LG, Bazzano LA, et al. Risk factors for congestive heart failure in US men and women: NHANES I epidemiologic follow-up study. Arch Intern Med 2001;161(7):996–1002.

15. Nicola PJ, Maradit-Kremers H, Roger VL, et al. The risk of congestive heart failure in rheumatoid arthritis: a population-based study over 46 years. Arthritis Rheum 2005;52(2):412–20.

16. Davis JM 3rd, Roger VL, Crowson CS, et al. The presentation and outcome of heart failure in patients with rheumatoid arthritis differs from that in the general population. Arthritis Rheum 2008; 58(9):2603–11.

17. Wolfe F, Michaud K. Heart failure in rheumatoid arthritis: rates, predictors, and the effect of antitumor necrosis factor therapy. Am J Med 2004; 116(5):305–11.

18. Crowson CS, Nicola PJ, Kremers HM, et al. How much of the increased incidence of heart failure in rheumatoid arthritis is attributable to traditional cardiovascular risk factors and ischemic heart disease? Arthritis Rheum 2005;52(10):3039–44.

19. Alpaslan M, Onrat E, Evcik D. Doppler echocardiographic evaluation of ventricular function in patients with rheumatoid arthritis. Clin Rheumatol 2003;22(2):84–8.

20. Di Franco M, Paradiso M, Mammarella A, et al. Diastolic function abnormalities in rheumatoid arthritis. Evaluation By echo Doppler transmitral flow and pulmonary venous flow: relation with duration of disease. Ann Rheum Dis 2000;59(3):227–9.

21. Myasoedova E, Crowson CS, Nicola PJ, et al. The influence of rheumatoid arthritis disease characteristics on heart failure. J Rheumatol 2011;38(8): 1601–6.

22. Kane GC, Karon BL, Mahoney DW, et al. Progression of left ventricular diastolic dysfunction and risk of heart failure. JAMA 2011;306(8):856–63.

23. Lam CS, Lyass A, Kraigher-Krainer E, et al. Cardiac dysfunction and noncardiac dysfunction as precursors of heart failure with reduced and preserved ejection fraction in the community. Circulation 2011;124(1):24–30.

24. Redfield MM, Jacobsen SJ, Burnett JC Jr, et al. Burden of systolic and diastolic ventricular dysfunction in the community: appreciating the scope of the heart failure epidemic. JAMA 2003; 289(2):194–202.

25. Aurigemma GP, Gottdiener JS, Shemanski L, et al. Predictive value of systolic and diastolic function

26. Bella JN, Palmieri V, Roman MJ, et al. Mitral ratio of peak early to late diastolic filling velocity as a predictor of mortality in middle-aged and elderly adults: the Strong Heart Study. Circulation 2002; 105(16):1928–33.

27. Solomon DH, Curhan GC, Rimm EB, et al. Cardiovascular risk factors in women with and without rheumatoid arthritis. Arthritis Rheum 2004;50(11): 3444–9.

28. Crowson CS, Therneau TM, Davis JM 3rd, et al. Accelerated aging influences cardiovascular disease risk in rheumatoid arthritis. Arthritis Rheum 2013;65:2562–6.

29. Gonzalez A, Maradit Kremers H, Crowson CS, et al. Do cardiovascular risk factors confer the same risk for cardiovascular outcomes in rheumatoid arthritis patients as in non-rheumatoid arthritis patients? Ann Rheum Dis 2008;67(1):64–9.

30. Boyer JF, Gourraud PA, Cantagrel A, et al. Traditional cardiovascular risk factors in rheumatoid arthritis: a meta-analysis. Joint Bone Spine 2011; 78(2):179–83.

31. Escalante A, Haas RW, del Rincon I. Paradoxical effect of body mass index on survival in rheumatoid arthritis: role of comorbidity and systemic inflammation. Arch Intern Med 2005;165(14):1624–9.

32. Myasoedova E, Crowson CS, Kremers HM, et al. Lipid paradox in rheumatoid arthritis: the impact of serum lipid measures and systemic inflammation on the risk of cardiovascular disease. Ann Rheum Dis 2011;70(3):482–7.

33. Choy E, Sattar N. Interpreting lipid levels in the context of high-grade inflammatory states with a focus on rheumatoid arthritis: a challenge to conventional cardiovascular risk actions. Ann Rheum Dis 2009;68(4):460–9.

34. Steiner G, Urowitz MB. Lipid profiles in patients with rheumatoid arthritis: mechanisms and the impact of treatment. Semin Arthritis Rheum 2009; 38(5):372–81.

35. Lazarevic MB, Vitic J, Mladenovic V, et al. Dyslipoproteinemia in the course of active rheumatoid arthritis. Semin Arthritis Rheum 1992;22(3):172–8.

36. Myasoedova E, Gabriel SE, Green AB, et al. The impact of statin use on lipid levels in statin-naive patients with rheumatoid arthritis (RA) vs. non-RA subjects: results from a population-based study. Arthritis Care Res (Hoboken) 2013;65:1592–9.

37. Scott IC, Ibrahim F, Johnson D, et al. Current limitations in the management of cardiovascular risk in rheumatoid arthritis. Clin Exp Rheumatol 2012; 30(2):228–32.

38. Toms TE, Panoulas VF, Douglas KM, et al. Statin use in rheumatoid arthritis in relation to actual

cardiovascular risk: evidence for substantial under-treatment of lipid-associated cardiovascular risk? Ann Rheum Dis 2010;69(4):683–8.

39. Panoulas VF, Douglas KM, Milionis HJ, et al. Prevalence and associations of hypertension and its control in patients with rheumatoid arthritis. Rheumatology (Oxford) 2007;46(9):1477–82.

40. van Halm VP, Peters MJ, Voskuyl AE, et al. Rheumatoid arthritis versus diabetes as a risk factor for cardiovascular disease: a cross-sectional study, the CARRE Investigation. Ann Rheum Dis 2009; 68(9):1395–400.

41. Peters MJ, van Halm VP, Voskuyl AE, et al. Does rheumatoid arthritis equal diabetes mellitus as an independent risk factor for cardiovascular disease? A prospective study. Arthritis Rheum 2009; 61(11):1571–9.

42. Peters MJ, Symmons DP, McCarey D, et al. EULAR evidence-based recommendations for cardiovascular risk management in patients with rheumatoid arthritis and other forms of inflammatory arthritis. Ann Rheum Dis 2010;69(2):325–31.

43. Solomon DH, Peters MJ, Nurmohamed MT, et al. Unresolved questions in rheumatology: motion for debate: the data support evidence-based management recommendations for cardiovascular disease in rheumatoid arthritis. Arthritis Rheum 2013; 65(7):1675–83.

44. Van Doornum S, Brand C, King B, et al. Increased case fatality rates following a first acute cardiovascular event in patients with rheumatoid arthritis. Arthritis Rheum 2006;54(7):2061–8.

45. Sodergren A, Stegmayr B, Lundberg V, et al. Increased incidence of and impaired prognosis after acute myocardial infarction among patients with seropositive rheumatoid arthritis. Ann Rheum Dis 2007;66(2):263–6.

46. McCoy SS, Crowson CS, Maradit-Kremers H, et al. Long-term outcomes and treatment after myocardial infarction in patients with rheumatoid arthritis. J Rheumatol 2013;40(5):605–10.

47. Van Doornum S, Brand C, Sundararajan V, et al. Rheumatoid arthritis patients receive less frequent acute reperfusion and secondary prevention therapy after myocardial infarction compared with the general population. Arthritis Res Ther 2010;12(5): R183.

48. Francis ML, Varghese JJ, Mathew JM, et al. Outcomes in patients with rheumatoid arthritis and myocardial infarction. Am J Med 2010;123(10): 922–8.

49. Monaco C, Terrando N, Midwood KS. Toll-like receptor signaling: common pathways that drive cardiovascular disease and rheumatoid arthritis. Arthritis Care Res (Hoboken) 2011;63(4):500–11.

50. Bjorkbacka H, Lavant EH, Fredrikson GN, et al. Weak associations between human leucocyte antigen genotype and acute myocardial infarction. J Intern Med 2010;268(1):50–8.

51. Palikhe A, Sinisalo J, Seppanen M, et al. Human MHC region harbors both susceptibility and protective haplotypes for coronary artery disease. Tissue Antigens 2007;69(1):47–55.

52. Paakkanen R, Lokki ML, Seppanen M, et al. Proinflammatory HLA-DRB1*01-haplotype predisposes to ST-elevation myocardial infarction. Atherosclerosis 2012;221(2):461–6.

53. Martens PB, Goronzy JJ, Schaid D, et al. Expansion of unusual CD4+ T cells in severe rheumatoid arthritis. Arthritis Rheum 1997;40(6):1106–14.

54. Gerli R, Schillaci G, Giordano A, et al. CD4+CD28- T lymphocytes contribute to early atherosclerotic damage in rheumatoid arthritis patients. Circulation 2004;109(22):2744–8.

55. Nakajima T, Schulte S, Warrington KJ, et al. T-cell-mediated lysis of endothelial cells in acute coronary syndromes. Circulation 2002;105(5):570–5.

56. Masiha S, Sundstrom J, Lind L. Inflammatory markers are associated with left ventricular hypertrophy and diastolic dysfunction in a population-based sample of elderly men and women. J Hum Hypertens 2013;27(1):13–7.

57. Cesari M, Penninx BW, Newman AB, et al. Inflammatory markers and onset of cardiovascular events: results from the Health ABC study. Circulation 2003;108(19):2317–22.

58. Vasan RS, Sullivan LM, Roubenoff R, et al. Inflammatory markers and risk of heart failure in elderly subjects without prior myocardial infarction: the Framingham Heart Study. Circulation 2003; 107(11):1486–91.

59. Deswal A, Petersen NJ, Feldman AM, et al. Cytokines and cytokine receptors in advanced heart failure: an analysis of the cytokine database from the Vesnarinone trial (VEST). Circulation 2001; 103(16):2055–9.

60. Liang KP, Myasoedova E, Crowson CS, et al. Increased prevalence of diastolic dysfunction in rheumatoid arthritis. Ann Rheum Dis 2010;69(9): 1665–70.

61. Maradit-Kremers H, Nicola PJ, Crowson CS, et al. Cardiovascular death in rheumatoid arthritis: a population-based study. Arthritis Rheum 2005; 52(3):722–32.

62. Maradit-Kremers H, Nicola PJ, Crowson CS, et al. Raised erythrocyte sedimentation rate signals heart failure in patients with rheumatoid arthritis. Ann Rheum Dis 2007;66(1):76–80.

63. Rudominer RL, Roman MJ, Devereux RB, et al. Independent association of rheumatoid arthritis with increased left ventricular mass but not with reduced ejection fraction. Arthritis Rheum 2009;60(1):22–9.

64. Bluemke DA, Kronmal RA, Lima JA, et al. The relationship of left ventricular mass and geometry to

incident cardiovascular events: the MESA (Multi-Ethnic Study of Atherosclerosis) study. J Am Coll Cardiol 2008;52(25):2148–55.

65. Myasoedova E, Davis JM 3rd, Crowson CS, et al. Brief report: rheumatoid arthritis is associated with left ventricular concentric remodeling: results of a population-based cross-sectional study. Arthritis Rheum 2013;65(7):1713–8.

66. Amundsen BH, Helle-Valle T, Edvardsen T, et al. Noninvasive myocardial strain measurement by speckle tracking echocardiography: validation against sonomicrometry and tagged magnetic resonance imaging. J Am Coll Cardiol 2006;47(4): 789–93.

67. Sitia S, Tomasoni L, Cicala S, et al. Detection of preclinical impairment of myocardial function in rheumatoid arthritis patients with short disease duration by speckle tracking echocardiography. Int J Cardiol 2012;160(1):8–14.

68. Fine N, Crowson CS, Lin G. Evaluation of myocardial function in patients with rheumatoid arthritis using strain imaging by speckle-tracking echocardiography. Ann Rheum Dis 2013. [Epub ahead of print].

69. Tomasson G, Aspelund T, Jonsson T, et al. Effect of rheumatoid factor on mortality and coronary heart disease. Ann Rheum Dis 2010;69(9):1649–54.

70. Liang KP, Kremers HM, Crowson CS, et al. Autoantibodies and the risk of cardiovascular events. J Rheumatol 2009;36(11):2462–9.

71. Kerola AM, Kauppi MJ, Kerola T, et al. How early in the course of rheumatoid arthritis does the excess cardiovascular risk appear? Ann Rheum Dis 2012; 71(10):1606–15.

72. Holmqvist ME, Wedren S, Jacobsson LT, et al. No increased occurrence of ischemic heart disease prior to the onset of rheumatoid arthritis: results from two Swedish population-based rheumatoid arthritis cohorts. Arthritis Rheum 2009;60(10): 2861–9.

73. Holmqvist ME, Wedren S, Jacobsson LT, et al. Rapid increase in myocardial infarction risk following diagnosis of rheumatoid arthritis amongst patients diagnosed between 1995 and 2006. J Intern Med 2010;268(6):578–85.

74. Yavasoglu I, Senturk T, Onbasili A. Diastolic dysfunction in rheumatoid arthritis and duration of disease. Rheumatol Int 2008;29(1):113–4.

75. Levendoglu F, Temizhan A, Ugurlu H, et al. Ventricular function abnormalities in active rheumatoid arthritis: a Doppler echocardiographic study. Rheumatol Int 2004;24(3):141–6.

76. Maisel AS, Koon J, Krishnaswamy P, et al. Utility of B-natriuretic peptide as a rapid, point-of-care test for screening patients undergoing echocardiography to determine left ventricular dysfunction. Am Heart J 2001;141(3):367–74.

77. Crowson CS, Myasoedova E, Davis JM 3rd, et al. Use of B-type natriuretic peptide as a screening tool for left ventricular diastolic dysfunction in rheumatoid arthritis patients without clinical cardiovascular disease. Arthritis Care Res (Hoboken) 2011; 63(5):729–34.

78. Provan SA, Angel K, Odegard S, et al. The association between disease activity and NT-proBNP in 238 patients with rheumatoid arthritis: a 10-year longitudinal study. Arthritis Res Ther 2008;10(3): R70.

79. Crowson CS, Matteson EL, Roger VL, et al. Usefulness of risk scores to estimate the risk of cardiovascular disease in patients with rheumatoid arthritis. Am J Cardiol 2012;110(3):420–4.

80. Souverein PC, Berard A, Van Staa TP, et al. Use of oral glucocorticoids and risk of cardiovascular and cerebrovascular disease in a population based case-control study. Heart 2004;90(8):859–65.

81. Wei L, MacDonald TM, Walker BR. Taking glucocorticoids by prescription is associated with subsequent cardiovascular disease. Ann Intern Med 2004;141(10):764–70.

82. Davis JM 3rd, Maradit Kremers H, Crowson CS, et al. Glucocorticoids and cardiovascular events in rheumatoid arthritis: a population-based cohort study. Arthritis Rheum 2007;56(3):820–30.

83. Crowson CS, Roger VL, Matteson EL, et al. Hospitalizations following heart failure diagnosis in rheumatoid arthritis. Arthritis Rheum 2010; 62(Suppl 10):67.

84. Antman EM, Bennett JS, Daugherty A, et al. Use of nonsteroidal antiinflammatory drugs: an update for clinicians: a scientific statement from the American Heart Association. Circulation 2007;115(12): 1634–42.

85. Aw TJ, Haas SJ, Liew D, et al. Meta-analysis of cyclooxygenase-2 inhibitors and their effects on blood pressure. Arch Intern Med 2005;165(5): 490–6.

86. Bernatsky S, Hudson M, Suissa S. Anti-rheumatic drug use and risk of hospitalization for congestive heart failure in rheumatoid arthritis. Rheumatology (Oxford) 2005;44(5):677–80.

87. Choi HK, Hernan MA, Seeger JD, et al. Methotrexate and mortality in patients with rheumatoid arthritis: a prospective study. Lancet 2002; 359(9313):1173–7.

88. Westlake SL, Colebatch AN, Baird J, et al. The effect of methotrexate on cardiovascular disease in patients with rheumatoid arthritis: a systematic literature review. Rheumatology (Oxford) 2010;49(2): 295–307.

89. Micha R, Imamura F, Wyler von Ballmoos M, et al. Systematic review and meta-analysis of methotrexate use and risk of cardiovascular disease. Am J Cardiol 2011;108(9):1362–70.

90. Suissa S, Bernatsky S, Hudson M. Antirheumatic drug use and the risk of acute myocardial infarction. Arthritis Rheum 2006;55(4):531–6.

91. Naranjo A, Sokka T, Descalzo MA, et al. Cardiovascular disease in patients with rheumatoid arthritis: results from the QUEST-RA study. Arthritis Res Ther 2008;10(2):R30.

92. Anker SD, Coats AJ. How to RECOVER from RENAISSANCE? The significance of the results of RECOVER, RENAISSANCE, RENEWAL and ATTACH. Int J Cardiol 2002;86(2–3):123–30.

93. Mann DL, McMurray JJ, Packer M, et al. Targeted anticytokine therapy in patients with chronic heart failure: results of the Randomized Etanercept Worldwide Evaluation (RENEWAL). Circulation 2004;109(13):1594–602.

94. Coletta AP, Clark AL, Banarjee P, et al. Clinical trials update: RENEWAL (RENAISSANCE and RECOVER) and ATTACH. Eur J Heart Fail 2002; 4(4):559–61.

95. Chung ES, Packer M, Lo KH, et al. Randomized, double-blind, placebo-controlled, pilot trial of infliximab, a chimeric monoclonal antibody to tumor necrosis factor-alpha, in patients with moderate-to-severe heart failure: results of the anti-TNF Therapy Against Congestive Heart Failure (ATTACH) trial. Circulation 2003;107(25):3133–40.

96. Listing J, Strangfeld A, Kekow J, et al. Does tumor necrosis factor alpha inhibition promote or prevent heart failure in patients with rheumatoid arthritis? Arthritis Rheum 2008;58(3):667–77.

97. Gabriel SE. Tumor necrosis factor inhibition: a part of the solution or a part of the problem of heart failure in rheumatoid arthritis? Arthritis Rheum 2008; 58(3):637–40.

98. Singh JA, Furst DE, Bharat A, et al. 2012 update of the 2008 American College of Rheumatology recommendations for the use of disease-modifying antirheumatic drugs and biologic agents in the treatment of rheumatoid arthritis. Arthritis Care Res (Hoboken) 2012;64(5):625–39.

99. Bulkley BH, Roberts WC. The heart in systemic lupus erythematosus and the changes induced in it by corticosteroid therapy. A study of 36 necropsy patients. Am J Med 1975;58(2): 243–64.

100. Haider YS, Roberts WC. Coronary arterial disease in systemic lupus erythematosus; quantification of degrees of narrowing in 22 necropsy patients (21 women) aged 16 to 37 years. Am J Med 1981; 70(4):775–81.

101. Hak AE, Karlson EW, Feskanich D, et al. Systemic lupus erythematosus and the risk of cardiovascular disease: results from the nurses' health study. Arthritis Rheum 2009;61(10):1396–402.

102. Jonsson H, Nived O, Sturfelt G. Outcome in systemic lupus erythematosus: a prospective study of patients from a defined population. Medicine (Baltimore) 1989;68(3):141–50.

103. Asanuma Y, Oeser A, Shintani AK, et al. Premature coronary-artery atherosclerosis in systemic lupus erythematosus. N Engl J Med 2003;349(25): 2407–15.

104. Roman MJ, Shanker BA, Davis A, et al. Prevalence and correlates of accelerated atherosclerosis in systemic lupus erythematosus. N Engl J Med 2003;349(25):2399–406.

105. Manzi S, Meilahn EN, Rairie JE, et al. Age-specific incidence rates of myocardial infarction and angina in women with systemic lupus erythematosus: comparison with the Framingham Study. Am J Epidemiol 1997;145(5):408–15.

106. Pons-Estel GJ, Gonzalez LA, Zhang J, et al. Predictors of cardiovascular damage in patients with systemic lupus erythematosus: data from LUMINA (LXVIII), a multiethnic US cohort. Rheumatology (Oxford) 2009;48(7):817–22.

107. Knight JS, Kaplan MJ. Cardiovascular disease in lupus: insights and updates. Curr Opin Rheumatol 2013;25:597–605.

108. Thacker SG, Zhao W, Smith CK, et al. Type I interferons modulate vascular function, repair, thrombosis, and plaque progression in murine models of lupus and atherosclerosis. Arthritis Rheum 2012;64(9):2975–85.

109. Ward MM. Premature morbidity from cardiovascular and cerebrovascular diseases in women with systemic lupus erythematosus. Arthritis Rheum 1999;42(2):338–46.

110. Buss SJ, Wolf D, Korosoglou G, et al. Myocardial left ventricular dysfunction in patients with systemic lupus erythematosus: new insights from tissue Doppler and strain imaging. J Rheumatol 2010; 37(1):79–86.

111. Pieretti J, Roman MJ, Devereux RB, et al. Systemic lupus erythematosus predicts increased left ventricular mass. Circulation 2007;116(4):419–26.

112. Bruce IN, Urowitz MB, Gladman DD, et al. Risk factors for coronary heart disease in women with systemic lupus erythematosus: the Toronto Risk Factor Study. Arthritis Rheum 2003;48(11): 3159–67.

113. Petri M, Spence D, Bone LR, et al. Coronary artery disease risk factors in the Johns Hopkins Lupus Cohort: prevalence, recognition by patients, and preventive practices. Medicine (Baltimore) 1992; 71(5):291–302.

114. Rahman P, Urowitz MB, Gladman DD, et al. Contribution of traditional risk factors to coronary artery disease in patients with systemic lupus erythematosus. J Rheumatol 1999;26(11):2363–8.

115. Bruce IN, Gladman DD, Urowitz MB. Premature atherosclerosis in systemic lupus erythematosus. Rheum Dis Clin North Am 2000;26(2):257–78.

116. Esdaile JM, Abrahamowicz M, Grodzicky T, et al. Traditional Framingham risk factors fail to fully account for accelerated atherosclerosis in systemic lupus erythematosus. Arthritis Rheum 2001; 44(10):2331–7.

117. Frostegard J. Rheumatic diseases: insights into inflammation and atherosclerosis. Arterioscler Thromb Vasc Biol 2010;30(5):892–3.

118. Bremander A, Petersson IF, Bergman S, et al. Population-based estimates of common comorbidities and cardiovascular disease in ankylosing spondylitis. Arthritis Care Res (Hoboken) 2011; 63(4):550–6.

119. Szabo SM, Levy AR, Rao SR, et al. Increased risk of cardiovascular and cerebrovascular diseases in individuals with ankylosing spondylitis: a population-based study. Arthritis Rheum 2011; 63(11):3294–304.

120. McCarey D, Sturrock RD. Comparison of cardiovascular risk in ankylosing spondylitis and rheumatoid arthritis. Clin Exp Rheumatol 2009;27(4 Suppl 55):S124–6.

121. Han C, Robinson DW Jr, Hackett MV, et al. Cardiovascular disease and risk factors in patients with rheumatoid arthritis, psoriatic arthritis, and ankylosing spondylitis. J Rheumatol 2006;33(11):2167–72.

122. Prodanovich S, Kirsner RS, Kravetz JD, et al. Association of psoriasis with coronary artery, cerebrovascular, and peripheral vascular diseases and mortality. Arch Dermatol 2009;145(6):700–3.

123. Kaye JA, Li L, Jick SS. Incidence of risk factors for myocardial infarction and other vascular diseases in patients with psoriasis. Br J Dermatol 2008; 159(4):895–902.

124. Gelfand JM, Neimann AL, Shin DB, et al. Risk of myocardial infarction in patients with psoriasis. JAMA 2006;296(14):1735–41.

125. Tobin AM, Veale DJ, Fitzgerald O, et al. Cardiovascular disease and risk factors in patients with psoriasis and psoriatic arthritis. J Rheumatol 2010; 37(7):1386–94.

126. Kimhi O, Caspi D, Bornstein NM, et al. Prevalence and risk factors of atherosclerosis in patients with psoriatic arthritis. Semin Arthritis Rheum 2007; 36(4):203–9.

127. Jamnitski A, Symmons D, Peters MJ, et al. Cardiovascular comorbidities in patients with psoriatic arthritis: a systematic review. Ann Rheum Dis 2013;72(2):211–6.

128. Gladman DD, Ang M, Su L, et al. Cardiovascular morbidity in psoriatic arthritis. Ann Rheum Dis 2009;68(7):1131–5.

The Role of Coronary Artery Disease in Heart Failure

Anuradha Lala, MD[a,b], Akshay S. Desai, MD, MPH[a,*]

KEYWORDS

• Coronary artery disease • Heart failure • Myocardial infarction • Coronary revascularization

KEY POINTS

• Coronary disease is the most common cause of heart failure (HF) and an important therapeutic target for improving HF-associated morbidity and mortality.

• The role of coronary revascularization in improving heart failure associated morbidity and mortality remains controversial.

• Recent data suggests that for many patients with coronary artery disease (CAD), HF, and reduced ejection fraction without angina, medical therapy may be equivalent to surgical revascularization as an initial management strategy.

• Patients with significant CAD and HF who are at a high risk for conventional surgical revascularization may be candidates for advanced therapies including mechanical circulatory support.

• The optimal strategy for revascularization in patients with HF with severe CAD who are surgical candidates continues to require careful consideration of the specific balance of risks and benefits for individual patients as well as incorporation of patient preferences.

INTRODUCTION

Enhanced survival following acute myocardial infarction (MI) and the declining prevalence of hypertension and valvular heart disease as contributors to incident heart failure (HF) have fueled the emergence of coronary artery disease (CAD) as the primary risk factor for HF development.[1] Nearly two-thirds of HF cases are attributed to underlying CAD.[2] Because myocardial ischemia may in some cases represent a treatable cause of HF, current HF guidelines[3] recommend invasive or noninvasive assessment for CAD in all newly diagnosed cases among patients at risk. Despite the acknowledged role of CAD in the development of HF, however, the role of coronary revascularization in reducing HF-associated morbidity and mortality remains controversial. In the discussion that follows, the authors review key features of the epidemiology and pathophysiology of CAD in patients with HF as well as the emerging data from recent clinical trials that inform the modern approach to management.

EPIDEMIOLOGY/PROGNOSIS OF CAD IN HF

• CAD is the most common cause of HF in developed countries.
• The incidence of HF after MI is significant and is associated with poor outcomes.
• CAD is common in both HF with reduced ejection fraction (EF) (HFREF) and HF with preserved EF (HFPEF).

Americans older than 40 years face a 20% lifetime risk of developing HF, with more than 650 000 new HF cases diagnosed in the United States

[a] Division of Cardiology, Department of Medicine, Brigham and Women's Hospital, Harvard Medical School, 75 Francis Street, Boston, MA 02115, USA; [b] Division of Cardiology, Department of Medicine, New York University School of Medicine, New York, NY, USA
* Corresponding author.
E-mail address: ADESAI@PARTNERS.ORG

Heart Failure Clin 10 (2014) 353–365
http://dx.doi.org/10.1016/j.hfc.2013.10.002
1551-7136/14/$ – see front matter © 2014 Elsevier Inc. All rights reserved.

annually.[3,4] HF is the most common cause of hospitalization in the elderly, with projected related annual health care costs exceeding $40 billion. Given the secular trends in the aging of the population that threaten a growing HF burden, HF prevention and management are a major public health concern.[5]

Although data from the Framingham Heart Study have historically identified hypertension as the primary cause of HF,[1] more recent data suggest that CAD and its complications are the dominant risk factors, particularly in developed countries. In a recent systematic literature review of HF epidemiology, ischemic heart disease was a factor for HF in more than 50% of incident cases in North America and Europe; 30% to 40% in Asia, Latin America, and the Caribbean; and less than 10% in sub-Saharan Africa.[6]

MI is the primary clinical intermediate between CAD and HF. The incidence of HF after MI depends on a variety of factors, including the size and location of the infarct, the severity of CAD, and the development of ischemic mitral regurgitation (MR). Of nearly 8000 patients in the Framingham Heart Study without a prior history of MI or congestive heart failure (CHF), 27% of patients died or had an incident MI before the development of CHF compared with 5% of patients who developed CHF without an antecedent MI during the follow-up of 118,000 person-years.[1] In another community-based study of 1915 higher-risk patients in Olmstead County with prior MI and no HF, 41% developed new-onset HF over a 7-year follow-up. Of these, 44% had reduced EF (<50%), 18% preserved (EF ≥50%), and 38% had no EF assessment within 60 days of the HF diagnosis.[7]

Once the diagnosis of HF is established, the presence of CAD also portends a poor prognosis.[2] Patients with previous MI at enrollment in the Survival and Ventricular Enlargement (SAVE) trial had an approximately 70% increased risk of cardiovascular death and/or left ventricular (LV) enlargement compared with those without prior MI.[8] Among 1000 patients hospitalized for acute MI studied by Suleiman and colleagues,[9] 112 patients (10.7%) were readmitted for HF at a median follow-up of 23 months. These patients who developed HF after MI were more likely to suffer recurrent infarction (15.2% vs 6.0%) and death (27.7% vs 8.8%) during the follow-up compared with those without HF. Patients who develop MR following MI may be at a particularly high risk for HF. Among 770 patients after an MI, 50% of whom had MR on echocardiography within 30 days after the infarct, the presence of moderate or severe MR was associated with a more than 3-fold increase in the risk of HF (hazard ratio [HR] 3.44, 95% confidence interval [CI] 1.74–6.82) and death (relative risk [RR] 1.55, 95% CI 1.08–2.22).[10]

Most epidemiologic studies examining incident HF do not differentiate between HFREF and HFPEF.[5,11] CAD is implicated in both clinical syndromes and may contribute to both systolic and diastolic ventricular dysfunction. Because in many cohorts a similar proportion of patients with reduced and preserved EF have CAD,[12] the diagnosis and management of CAD may have relevance for clinical HF management independent of EF.

DIAGNOSIS OF CAD IN HF

- CAD in HF may be present without a history of angina.
- CAD may be detected by coronary angiography or noninvasive imaging.
- Angiographic findings of CAD must be interpreted within the clinical context of patients and may not be the sole contributor to LV dysfunction.

Given the high prevalence of CAD, all patients with HF should undergo a complete history and physical examination to assess for atherosclerosis risk factors and symptoms of ischemia or infarction. However, CAD may not always be clinically apparent because typical anginal symptoms are frequently absent in those presenting with new-onset HF.[13] In the seminal Johns Hopkins study of 1230 patients with initially unexplained cardiomyopathy, CAD was identified in 7% of cases by coronary angiography.[14] Because the presence of CAD may have important implications for treatment, the Heart Failure Society of America's guidelines[15] recommend invasive or noninvasive testing in all patients at a high risk for CAD to assess for ischemia and or severity of CAD.

Coronary Angiography

CAD may be detected via coronary angiography when ischemia is suspected and coronary anatomy is unknown or when angina is not present with a known history of CAD, as indicated by the 2013 guidelines from the American College of Cardiology (ACC)/American Heart Association (AHA) on the management of HF (class IIa recommendation, level of evidence [LOE] C).[3] In accordance with the guidelines for revascularization,[16] coronary angiography should only be performed in those patients in whom revascularization is a potentially feasible option.

Noninvasive Imaging

It is reasonable to perform noninvasive stress testing (either exercise or pharmacologic) often with imaging to detect myocardial ischemia and viability in patients with de novo HF and known coronary disease with no angina (class IIa, LOE C).[3] Current guidelines also mention the utility of magnetic resonance imaging to assess for the burden of scar as measured by the presence of late gadolinium enhancement or infiltrative processes. Although multidetector row or electron beam computed tomography (CT) for the detection of calcium/calcification[17] and cardiac magnetic resonance angiography[18] have been used to diagnose CAD, scintigraphic and echocardiographic modalities have typically been the ischemia tests most routinely used.[19] Improvements in temporal and spatial resolution have allowed cardiac CT angiography (CTA) to become an attractive alternative as a noninvasive means for visualizing coronary anatomy. In general for those patients at low to intermediate risk, noninvasive assessment for CAD using either CTA or stress testing is an acceptable initial diagnostic strategy. In higher-risk patients (with symptoms of angina, history of sudden cardiac death [SCD], or multiple risk factors), however, invasive coronary angiography should be considered for the evaluation of possible revascularization.[20]

The term *ischemic cardiomyopathy*, which is often used to describe impaired LV function (LVEF ≤40%) caused by coronary disease, is defined as one of the following[21]:

- History of MI or revascularization, either percutaneous coronary intervention (PCI) or coronary artery bypass grafting (CABG) surgery
- ≥75% stenosis of the left main coronary artery or proximal left anterior descending (LAD) artery
- ≥75% stenosis of 2 or more epicardial vessels

The demonstration of CAD on an angiogram must be interpreted within the clinical context of the patients' history and supporting data. The presence of asymptomatic coronary artery atherosclerosis in the setting of reduced EF does not imply a causal relationship unless there is evidence of prior myocardial injury. An analysis of more than 1900 patients seeking to standardize the definition of ischemic cardiomyopathy suggested that those patients with single-vessel coronary disease (other than left main or LAD) and no history of MI or revascularization be characterized as nonischemic, acknowledging that CAD may be present in patients with HF from other causes.[21]

CONTRIBUTIONS OF CAD TO THE PATHOGENESIS OF HF

- MI leads to a series of changes in infarcted and noninfarcted tissue, encompassed in the term *LV remodeling*.
- The progression of HF is related to the degree of LV remodeling.
- Chronic ischemia leads to LV dysfunction.
- The degree of MR as a consequence of ischemia is directly related to survival in HF.
- Patients with CAD and LV dysfunction are at risk for SCD.

LV Remodeling and Systolic Dysfunction

Following MI, there is a sudden change in loading conditions caused by the acute myocardial injury that initiates a cascade of neurohormonal activation and pathologic changes, including myocyte hypertrophy and myocardial fibrosis, in the infarcted tissue and the surrounding noninfarcted myocardium. Progressive ventricular remodeling as a result of these changes results in cavity dilation, MR, and systolic dysfunction that provide the substrate for HF development.[22] The scope of these changes is determined by the size and extent of the infarct, the degree of stunned myocardium, and the severity of local inflammation.[23] Although timely restoration of blood flow in the infarct-related artery by thrombolysis or PCI has produced remarkable reductions in mortality rates after MI, ventricular remodeling may still ensue, particularly in patients who present late after the symptom onset to clinical attention.[24]

Myocardial Stunning and Hibernation

HF and ventricular remodeling may also develop in the absence of extensive MI. In some cases, chronic hypoperfusion related to significant flow-limiting CAD leads to decreased oxygen delivery and sympathetic nervous system activation. In particular, the surge of catecholamines in this context may impact the function of still-viable myocytes and impair contractility in both the acute and chronic setting.

Viable myocardium refers to myocardium that is not irreversibly scarred or damaged and is often used interchangeably with the terms *stunned myocardium* and *hibernating myocardium*. Stunned myocardium is myocardium with impaired contractility as a result of acute ischemia followed by spontaneous restoration of perfusion. The impaired contractility may persist for hours or days but returns to normal if perfusion is maintained. Hibernating myocardium refers to viable but noncontractile myocardium in the setting of chronic ischemia, for which function may be restored by revascularization or medical therapy.[25,26] The recognition of viable myocardium and the differentiation from scar or irreversibly damaged myocardium may be clinically important because it suggests the potential for partial recovery of ventricular function with the restoration of blood flow through coronary revascularization.[27]

Ischemic MR

Myocardial ischemia can also contribute to transient papillary muscle dysfunction resulting in acute, transient MR abrupt (flash) pulmonary edema.[28,29] In the extreme, MI may result in papillary muscle rupture and refractory HF that requires emergent surgical intervention.[30] More commonly, ischemic MR refers to chronic MR, which develops as a consequence of progressive ventricular remodeling following MI (particularly of the inferoposterior wall). In this case, leaflet tethering caused by distortion of the papillary muscle architecture results in incomplete coaptation and eccentric MR. The severity of MR in this context is closely correlated with the risk for subsequent HF and mortality.[10]

Sudden Cardiac Death

Patients with CAD and MI complicated by LV dysfunction are at a high risk for sudden death, particularly in the early post-MI period.[31] The mechanism of sudden death is frequently related to recurrent myocardial injury or to the abrupt onset of ventricular arrhythmias. Ongoing myocardial ischemia may provoke ventricular fibrillation or polymorphic ventricular tachycardia, whereas scarred myocardium may provide a substrate for reentry and sustained ventricular tachycardia.[32]

TREATMENT OF CAD AND HF
CAD and HFPEF

CAD is an important contributor to HF, independent of EF. Patients with HFPEF comprise a heterogeneous group in which few evidence-based treatments are available. It is thought that the dominant pathophysiology is related to abnormal diastolic function as a consequence of increased passive stiffness and impaired myocardial relaxation.[33,34] Myocardial ischemia is an important contributor to diastolic dysfunction and functional limitation in patients with HFPEF and may be an important reversible cause of HF in this context.[35] The current treatment guidelines recommend consideration of coronary revascularization in patients with HFPEF and significant CAD, particularly those with anginal symptoms.[3,36] Attention to risk factor management is important in stalling CAD progression, though few specific medical treatments have shown a benefit in reducing morbidity and mortality in this population.[37–40]

CAD and HFREF

In contrast to HFPEF, there is a substantial evidence base for guiding the management of patients with ventricular dysfunction and HF complicating MI. Several landmark, prospective, randomized clinical trials have informed the design of strategies for optimal pharmacologic and device therapy in this population (**Table 1**). Although a detailed discussion of the rationale for each is beyond the scope of this review, the elements of effective therapy include the following:

- Angiotensin-converting enzyme inhibitors (ACEI) are appropriate to consider in most hemodynamically stable patients post-MI with an LVEF of 40% or less. These drugs are effective inhibitors of the renin-angiotensin-aldosterone axis and reduce the incidence of HF and mortality after MI by preventing LV remodeling, reinfarction, and SCD. Because benefits seem to be dose dependent, doses should be titrated to the targets established by clinical trials or the maximum tolerated dose.
- Angiotensin receptor blockers (ARBs) are suitable substitutes for ACEI when ACEI are not tolerated (most commonly caused by cough) both after MI and in chronic HF to reduce HF morbidity and mortality.
- Beta-blockers improve mortality across the spectrum of HF with reduced EF, including those with HF after MI by reducing hospitalizations, sudden death, and recurrent MI. In contrast to ACEI and ARBs, drugs within this class vary in efficacy, with a proven benefit only for bisoprolol, carvedilol, and metoprolol succinate.
- Aldosterone antagonists improve mortality after MI as well as in the chronic HF setting with symptoms on background therapy of beta-blocker and ACEI/ARB therapy, with an estimated glomerular filtration rate greater than 30 mL/min/1.73 m^2 and potassium of 5.0 mEq/L or less. Although the best-studied agent in the post-MI context is eplerenone,[41] data in unselected patients with advanced HF suggest that spironolactone is likely to be equivalent if administered at the appropriate dose. Treatment with aldosterone antagonists is associated with a high risk for hyperkalemia[42] and should be undertaken only in the context of careful surveillance of potassium and creatinine.

Table 1
Relevant trials of medical therapy for CAD and HF

Trial	Study Setting	Intervention	Follow-up (mo)	Primary End Point	Results
ACEI					
SAVE	3 d after MI, LVEF ≤40% without overt HF	Captopril vs placebo	42	ACM	20.0% in captopril group and 20.1% in placebo group (RR 0.79 [0.65–0.95] P = .014)
TRACE	3–7 d after MI, LVEF ≤35% after MI	Trandolapril vs placebo	24	ACM	35% in trandolapril group vs 42% in placebo (P = .001)
AIRE	3–10 d after MI with HF, LVEF not obtained in all pts	Ramipril vs placebo	15	ACM	17% in ramipril group vs 23% in placebo (HR 0.73, 0.60–0.89) P = .002
Angiotensin Receptor Blockers					
OPTIMAAL	Up to 10 d after MI with HF, or LVEF ≤35%	Losartan vs captopril	30	ACM	18% in losartan group vs 16% in captopril group (RR 1.13 [0.99–1.28] P = .07) but did not meet criteria for noninferiority
VALIANT	Up to 10 d after MI, with HF or LVEF ≤35%	Valsartan vs captopril	25	ACM	20% in valsartan group vs 20% in captopril group. (HR 1.0 [0.90–1.09] P = .73)
Beta-Blockers					
CAPRICORN	3–21 d after MI, LVEF <40%	Carvedilol vs placebo (on background of ACEI)	16	ACM	12% in carvedilol group vs 15% in placebo group (HR 0.77 [0.6–0.98] P = .03)
Aldosterone Antagonists					
EPHESUS	3–14 d after MI, LVEF <40% + HF sign or symptoms	Eplerenone vs placebo	16	ACM	14% in eplerenone group vs 17% in placebo group (RR 0.85 [0.75–0.96] P = .008)
HMG-CoA Reductase Inhibitors (Statins)					
CORONA	NYHA class II–IV, LVEF <40%, >6 mo after MI	Rosuvastatin vs placebo	33	Composite of CV death, nonfatal MI, nonfatal stroke	11 in rosuvastatin group vs 12 in placebo group per 100 patient-years (HR 0.92 [0.83–1.02] P = .12)
GISSI-HF	NYHA class II–IV, chronic HF, no EF criteria	Rosuvastatin vs placebo	47	1. ACM 2. ACM or CV hospitalization	1. 29% in rosuvastatin group vs 28% in placebo group (HR 1.00 [0.90–1.12] P = .943) 2. 57% in rosuvastatin group and 56% in placebo group (HR 1.01 (0.91–1.11])

Abbreviations: ACEI, angiotensin-converting enzyme inhibitors; ACM, all-cause mortality; AIRE, Acute Infarction Ramipril Efficacy; CV, cardiovascular; HMG-CoA, 3-hydroxy-3-meth-ylglutaryl-coenzyme A; NYHA, New York Heart Association; pts, patients; TRACE, Trandolapril Cardiac Evaluation.
Data from Refs.[8,31,41,43–48]

The 3-hydroxy-3-methylglutaryl-coenzyme A reductase inhibitors (statins) are effective in reducing the incidence of MI and cardiovascular death in a broad range of primary and secondary prevention contexts. In high-risk patients with HF and CAD, however, the incremental benefits of statin therapy have been difficult to demonstrate.[47,48] Accordingly, statin therapy is not recommended for the sole purpose of improving HF-related outcomes.[3]

Antiplatelet therapy with aspirin is often used for secondary prevention in patients after MI with HF with no specific recommendations made with regard to independently improving HF-related outcomes.[49] Anticoagulation is only recommended in HFREF in the presence of atrial fibrillation and one additional risk factor and/or a prior thromboembolic event.[3,50]

Although calcium channel blockers have antiischemic properties, studies of nifedipine and diltiazem suggested increased mortality with the use of these agents in the HF population.[51] Amlodipine was studied in the Prospective Randomized Amlodipine Survival Evaluation trial, which revealed a neutral effect in patients with CAD with respect to HF or cardiovascular hospitalizations.[52] Given the lack of apparent benefit and their negative inotropic effects, the use of these agents in patients with HF should be reserved for the management of refractory anginal symptoms despite maximal treatment with beta-blockers and other evidence-based therapies.

Device Therapy

Because of the high risk of sudden death in patients with HF or LV dysfunction following MI, there has been considerable interest in the use of defibrillator therapy in this population. The optimal timing of implantable cardioverter-defibrillator (ICD) implantation following acute MI remains controversial because trials of implantation in the early post-MI period have been associated with no net benefit.[53] Current guidelines[3,54] recommend implantation of an ICD for the primary prevention of SCD in patients with ischemic cardiomyopathy and an LVEF of 35% or less with New York Heart Association (NYHA) class II or greater symptoms or an LVEF of 30% or less with NYHA class I or greater symptoms, who are at least 40 days after MI. This class I recommendation is informed by the results of large randomized controlled trials:

- The Multicenter Automatic Defibrillator Implantation Trial (MADIT I) compared ICD implantation with conventional medical therapy in patients with a prior MI, an LVEF of 35%

or less, and inducible ventricular arrhythmias during an electrophysiologic study (EPS). This trial was the first trial to show a mortality benefit with ICDs (16% all-cause mortality) compared with medical therapy alone (39%) in 196 patients (HR 0.46, 95% CI 0.26–0.82).[55]
- MADIT II established that patients with a prior MI and an LVEF of 30% or less and NYHA class I to III symptoms sustained a 31% reduction in the relative risk of death as compared with medical therapy alone. EPS was not required; however, patients had to be 1 month after MI and at least 3 months after revascularization.[56]
- The Defibrillator in Acute MI Trial studied the benefit of ICD implantation early after MI. Patients with an LVEF of 35% or less were enrolled 6 to 40 days after MI with no improvement in the overall mortality in the ICD group because the reduction of arrhythmic events was offset by an increase in nonarrhythmic events.[53]

There does not seem to be a differential rate of SCD in patients with ischemic versus nonischemic cardiomyopathy. Analyses from the Sudden Cardiac Death in Heart Failure Trial[57] demonstrated a similar reduction in ventricular tachyarrhythmias in the ischemic and nonischemic cardiomyopathy groups: HR 0.43, 95% CI 0.27 to 0.67 in the ischemic group and HR 0.34, 95% CI 0.17 to 0.70 in the nonischemic group, with similar trends observed in smaller studies.[58]

Cardiac Resynchronization Therapy

Cardiac resynchronization therapy (CRT) has been shown to be of benefit in patients with an LVEF of 35% or less, in sinus rhythm, who have a left bundle branch block on surface electrocardiogram with a QRS duration of 150 ms or more, and with NYHA class II symptoms or greater on optimal medical therapy (OMT).[3,54] The benefits of CRT include improved survival, 6-minute walk distance, MR, LVEF, LV remodeling, maximum oxygen consumption (Vo_2 max), and reduced ventricular arrhythmias and HF hospitalizations.[59–61] These benefits seem to accrue equally to patients with and without CAD, with no treatment interaction noted by the HF cause in any of the large randomized trials. Although the treatment guidelines do not discriminate between patients with HF with and without CAD, patients with underlying ischemic cardiomyopathy tend to have less improvement of LVEF and less reversal of LV remodeling compared with those with a nonischemic cause.[59] The delivery of effective CRT may also be challenging in patients with CAD because optimal lead placement may be compromised by myocardial scar.[58] Transvenous access through the coronary sinus may occasionally be compromised in patients with prior coronary bypass surgery, necessitating an epicardial approach to LV lead implantation.[62,63]

SELECTION OF PATIENTS FOR REVASCULARIZATION

Early randomized controlled trials of more than 2200 patients established the safety and efficacy of proceeding with CABG for surgical revascularization in patients with HF with chronic stable angina and preserved EF.[64] The largest of these, the Coronary Artery Surgery Study[65] (CASS), randomized 780 patients with stable ischemic heart disease to receive surgical (CABG) or nonsurgical treatment (medical therapy); randomization was stratified based on LVEF (35%–50% vs >50%), extent of CAD on angiography, and the presence or absence of angina, with 10-year follow-up. Of the 390 patients on medical therapy alone, 21% died compared with 18% of 390 patients treated with medical therapy as well as CABG ($P = .25$). In a subgroup analyses, patients with EF between 35% and 50% seemed to derive an incremental benefit from surgical revascularization over medical therapy. Of the 160 patients in this low-EF subgroup, 32 out of 82 (38%) died on medical therapy alone as compared with 16 out of 78 (21%) who underwent CABG ($P = .01$). Of note, the smaller subset of patients (54 out of 78) with systolic dysfunction but no angina did not demonstrate the same benefit ($P = .12$). The results of the primary CASS study do not inform the management of patients with LVEF less than 35%, who were systematically excluded.

Nearly 25,000 patients screened for entry into the CASS trial but not randomized were followed in a registry. Of these, 651 patients had an LVEF less than 35%, with 231 who underwent CABG and 420 medical therapy alone. The overall 5-year survival favored surgical intervention. This finding was attributed to the subset of 254 patients with an LVEF less than 26%, in which the 82 patients who underwent CABG seemed to derive a survival advantage as compared with 172 patients treated medically ($P = .006$).[66] In an observational study from Duke of less than 1400 patients with CAD and an LVEF of less than 40%, the 339 patients who received surgical revascularization with CABG had improved mortality when compared with the 1052 patients who received medical therapy alone, regardless of LVEF or HF symptoms.[67]

The results of these early trials must be interpreted in the light of medical therapy available in that era, which consisted primarily of digoxin and diuretics, both which have since been shown to have a neutral or even adverse effect on mortality.[2] Improvements in medical therapy as well as advances in contemporary cardiac surgical techniques have made it difficult to extrapolate results from the early trials to treatment in the modern era. Nevertheless based on this subset of patients in CASS and other older observational studies, there is a general consensus that patients with HF with angina, severe coronary disease, and an LVEF greater than 35% should be referred for revascularization for improvement in mortality and symptoms.[3,68,69] Although the data are limited, these results are often extrapolated to the population with anginal symptoms and EF less than 35% in whom the presence of angina is frequently used as a clinical surrogate for viability. However, the long-term benefits of this approach, particularly in patients who have already experienced significant ventricular remodeling, remains unclear.

In select patients whereby complete revascularization with PCI is possible, multivessel PCI may be a reasonable alternative to surgery, particularly in those who are thought to be at a high risk for surgical complications.[70] Patients with HF and/or patients with LV dysfunction have been largely underrepresented in studies comparing the efficacy of multivessel PCI with CABG, however, and warrant further study as to the optimal revascularization approach.[71]

The role of revascularization in patients with CAD, reduced LV function, and no anginal symptoms is even less certain. The argument in favor of revascularization in these patients follows on the open artery hypothesis, which suggests that effective and complete restoration of coronary blood will rescue the function of viable but hypoperfused myocardium and retard HF progression and progressive ventricular remodeling.[72] Because the up-front risk with coronary bypass surgery in patients with LV dysfunction is high, the balance of risks and benefits in this population has long been an issue of debate. Mortality can range from 5% to 20%, with morbidity including reinfarction and stroke in the early perioperative period.[26] Therefore, to justify the early risk of surgery, long-term benefits in terms of survival and symptoms must be demonstrated. Recent data from the Occluded Artery Trial[73] and Clinical Outcomes Utilizing Revascularization and Aggressive Drug Evaluation[74] trial have called the open artery hypothesis into question and raised concern about the value of reperfusion in stable, asymptomatic CAD.

To address this uncertainty, the STICH (Surgical Treatment for Ischemic Heart Failure) trial[75] randomized 1212 patients with an EF less than or equal to 35% and coronary disease appropriate for surgical revascularization to OMT alone or OMT and CABG in a nonblinded fashion. Signs and symptoms of HF were not required for enrollment; however, patients with significant left main disease were excluded. Rigorous care was taken to ensure excellent surgical practice; nearly all patients were on ACEI or ARB, beta-blockers, aspirin, and statin therapy. Over a 5-year follow-up using an intention-to-treat analysis, there was no significant difference with regard to the primary end point of all-cause mortality between the 2 groups (41% in the medical therapy group as compared with 36% in the revascularization group [HR 0.86, 0.72–1.04, $P = .12$]). Prespecified secondary end points of cardiovascular death, hospitalizations, and HF hospitalizations seemed to be decreased by the addition of CABG to OMT.

Viability

Several imaging modalities have been used for the detection of viable myocardium. Because of the relative feasibility and widespread availability, thallium or technetium-based nuclear scintigraphy and dobutamine stress echocardiography are more commonly used than positron emission tomography (PET) and/or delayed contrast enhancement on cardiovascular magnetic resonance (CMR) scanning. Several studies suggest that the presence of myocardial viability is associated with improved outcomes[19]; however, the substudy of the STICH trial was the first large prospective study to evaluate the impact of viability testing on revascularization and subsequent outcomes. Viability testing did not seem to predict improved survival with an initial strategy of revascularization. Several potential limitations of this substudy have been pointed out[76]:

- Viability testing was performed at the discretion of the investigators in a nonrandomized fashion, which may have introduced bias, similar to limitations of previous observational studies.
- There were considerable differences in the clinical characteristics of patients in each of the viability groups (CABG vs medical therapy alone) in accordance with a nonrandomized approach.
- Dobutamine echocardiography and single-photon emission CT (SPECT) were used interchangeably even though there are differences in the performance characteristics of each test. SPECT has higher sensitivity while

dobutamine echocardiography has a higher specificity.
- Prior viability studies have reported the ability of SPECT and dobutamine echocardiography to predict reduction in LV systolic volumes and dimensions following revascularization; however, this information was not provided in STICH.
- Newer techniques using CMR and PET imaging may have a higher sensitivity and negative predictive value when compared with SPECT and dobutamine echocardiography.

Although the presence of viable myocardium did not impact the treatment strategy used, those with viable myocardium did experience better overall survival than those without viability.

Clinical Practice

How is the clinician to interpret the results of this well-conducted modern-era randomized controlled trial into clinical practice? Opinions and understanding of the STICH data have varied widely among the medical community. Many have argued that the favorable impact on outcomes, including cardiovascular-related death and hospitalizations, and ventricular remodeling support the routine use of surgical revascularization in patients with low EF and multivessel CAD. The neutral overall results of the STICH trial, however, make it challenging to draw definitive conclusions from these secondary analyses. Moreover, the lack of blinding in STICH may have biased these secondary results in favor of the CABG arm because patients assigned to surgery may have received more intensive follow-up.

How does the STICH population compare with the population encountered in clinical practice? Trial recruitment for STICH was delayed because many investigators had trouble finding a population in which there was sufficient equipoise about the benefits of revascularization to permit randomization in a clinical trial. Accordingly, STICH patients tended to be younger (mean age of 60 years), had more angina (>60%), and less severe symptoms of HF (NYHA class 1–2) than those enrolled in HF trials. Whether a sicker cohort (more LV enlargement and/or severe symptoms of HF) with higher surgical risk would have experienced a similar balance of risks and benefits with surgery and medical treatment remains unclear. For some patients with severe HF and CAD, the risks of conventional surgery may be prohibitive; advanced therapies, such as LV assist devices and/or cardiac transplantation, may be a better option. The STICH trial results are best interpreted in the context of the specific patient population randomized. Accordingly, it is important to recall that those randomized were patients who had the following:

- Suitable anatomy for surgical revascularization and favorable comorbidity profile
- Clinical equipoise on the part of the physician and/or patients about the incremental benefit of surgery as compared with medical therapy alone
- EF less than 35%

Patients did NOT have the following:

- Significant left main disease or equivalent (ostial LAD or circumflex disease)
- Severe or refractory HF symptoms (NYHA class III-IV) or angina (Canadian Cardiovascular Society III angina or greater)
- Significant LV enlargement

Nearly 1 out of 5 patients (17%) in the medical-therapy-alone group crossed over to the added surgical revascularization group and faired just as well as those who had surgery up front. Therefore, a reasonable interpretation of this trial is that in STICH patients with coronary disease and reduced LV function, an initial strategy of medical therapy alone is appropriate and that a strategy of surgical revascularization with CABG can safely be deferred and reconsidered if necessary over time.

The authors' approach to the selection of patients with HF and CAD for revascularization is outlined in **Fig. 1**. In patients with coronary disease (no left main coronary artery stenosis or equivalent disease) and reduced EF for whom there is uncertainty about the relative benefits of medical therapy alone and surgical revascularization, the nature and severity of the patients' symptoms may help to tip the balance. If symptoms of severe angina are present, CABG may be indicated for the relief of symptoms alone in patients who carry acceptable surgical risk. Although no strict parameters exist to define the extensive LV cavity dilation, change in EF has been linearly correlated to baseline LV end-systolic volume, with higher volumes associated with a lower likelihood of improvement in LV function after revascularization.[77] Significant LV dilation may, therefore, identify patients for whom HF is likely to progress despite revascularization and for whom the incremental benefit of revascularization may be limited for the up-front risk.[24] In the absence of severe symptoms or significant LV dilation, the decision regarding surgical revascularization or medical therapy must be individualized. Despite the negative overall results of the STICH viability substudy, this is a population whereby viability testing may help to inform the decision regarding treatment. Many would favor revascularization in patients with a large burden of ischemia or viable myocardium because of the potential for segmental

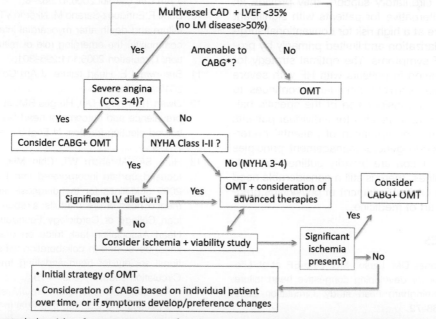

Fig. 1. Suggested algorithm for management of patients with multivessel CAD and LV dysfunction. * Multivessel PCI may be an alternative in patients who are at a high risk for surgery. LM, left main coronary artery.

recovery of function as long as significant remodeling has not already occurred. If there is no significant ischemia or viability, the risks of surgery may be unacceptable and an initial strategy of medical therapy alone is certainly safe and effective. Should symptoms develop over time or patients' preferences change, surgical revascularization remains an excellent therapeutic option. For patients with severe HF symptoms (NYHA III-IV) despite optimal medical therapy and advanced LV remodeling, the benefits of surgical revascularization should be considered in the context of alternative advanced therapies, such as mechanical circulatory support or cardiac transplantation.

SUMMARY

Coronary disease is the most common cause of HF and an important therapeutic target for improving HF-associated morbidity and mortality. Modern medical pharmacologic and device therapy for HF has evolved considerably in the era since the original trials favoring early surgical revascularization were conducted and may have altered the balance of risks and benefits. Recent data suggest that for many patients with CAD, HF, and reduced EF without angina, an initial conservative strategy of medical treatment with selective use of revascularization among those who develop progressive symptoms of angina or HF may be equivalent to an up-front strategy of surgical revascularization for all. An expanding array of advanced therapies, including options for durable mechanical circulatory support, may provide an important alternative for patients with significant CAD who are at a high risk for conventional surgical revascularization and limited primarily by progressive HF symptoms. The optimal strategy for revascularization in patients with HF with severe CAD who are surgical candidates continues to require careful consideration of the specific balance of risks and benefits for individual patients as well as the incorporation of patients' preferences. Although general management principles for this population are broadly outlined in treatment guidelines, there is still a considerable need for the best clinical judgment of physicians practiced in the art of medicine.

REFERENCES

1. Lloyd-Jones DM, Larson MG, Leip EP, et al. Lifetime risk for developing congestive heart failure: the Framingham heart study. Circulation 2002; 106:3068–72.
2. Gheorghiade M, Sopko G, De Luca L, et al. Navigating the crossroads of coronary artery disease and heart failure. Circulation 2006;114: 1202–13.
3. Yancy CW, Jessup M, Bozkurt B, et al. 2013 ACCF/AHA guideline for the management of heart failure: a report of the American College of Cardiology Foundation/American Heart Association Task Force on Practice Guidelines. J Am Coll Cardiol 2013;62: e147–239.
4. Djousse L, Driver JA, Gaziano JM. Relation between modifiable lifestyle factors and lifetime risk of heart failure. JAMA 2009;302:394–400.
5. Go AS, Mozaffarian D, Roger VL, et al. Heart disease and stroke statistics–2013 update: a report from the American Heart Association. Circulation 2013;127:e6–245.
6. Khatibzadeh S, Farzadfar F, Oliver J, et al. Worldwide risk factors for heart failure: a systematic review and pooled analysis. Int J Cardiol 2012;168: 1186–94.
7. Hellermann JP, Jacobsen SJ, Redfield MM, et al. Heart failure after myocardial infarction: clinical presentation and survival. Eur J Heart Fail 2005;7: 119–25.
8. Pfeffer MA, Braunwald E, Moye LA, et al. Effect of captopril on mortality and morbidity in patients with left ventricular dysfunction after myocardial infarction. Results of the survival and ventricular enlargement trial. The save investigators. N Engl J Med 1992;327:669–77.
9. Suleiman M, Khatib R, Agmon Y, et al. Early inflammation and risk of long-term development of heart failure and mortality in survivors of acute myocardial infarction predictive role of c-reactive protein. J Am Coll Cardiol 2006;47:962–8.
10. Bursi F, Enriquez-Sarano M, Nkomo VT, et al. Heart failure and death after myocardial infarction in the community: the emerging role of mitral regurgitation. Circulation 2005;111:295–301.
11. Braunwald E. Heart failure. J Am Coll Cardiol HF 2013;1:1–20.
12. Owan TE, Hodge DO, Herges RM, et al. Trends in prevalence and outcome of heart failure with preserved ejection fraction. N Engl J Med 2006;355: 251–9.
13. Hunt SA, Abraham WT, Chin MH, et al. 2009 focused update incorporated into the ACC/AHA 2005 guidelines for the diagnosis and management of heart failure in adults: a report of the American College of Cardiology Foundation/American Heart Association task force on practice guidelines: developed in collaboration with the international society for heart and lung transplantation. Circulation 2009;119:e391–479.
14. Felker GM, Thompson RE, Hare JM, et al. Underlying causes and long-term survival in patients with initially unexplained cardiomyopathy. N Engl J Med 2000;342:1077–84.

15. Ghali JK, Massie BM, Mann DL, et al. Guidelines, performance measures, and the practice of medicine: mind the gap. J Card Fail 2010;16:915–8.

16. Hillis LD, Smith PK, Anderson JL, et al. 2011 ACCF/AHA guideline for coronary artery bypass graft surgery: a report of the American College Of Cardiology Foundation/American Heart Association Task Force On Practice Guidelines. Circulation 2011;124:e652–735.

17. Butler J. The emerging role of multi-detector computed tomography in heart failure. J Card Fail 2007;13:215–26.

18. Valle-Munoz A, Estornell-Erill J, Soriano-Navarro CJ, et al. Late gadolinium enhancement-cardiovascular magnetic resonance identifies coronary artery disease as the aetiology of left ventricular dysfunction in acute new-onset congestive heart failure. Eur J Echocardiogr 2009;10:968–74.

19. Asrani NS, Chareonthaitawee P, Pellikka PA. Viability by MRI or PET would not have changed the results of the STICH trial. Prog Cardiovasc Dis 2013;55:494–7.

20. McMurray JJ, Adamopoulos S, Anker SD, et al. ESC guidelines for the diagnosis and treatment of acute and chronic heart failure 2012: the task force for the diagnosis and treatment of acute and chronic heart failure 2012 of the European Society Of Cardiology. Developed in collaboration with the Heart Failure Association (HFA) of the ESC. Eur Heart J 2012;33:1787–847.

21. Felker GM, Shaw LK, O'Connor CM. A standardized definition of ischemic cardiomyopathy for use in clinical research. J Am Coll Cardiol 2002;39:210–8.

22. Sutton MG, Sharpe N. Left ventricular remodeling after myocardial infarction: pathophysiology and therapy. Circulation 2000;101:2981–8.

23. Pfeffer MA, Braunwald E. Ventricular remodeling after myocardial infarction. Experimental observations and clinical implications. Circulation 1990;81:1161–72.

24. Bolognese L, Neskovic AN, Parodi G, et al. Left ventricular remodeling after primary coronary angioplasty: patterns of left ventricular dilation and long-term prognostic implications. Circulation 2002;106:2351–7.

25. Underwood SR, Bax JJ, vom Dahl J, et al. Imaging techniques for the assessment of myocardial hibernation. Report of a study group of the European Society of Cardiology. Eur Heart J 2004;25:815–36.

26. Elamm C, Fang JC. The world post-stich: is this a "game changer?" A non-invasive cardiologist's perspective-revascularization is the treatment of choice only in patients who fail medical therapy. Prog Cardiovasc Dis 2013;55:466–9.

27. Mann DL. Left ventricular size and shape: determinants of mechanical signal transduction pathways. Heart Fail Rev 2005;10:95–100.

28. Grigioni F, Enriquez-Sarano M, Zehr KJ, et al. Ischemic mitral regurgitation: long-term outcome and prognostic implications with quantitative Doppler assessment. Circulation 2001;103:1759–64.

29. Levine RA, Schwammenthal E. Ischemic mitral regurgitation on the threshold of a solution: from paradoxes to unifying concepts. Circulation 2005;112:745–58.

30. Nishimura RA, Gersh BJ, Schaff HV. The case for an aggressive surgical approach to papillary muscle rupture following myocardial infarction: "from paradise lost to paradise regained". Heart 2000;83:611–3.

31. Pfeffer MA, McMurray JJ, Velazquez EJ, et al. Valsartan, captopril, or both in myocardial infarction complicated by heart failure, left ventricular dysfunction, or both. N Engl J Med 2003;349:1893–906.

32. Koplan BA, Stevenson WG. Ventricular tachycardia and sudden cardiac death. Mayo Clin Proc 2009;84:289–97.

33. Zile MR, Brutsaert DL. New concepts in diastolic dysfunction and diastolic heart failure: part II: causal mechanisms and treatment. Circulation 2002;105:1503–8.

34. Zile MR, Brutsaert DL. New concepts in diastolic dysfunction and diastolic heart failure: part I: diagnosis, prognosis, and measurements of diastolic function. Circulation 2002;105:1387–93.

35. Shah SJ. Evolving approaches to the management of heart failure with preserved ejection fraction in patients with coronary artery disease. Curr Treat Options Cardiovasc Med 2010;12:58–75.

36. Fox K, Garcia MA, Ardissino D, et al. Guidelines on the management of stable angina pectoris: executive summary: the task force on the management of stable angina pectoris of the European Society of Cardiology. Eur Heart J 2006;27:1341–81.

37. Yusuf S, Pfeffer MA, Swedberg K, et al. Effects of candesartan in patients with chronic heart failure and preserved left-ventricular ejection fraction: the CHARM-Preserved Trial. Lancet 2003;362:777–81.

38. Massie BM, Carson PE, McMurray JJ, et al. Irbesartan in patients with heart failure and preserved ejection fraction. N Engl J Med 2008;359:2456–67.

39. van Veldhuisen DJ, Cohen-Solal A, Bohm M, et al. Beta-blockade with nebivolol in elderly heart failure patients with impaired and preserved left ventricular ejection fraction: data from seniors (study of effects of nebivolol intervention on outcomes and rehospitalization in seniors with heart failure). J Am Coll Cardiol 2009;53:2150–8.

40. Cleland JG, Tendera M, Adamus J, et al. The perindopril in elderly people with chronic heart failure (PEP-CHF) study. Eur Heart J 2006;27:2338–45.

41. Pitt B, Remme W, Zannad F, et al. Eplerenone, a selective aldosterone blocker, in patients with left ventricular dysfunction after myocardial infarction. N Engl J Med 2003;348:1309–21.

42. Juurlink DN, Mamdani MM, Lee DS, et al. Rates of hyperkalemia after publication of the Randomized Aldactone Evaluation Study. N Engl J Med 2004; 351:543–51.

43. Kober L, Torp-Pedersen C, Carlsen JE, et al. A clinical trial of the angiotensin-converting-enzyme inhibitor trandolapril in patients with left ventricular dysfunction after myocardial infarction. Trandolapril Cardiac Evaluation (TRACE) study group. N Engl J Med 1995;333:1670–6.

44. Effect of ramipril on mortality and morbidity of survivors of acute myocardial infarction with clinical evidence of heart failure. The Acute Infarction Ramipril Efficacy (AIRE) Study investigators. Lancet 1993;342:821–8.

45. Dickstein K, Kjekshus J. Effects of losartan and captopril on mortality and morbidity in high-risk patients after acute myocardial infarction: the OPTIMAAL randomised trial. Optimal trial in myocardial infarction with angiotensin II antagonist losartan. Lancet 2002;360:752–60.

46. Dargie HJ. Effect of carvedilol on outcome after myocardial infarction in patients with left-ventricular dysfunction: the CAPRICORN randomised trial. Lancet 2001;357:1385–90.

47. Kjekshus J, Apetrei E, Barrios V, et al. Rosuvastatin in older patients with systolic heart failure. N Engl J Med 2007;357:2248–61.

48. Tavazzi L, Maggioni AP, Marchioli R, et al. Effect of rosuvastatin in patients with chronic heart failure (the GISSI-HF trial): a randomised, double-blind, placebo-controlled trial. Lancet 2008;372:1231–9.

49. Homma S, Thompson JL, Pullicino PM, et al. Warfarin and aspirin in patients with heart failure and sinus rhythm. N Engl J Med 2012;366: 1859–69.

50. Loh E, Sutton MS, Wun CC, et al. Ventricular dysfunction and the risk of stroke after myocardial infarction. N Engl J Med 1997;336:251–7.

51. Goldstein RE, Boccuzzi SJ, Cruess D, et al. Diltiazem increases late-onset congestive heart failure in postinfarction patients with early reduction in ejection fraction. The adverse experience committee; and the multicenter diltiazem postinfarction research group. Circulation 1991;83:52–60.

52. Packer M, O'Connor CM, Ghali JK, et al. Effect of amlodipine on morbidity and mortality in severe chronic heart failure. Prospective randomized amlodipine survival evaluation study group. N Engl J Med 1996;335:1107–14.

53. Hohnloser SH, Kuck KH, Dorian P, et al. Prophylactic use of an implantable cardioverter-defibrillator after acute myocardial infarction. N Engl J Med 2004;351:2481–8.

54. Tracy CM, Epstein AE, Darbar D, et al. 2012 ACCF/AHA/HRS focused update of the 2008 guidelines for device-based therapy of cardiac rhythm abnormalities: a report of the American College Of Cardiology Foundation/American Heart Association Task Force on Practice Guidelines and the Heart Rhythm Society. [corrected]. Circulation 2012;126:1784–800.

55. Moss AJ, Hall WJ, Cannom DS, et al. Improved survival with an implanted defibrillator in patients with coronary disease at high risk for ventricular arrhythmia. Multicenter automatic defibrillator implantation trial investigators. N Engl J Med 1996; 335:1933–40.

56. Moss AJ, Zareba W, Hall WJ, et al. Prophylactic implantation of a defibrillator in patients with myocardial infarction and reduced ejection fraction. N Engl J Med 2002;346:877–83.

57. Bardy GH, Lee KL, Mark DB, et al. Amiodarone or an implantable cardioverter-defibrillator for congestive heart failure. N Engl J Med 2005;352: 225–37.

58. McLeod CJ, Shen WK, Rea RF, et al. Differential outcome of cardiac resynchronization therapy in ischemic cardiomyopathy and idiopathic dilated cardiomyopathy. Heart Rhythm 2011;8:377–82.

59. Cleland JG, Daubert JC, Erdmann E, et al. The effect of cardiac resynchronization on morbidity and mortality in heart failure. N Engl J Med 2005;352: 1539–49.

60. Moss AJ, Hall WJ, Cannom DS, et al. Cardiac-resynchronization therapy for the prevention of heart-failure events. N Engl J Med 2009;361: 1329–38.

61. Tang AS, Wells GA, Talajic M, et al. Cardiac-resynchronization therapy for mild-to-moderate heart failure. N Engl J Med 2010;363:2385–95.

62. Gasparini M, Mantica M, Galimberti P, et al. Is the outcome of cardiac resynchronization therapy related to the underlying etiology? Pacing Clin Electrophysiol 2003;26:175–80.

63. Gasparini M, Mantica M, Galimberti P, et al. Is the left ventricular lateral wall the best lead implantation site for cardiac resynchronization therapy? Pacing Clin Electrophysiol 2003;26:162–8.

64. Yusuf S, Zucker D, Peduzzi P, et al. Effect of coronary artery bypass graft surgery on survival: overview of 10-year results from randomised trials by the coronary artery bypass graft surgery trialists collaboration. Lancet 1994;344:563–70.

65. Myocardial infarction and mortality in the coronary artery surgery study (CASS) randomized trial. N Engl J Med 1984;310:750–8.

66. Alderman EL, Fisher LD, Litwin P, et al. Results of coronary artery surgery in patients with poor left ventricular function (cass). Circulation 1983;68: 785–95.

67. O'Connor CM, Velazquez EJ, Gardner LH, et al. Comparison of coronary artery bypass grafting versus medical therapy on long-term outcome in patients with ischemic cardiomyopathy (a 25-year experience from the duke cardiovascular disease databank). Am J Cardiol 2002;90:101–7.

68. Hillis LD, Smith PK, Anderson JL, et al. 2011 ACCF/AHA guideline for coronary artery bypass graft surgery: executive summary: a report of the American College of Cardiology Foundation/American Heart Association Task Force on Practice Guidelines. Circulation 2011;124:2610–42.

69. Patel MR, Dehmer GJ, Hirshfeld JW, et al. ACCF/SCAI/STS/AATS/AHA/ASNC/HFSA/SCCT 2012 appropriate use criteria for coronary revascularization focused update: a report of the American College of Cardiology Foundation Appropriate Use Criteria Task Force, Society for Cardiovascular Angiography and Interventions, Society of Thoracic Surgeons, American Association for Thoracic Surgery, American Heart Association, American Society of Nuclear Cardiology, and the Society of Cardiovascular Computed Tomography. J Am Coll Cardiol 2012;59:857–81.

70. Hlatky MA, Boothroyd DB, Bravata DM, et al. Coronary artery bypass surgery compared with percutaneous coronary interventions for multivessel disease: a collaborative analysis of individual patient data from ten randomised trials. Lancet 2009;373:1190–7.

71. Hlatky MA, Boothroyd DB, Baker L, et al. Comparative effectiveness of multivessel coronary bypass surgery and multivessel percutaneous coronary intervention: a cohort study. Ann Intern Med 2013; 158:727–34.

72. Braunwald E. Myocardial reperfusion, limitation of infarct size, reduction of left ventricular dysfunction, and improved survival. Should the paradigm be expanded? Circulation 1989;79:441–4.

73. Hochman JS, Lamas GA, Buller CE, et al. Coronary intervention for persistent occlusion after myocardial infarction. N Engl J Med 2006;355:2395–407.

74. Boden WE, O'Rourke RA, Teo KK, et al. Optimal medical therapy with or without PCI for stable coronary disease. N Engl J Med 2007;356: 1503–16.

75. Velazquez EJ, Lee KL, Deja MA, et al. Coronary-artery bypass surgery in patients with left ventricular dysfunction. N Engl J Med 2011;364:1607–16.

76. Srichai MB, Jaber WA. Viability by MRI or pet would have changed the results of the STICH trial. Prog Cardiovasc Dis 2013;55:487–93.

77. Bax JJ, Schinkel AF, Boersma E, et al. Extensive left ventricular remodeling does not allow viable myocardium to improve in left ventricular ejection fraction after revascularization and is associated with worse long-term prognosis. Circulation 2004; 110:II18–22.

Comorbidities and Polypharmacy

Thomas G. von Lueder, MD, PhD[a,b],*, Dan Atar, MD, PhD[a,b]

KEYWORDS

- Heart failure • Comorbidities • Polypharmacy • Elderly

KEY POINTS

- Heart failure (HF) is predominantly a disease that affects the elderly population, a cohort in which comorbidities are common.
- The majority of comorbidities and the degree of their severity have prognostic implications in HF.
- Polypharmacy in HF is common, has increased throughout the past 2 decades, and may pose a risk for adverse drug interactions (ADRs), accidental overdosing, or medication nonadherence.
- Polypharmacy, in particular in the elderly, is rarely assessed in traditional clinical trials, highlighting a need for entirely novel HF research strategies.

INTRODUCTION

HF is predominantly a disease that affects the elderly population, with approximately 80% of HF patients age 65 or older. Projections are for a steep increase in HF prevalence in the elderly due to changing demographics. Like HF, many other chronic disorders are more common in the elderly and frequently coexist in patients with HF. These comorbidities, both cardiac and noncardiac, may share the same pathomechanisms as HF (for example, inflammation), develop at or after the onset of HF, or may represent distinct disease entities and antecede HF. In general, HF patients with comorbidities exhibit substantially greater morbidity and mortality compared with HF patients without comorbidities. Data from both community-dwelling and hospitalized patients with HF show that the average number of comorbidities in HF has been on the rise.

Contemporary medical therapy for HF dictates use of multiple medications with proved survival advantage. Comorbidities in HF further increase the number and, perhaps, dosage of drugs needed to achieve sufficient clinical efficacy for either condition. Polypharmacy (defined as the use of 4 or more concomitant drugs) is a growing concern in HF. Despite reductions in use of drugs without documented survival benefit in HF over the past decade, the average number of medications managed by individual HF patients has been increasing. Polypharmacy increases the risk of adverse drug effects, interactions, accidental overdosing, or nonadherence, particularly in frail and cognitively impaired HF patients. The steep increase in the prevalence of comorbidities together with expanding medication use continues to add to the complexity of HF care. This article reviews important comorbidities in HF and major issues related to polypharmacy and discusses how best to manage these complicating factors in HF care.

COMMON COMORBIDITIES AND TREATMENT IMPLICATIONS IN HF

HF can originate from multiple inherited or acquired cardiac or noncardiac diseases and usually converges into a clinical syndrome characterized by typical HF symptoms and evidence of reduced cardiac function. Given this vastly complex and

The authors have no disclosures to report.
[a] Department of Cardiology, Oslo University Hospital Ullevål, University of Oslo, Kirkeveien 166, Oslo 0407, Norway; [b] Institute of Clinical Sciences, University of Oslo, Kirkeveien 166, Oslo 0407, Norway
* Corresponding author.
E-mail address: tomvonoslo@yahoo.com

Heart Failure Clin 10 (2014) 367–372
http://dx.doi.org/10.1016/j.hfc.2013.12.001
1551-7136/14/$ – see front matter © 2014 Elsevier Inc. All rights reserved.

heterogenous spectrum of HF pathomechanisms, it is not surprising that numerous other conditions can coexist in HF. Some of these comorbidities may precede and even induce HF; others may occur independently, albeit with temporal overlap. Yet other conditions, such as anemia and renal failure, may occur as a consequence of HF. Despite robust evidence—some from large trials and others from databases—that comorbidities in HF indicate an unfavorable overall prognosis, little unifying information exists on how to approach comorbidities in HF. The paucity of scientific data is further illustrated by absence of rigorous evaluation and management recommendations issued by major guideline bodies. Very recent data, however, indicate that in HF with preserved ejection fraction, the burden of noncardiac comorbidities is not only higher than in HF with reduced ejection fraction but also associated with a higher rate of non-HF hospitalizations.[1] Some investigators even suggest that comorbidities drive coronary endothelial inflammation and cardiac remodeling.[2]

Common specific comorbidities are discussed and typical clinical dilemmas highlighted related to polypharmacy arising from medical treatment of multiple conditions.

Renal Dysfunction and Failure

Impaired renal function is present in many, if not most, patients with HF and thus represents a major clinical problem in HF patient care.[3,4] Traditionally, it has been assumed that cardiac pump failure leads to renal hypoperfusion or congestion and, thus, kidney dysfunction. Although hemodynamics may provide partial explanations, the mechanisms underlying comorbid heart–kidney failure are substantially more complex. There has been increasing recognition of a bidirectional relationship between HF and kidney dysfunction in recent years. Novel data suggest that systemic proinflammatory processes, neuroendocrine overdrive, preexisting renal disease, uremic toxins, and multiple other factors contribute, singly or in combination.[5] Also, pharmacotherapy for HF or comorbidities may adversely affect renal function[6] (see article elsewhere in this issue). Importantly, based on a large body of clinical trial data, the presence of renal dysfunction and failure is one of the strongest predictors of excessive morbidity and mortality in HF. Accordingly, major research efforts are directed toward preventing renal dysfunction and failure in HF.[7]

Anemia

Anemia is commonly defined as a blood hemoglobin concentration of less than 13 g/dL in men and less than 12 g/dL in women. Underappreciated by clinicians until recently, anemia is a significant and frequent comorbidity in patients with HF, in particular in the elderly and those with renal dysfunction or failure (see article elsewhere in this issue). Multiple pathomechanisms that are operative in HF may initiate and sustain anemia. For instance, activation of the *renin-angiotensin-aldosterone system* and other neurohormonal systems induces plasma volume expansion, leading to hemodilution and decreased hemoglobin levels. In addition, circulating factors, including cytokines and interleukin, may directly suppress erythropoiesis in bone marrow.[8] Experimental evidence suggests that distinct mechanisms drive bone marrow depression in HF of ischemic origin compared with HF of nonischemic origin.[9] Also, renal failure, such as in cardiorenal syndrome, may lead to reductions in erythropoietin levels and, thus, anemia. Together with volume expansion inherent to renal dysfunction and failure, several mechanisms underlie anemia in cardiorenal syndrome. The presence of anemia in HF seems to confer greater morbidity and adverse prognosis. Anemia may not, however, be an independent prognostic marker because recent registry data indicate an association with comorbid renal disease and more advanced HF.[10] Based on these considerations, it seems logical that correction of anemia may be of benefit in HF. Whether specific treatment (with erythropoietin analogues) may alter clinical outcomes in HF is only currently undergoing scientific scrutiny. General assessment, diagnostic work-up, and management of anemia have been encouraged in recent HF guidelines.[11,12]

Respiratory Disorders

Comorbid respiratory disorders are a common finding in HF patients and contribute to shortness of breath, poor exertional capacity, and low quality of life. These disorders include chronic airway diseases, such as chronic obstructive pulmonary disease (COPD), obstructive sleep apnea (OSA), and central sleep apnea.[13,14] Not only do symptoms overlap but also the underlying pathogenetic mechanisms may share similarities with those that are operative in HF. For example, in OSA patients, risk factors for HF, such as obesity, hypertension, and endothelial dysfunction, frequently coexist, although a causal relationship between OSA and HF remains to be conclusively shown.[15] Due to the nonspecific nature of respiratory and HF symptoms, it sometimes may be hard to establish the temporal sequence of these 2 disease entities within an individual patient. It has been shown that HF patients with OSA have increased after-load during sleep, which is normalized by therapy with continuous positive airway pressure.[16] The presence of OSA aggravates HF and thus may warrant specific management.

Tobacco smoking is an important exogenous factor that contributes to chronic airway and coronary artery disease. Although governmental interventions and public awareness campaigns on smoking have reduced the number of daily smokers in Western societies over the past decade, the prevalence of respiratory diseases in both HF and non-HF populations will continue to rise due to the long lag from exposure to clinical onset. The individual contribution of HF and comorbid COPD to dyspnea is often hard to determine for a clinician. Spirometry and other functional tests are unreliable in decompensated HF. Respiratory comorbidities are addressed further elsewhere in this issue.

Gout and Arthritis

Rheumatoid arthritis (RA), ankylosing spondylitis, psoriatic arthritis, and gout are important comorbidities in HF and highly prevalent conditions.[17,18] As with HF, the prevalence of arthritis increases with age.[19–21] In addition, the prevalence of HF is higher in patients with arthritis.[19] Patients with arthritis exhibit higher mortality and morbidity rates compared with the general population, which are essentially caused by excess in cardiovascular (CV) disease. In RA patients, plasma levels of the N-terminal prohormone of brain natriuretic peptide predicted mortality in a cohort that was followed for 10 years.[22] Traditional risk scores based on established CV risk factors have been validated and are commonly used in the general population but systematically underestimate CV risk in patients with RA.[23,24] HF patients with RA have substantially worse outcomes than HF patients without comorbid RA.[25]

In addition, anti-RA drugs often are little compatible with HF therapy, with immunomodulators perhaps making one exception: tumor necrosis factor (TNF)-α bockade has failed to improve outcomes in pure HF. Yet, recent work in patients with inflammatory arthropathies demonstrated improvements in peripheral vascular function and morphology by TNF-α blockade, typical surrogate markers of clinical outcomes.[26] Despite the significance of comorbid arthritis to HF, even the most recent HF guidelines do not address assessment, prevention, and management of CV disease in these patients.[12] Many investigators, therefore, suggest that in HF, comorbid arthritis is an aggravating factor and should be evaluated

and managed in a multidisciplinary health care setting.

Other Comorbidities with Relevance to HF

Patients with HF are more prone to suffer from depression and other affective disorders. Some may, understandably, merely reflect the poor overall quality of life in HF. Chronic cerebral hypoperfusion has been proposed as a contributing mechanism.[27] Alternatively, environmental (such as diet and lifestyle decisions), genetic, and other contributing factors may contribute both to HF and comorbid mood disorders. In addition, cerebrovascular diseases and stroke are more common in HF than in the general population and are associated with cognitive impairment and depression. Unintentional weight loss that may occur in depressed HF patients is an independent predictor of poor outcomes.[28] Whenever feasible, HF patients should be evaluated for the presence of affective disorders and cognitive impairment. These comorbidities not only may be alleviated through specific therapy but also may influence treatment decisions and help determine the appropriate level of care in an individual HF patient.

POLYPHARMACY IN HF—SCOPE OF THE PROBLEM

HF commands the use of several drugs, including angiotensin-converting enzyme inhibitors, β-blockers, and mineralocorticoid receptor antagonists.[12,29] There is a clear trend for an increasing number of drugs used in patients with HF. Recent data in a community-based HF population indicate that the average number of prescription drugs managed by HF patients increased from 4.1 to 6.4 over the past 2 decades, reflecting a significant increase in the number of comorbidities per patient (**Fig. 1**).[30] The same investigators also show

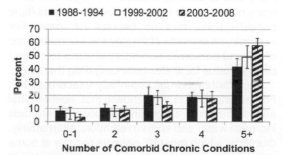

Fig. 1. Temporal changes of number of comorbidities in community-dwelling subjects with HF over a period of 2 decades. (*From* Wong CY, Chaudhry SI, Desai MM, et al. Trends in comorbidity, disability, and polypharmacy in heart failure. Am J Med 2011;124(2):140; with permission.)

that the proportion of HF patients above the age of 80 years almost doubled within the same period of time.[30] In elderly patients hospitalized with HF, mortality and readmission rates have not improved despite recent advances of pharmacologic therapy.[31]

The extent and severity of comorbidities in HF necessitate additional pharmacotherapy to control them, further adding to the complexity of HF management. Because HF patients with comorbidities are more likely to be frail and elderly, drug target doses and sufficient medication adherence may be harder to achieve than in younger HF patients. In this context, polypharmacy attenuates biologic responses to HF therapy and greatly increases the risk for ADRs. In the elderly, CV drugs seem the most common drug category implicated with ADRs.[32] Importantly, ADRs may be oligosymptomatic and thus difficult to diagnose. With aging populations and the rising prevalence of HF and of comorbidities, ADRs will continue to represent a significant reason for hospitalization.

SIGNIFICANCE OF POLYPHARMACY FOR HF PHARMACOTHERAPY

Interactions between specific drugs to treat HF and those to treat comorbidities are common and greatly augment the complexity of HF management.

Medical treatment of HF with comorbidities often faces the dilemma of mutually exclusive drugs, that is, drugs that improve one condition and deteriorate another or vice versa.

As an example, in HF and comorbid respiratory disease, β-blockers represent a cornerstone of contemporary HF pharmacotherapy but may have an adverse impact on pulmonary function. Conversely, glucocorticosteroids are sometimes warranted in episodes of COPD exacerbation but may increase sodium and water retention and, thus, lead to decompensated HF. In general, clinicians need to base treatment decisions on multiple considerations that go beyond HF care. For example, an estimate of the individual contributions of HF and comorbid respiratory disease to current clinical status facilitates balancing drug therapies.

Many arthritis drugs potentially exacerbate HF. For example, it is well known that nonsteroidal antiinflammatory drugs and glucocorticosteroids increase water and sodium retention. Alternatively, diuretics, which most HF patients receive at some stage, increase serum uric acid and predispose to acute episodes of gout.

With many HF patients managed in primary care and other nonspecialized settings, the true extent of excessive morbidity and mortality caused by polypharmacy in HF is difficult to quantify.

MANAGING POLYPHARMACY IN HF PATIENTS WITH COMORBIDITIES

Some fundamental principles in pharmacotherapy may inform treatment decisions in elderly HF patients with extensive comorbidities. In general, possible negative consequences of medical and nonpharmacologic interventions need to be considered. For instance, if renal function is impaired, angiography and other contrast-enhanced diagnostic procedures should be performed only if clear clinical benefit is expected. Drugs with known risk of interactions need to be carefully up-titrated, and medication should be reassessed regularly, in particular in the very elderly, in nonresponders, and in cognitively impaired patients. Data are scarce on how best to reintroduce and maintain HF pharmacotherapy after transient organ dysfunction, such as kidney failure.

Nurse-based administration of drug therapy to elderly, frail, and cognitively impaired patients likely enhances medication adherence and reduces polypharmacy and ADRs in HF. In those patients where focus has shifted from the hope of long-term survival benefits to optimal quality of life, palliation and withdrawal of effective HF drugs may be warranted.

SUMMARY AND CONCLUDING REMARKS

In patients with HF, the prevalence of comorbidities, the extent of polypharmacy, and the associated additional morbidity and mortality have increased significantly over recent years, although some uncertainty remains on the true prevalence of comorbidities as a result of varying disagreement between self-reported and clinically diagnosed comorbidities. HF patients with comorbidities more often are elderly, have more comorbidities, and exhibit increased risk of ADRs. Polypharmacy is becoming a major complicating factor in HF patients and represents a risk for ADRs, accidental drug overdosing, and medication nonadherence. Therefore, clinicians need to be vigilant about possible drug interactions. Finally, medical therapy for HF with comorbidities should not be considered in isolation but rather be an essential component of an overall patient-focused management plan, which is based on identifying the needs and the appropriate level of care of individual HF patients.

REFERENCES

1. Ather S, Chan W, Bozkurt B, et al. Impact of noncardiac comorbidities on morbidity and mortality in a predominantly male population with heart failure

and preserved versus reduced ejection fraction. J Am Coll Cardiol 2012;59(11):998–1005.

2. Paulus WJ, Tschope C. A novel paradigm for heart failure with preserved ejection fraction: comorbidities drive myocardial dysfunction and remodeling through coronary microvascular endothelial inflammation. J Am Coll Cardiol 2013;62(4):263–71.

3. Waldum B, Westheim AS, Sandvik L, et al. Renal function in outpatients with chronic heart failure. J Card Fail 2010;16(5):374–80.

4. Cleland JG, Carubelli V, Castiello T, et al. Renal dysfunction in acute and chronic heart failure: prevalence, incidence and prognosis. Heart Fail Rev 2012;17(2):133–49.

5. Lekawanvijit S, Kompa AR, Wang BH, et al. Cardiorenal syndrome: the emerging role of protein-bound uremic toxins. Circ Res 2012;111(11): 1470–83.

6. Weinfeld MS, Chertow GM, Stevenson LW. Aggravated renal dysfunction during intensive therapy for advanced chronic heart failure. Am Heart J 1999;138(2 Pt 1):285–90.

7. Dobre D, Rossignol P, Metra M, et al. Can we prevent or treat renal dysfunction in chronic heart failure? Heart Fail Rev 2012;17(2):283–90.

8. Shah R, Agarwal AK. Anemia associated with chronic heart failure: current concepts. Clin Interv Aging 2013;8:111–22.

9. Iversen PO, Andersson KB, Finsen AV, et al. Separate mechanisms cause anemia in ischemic vs. nonischemic murine heart failure. Am J Physiol Regul Integr Comp Physiol 2010;298(3): R808–14.

10. Waldum B, Westheim AS, Sandvik L, et al. Baseline anemia is not a predictor of all-cause mortality in outpatients with advanced heart failure or severe renal dysfunction. Results from the Norwegian Heart Failure Registry. J Am Coll Cardiol 2012; 59(4):371–8.

11. McMurray JJ, Anand IS, Diaz R, et al. Baseline characteristics of patients in the Reduction of Events with Darbepoetin alfa in Heart Failure trial (RED-HF). Eur J Heart Fail 2013;15(3):334–41.

12. McMurray JJ, Adamopoulos S, Anker SD, et al. ESC Guidelines for the diagnosis and treatment of acute and chronic heart failure 2012: the task force for the diagnosis and treatment of acute and chronic heart failure 2012 of the European Society of Cardiology. Developed in collaboration with the Heart Failure Association (HFA) of the ESC. Eur Heart J 2012;33(14): 1787–847.

13. Kasai T, Bradley TD. Obstructive sleep apnea and heart failure: pathophysiologic and therapeutic implications. J Am Coll Cardiol 2011;57(2):119–27.

14. Bhatt SP, Dransfield MT. Chronic obstructive pulmonary disease and cardiovascular disease. Transl Res 2013;162(4):237–51.

15. Wong CY, O'Moore-Sullivan T, Leano R, et al. Association of subclinical right ventricular dysfunction with obesity. J Am Coll Cardiol 2006;47(3):611–6.

16. Tkacova R, Rankin F, Fitzgerald FS, et al. Effects of continuous positive airway pressure on obstructive sleep apnea and left ventricular afterload in patients with heart failure. Circulation 1998;98(21): 2269–75.

17. Lawrence RC, Felson DT, Helmick CG, et al. Estimates of the prevalence of arthritis and other rheumatic conditions in the United States. Part II. Arthritis Rheum 2008;58(1):26–35.

18. Helmick CG, Felson DT, Lawrence RC, et al. Estimates of the prevalence of arthritis and other rheumatic conditions in the United States. Part I. Arthritis Rheum 2008;58(1):15–25.

19. Han C, Robinson DW Jr, Hackett MV, et al. Cardiovascular disease and risk factors in patients with rheumatoid arthritis, psoriatic arthritis, and ankylosing spondylitis. J Rheumatol 2006;33(11): 2167–72.

20. Zhu Y, Pandya BJ, Choi HK. Comorbidities of Gout and Hyperuricemia in the US General Population: NHANES 2007-2008. Am J Med 2012; 125(7):679–687 e1.

21. Doherty M. New insights into the epidemiology of gout. Rheumatology (Oxford) 2009;48(Suppl 2): ii2–8.

22. Provan SA, Angel K, Odegard S, et al. The association between disease activity and NT-proBNP in 238 patients with rheumatoid arthritis: a 10 year longitudinal study. Arthritis Res Ther 2008; 10(3):R70.

23. Crowson CS, Matteson EL, Roger VL, et al. Usefulness of risk scores to estimate the risk of cardiovascular disease in patients with rheumatoid arthritis. Am J Cardiol 2012;110(3):420–4.

24. Symmons DP, Gabriel SE. Epidemiology of CVD in rheumatic disease, with a focus on RA and SLE. Nat Rev Rheumatol 2011;7(7):399–408.

25. Davis JM III, Roger VL, Crowson CS, et al. The presentation and outcome of heart failure in patients with rheumatoid arthritis differs from that in the general population. Arthritis Rheum 2008; 58(9):2603–11.

26. Angel K, Provan SA, Gulseth HL, et al. Tumor necrosis factor alpha antagonists improve aortic stiffness in patients with inflammatory arthropathies: a controlled study. Hypertension 2010; 55(2):333–8.

27. Alosco ML, Spitznagel MB, Cohen R, et al. Reduced cerebral perfusion predicts greater depressive symptoms and cognitive dysfunction at a 1-year follow-up in patients with heart failure. Int J Geriatr Psychiatry 2013. [Epub ahead of print].

28. Song EK, Lee Y, Moser DK, et al. The link of unintentional weight loss to cardiac event-free survival in

patients with heart failure. J Cardiovasc Nurs 2013. [Epub ahead of print].

29. Krum H, von Lueder T. Advances in heart failure management. London, UK: Future Medicine Ltd; 2012.

30. Wong CY, Chaudhry SI, Desai MM, et al. Trends in comorbidity, disability, and polypharmacy in heart failure. Am J Med 2011;124(2):136–43.

31. Kosiborod M, Lichtman JH, Heidenreich PA, et al. National trends in outcomes among elderly patients with heart failure. Am J Med 2006;119(7): 616.e1–7.

32. Sikdar KC, Dowden J, Alaghehbandan R, et al. Adverse drug reactions in elderly hospitalized patients: a 12-year population-based retrospective cohort study. Ann Pharmacother 2012;46(7–8):960–71.

Index

Moving?

Make sure your subscription moves with you!

To notify us of your new address, find your **Clinics Account Number** (located on your mailing label above your name), and contact customer service at:

Email: journalscustomerservice-usa@elsevier.com

800-654-2452 (subscribers in the U.S. & Canada)
314-447-8871 (subscribers outside of the U.S. & Canada)

Fax number: 314-447-8029

Elsevier Health Sciences Division
Subscription Customer Service
3251 Riverport Lane
Maryland Heights, MO 63043

ELSEVIER

Moving?

Make sure your subscription moves with you!

To notify us of your new address, find your Clinics Account Number (located on your mailing label above your name), and contact customer service at:

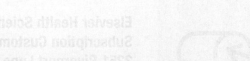

Email: journalscustomerservice-usa@elsevier.com

800-654-2452 (subscribers in the U.S. & Canada)
314-447-8871 (subscribers outside of the U.S. & Canada)

Fax number: 314-447-8029

Elsevier Health Sciences Division
Subscription Customer Service
3251 Riverport Lane
Maryland Heights, MO 63043

*To ensure uninterrupted delivery of your subscription, please notify us at least 4 weeks in advance of move.

Printed and bound by CPI Group (UK) Ltd, Croydon, CR0 4YY

03/10/2024

01040378-0013